Vascular and Intravascular Imaging Trends, Analysis, and Challenges, Volume 1

Stent applications

Vascular and Intravascular Imaging Trends, Analysis, and Challenges, Volume 1

Stent applications

Petia Radeva
Universitat de Barcelona, Barcelona, Spain
and
Computer Vision Center, Bellaterra (Barcelona), Spain

Jasjit S Suri
ATHEROPOINT, California, USA

IOP Publishing, Bristol, UK

ISBN 978-0-7503-1997-3 (ebook)
ISBN 978-0-7503-1995-9 (print)
ISBN 978-0-7503-1996-6 (mobi)

DOI 10.1088/2053-2563/ab01fa

Version: 20190801

IOP Expanding Physics
ISSN 2053-2563 (online)
ISSN 2054-7315 (print)

British Library Cataloguing-in-Publication Data: A catalogue record for this book is available from the British Library.

Published by IOP Publishing, wholly owned by The Institute of Physics, London

IOP Publishing, Temple Circus, Temple Way, Bristol, BS1 6HG, UK

US Office: IOP Publishing, Inc., 190 North Independence Mall West, Suite 601, Philadelphia, PA 19106, USA

To our families and friends for their infinite patience, love and support.

Contents

Preface

Cardiovascular diseases (CVDs) are responsible for a third of all deaths in women worldwide and more than a half in men. Mortality from coronary heart disease (CHD) is falling due to the continuous improvement in treatment devices and imaging, but morbidity appears to be rising every year. The aetiology of the CVDs is multifactorial; different factors play a role, such as environment, lifestyle and genetics. As they are the leading cause of morbidity and mortality worldwide, healthcare costs for the management of CVDs are predicted to increase by more than 40% by 2040 in developed countries (e.g. the USA). This fact underlines the importance of addressing different open questions, such as the following. What are the most appropriate diagnosis and interventional strategies? What are the optimal devices for treatment and how can they avoid secondary effects? Which imaging technique gives the most information about the morphology and the dynamics of the coronary vessels? How should one combine complementary information from multi-modal imaging? How does one best evaluate coronary interventions, perform follow-up on coronary lesion evolution, predict the outcomes of interventions, and make possible the retrieval and construction of clinical atlases on a huge scale, etc?

In this book, we are pleased to present several advanced clinical and medical imaging studies that cover a wide spectrum of clinical disease issues, clinical intervention techniques, imaging modalities for plaque visualization and inspection, automatic analysis and clinical parameter extraction techniques, and advanced tools for the navigation of and intervention for coronary lesions.

This book is organized into four sections. The first comprises two clinical papers that discuss the most commonly used clinical imaging techniques for coronary plaque detection and analysis (angiography, intravascular ultrasound, optical coherence tomography (OCT), etc) with their advantages and disadvantages. Special attention is paid to late stent pathology, restenosis, neoatherosclerosis and late malapposition, and their diagnosis in OCT images.

The second section is devoted to computer modeling and computational fluid hemodynamics for nonlinear stent deployment, modeling plaque formation and progression. Continuum-based methods for modeling the evolution of plaque are derived. Low-density lipoprotein (LDL) penetration is defined using a convection–diffusion equation, while endothelial permeability is shear stress dependent. The inflammatory process is modeled using reaction–diffusion partial differential equations. The predictive value of computational models is of high interest in the clinical context. The ability to plan one or more treatment alternatives and being able to assess their outcomes can help in identifying potentially harmful or dangerous situations. Also, the fact that such tools can be used within the intervention room or, equivalently, obtain a response in real time, opens the possibility of their being used in day-to-day clinical practice.

The third section covers different works on image analysis of coronary and carotid vessels: segmentation of vessels and stents in intravascular ultrasound

(IVUS) and OCT using advanced computer vision techniques such as graph-cuts and active shape models; advanced medical imaging and computer vision techniques for automatic plaque characterization in coronary and carotid vessels; computer models for blood and plaque growth, robust techniques for IVUS, and histological tissue characterization and registration; calcium real-time analysis; novel methods to combine dynamic and morphological features for robust plaque characterization in the carotid; and robust methods for 2D and 3D image registration followed by different strategies to be used for better image-guided intervention. Here we can also find methods that go beyond the more 'classical' problems to analyze coronary lesions, proposing models for extraluminal blood perfusion, studying the relation between carotid–coronary plaque progression and extending the discussions to neural aneurysm, proposing a complete overview from neurovascular images to morphology analysis, diagnosis and treatment.

The last section is devoted to disease risk stratification, which is considered from different sources such as the intima–media thickness of the carotid, the wall morphology of the carotid, as well as fusing wall-based and texture-based features within a machine learning paradigm. All these techniques and methodologies are very important in order to predict the risk of an increase in stenosis and stress on the fibrous cap thickness, which can cause the risk of rupture leading to myocardial infarction. Rupture of the arterial wall cap can cause calcium to dislodge, blocking the oxygen-rich blood flow in the arteries, leading to myocardial infarction or stroke. Prior to stenting and percutaneous interventional procedures, cardiologists can be aided by performing pre-screening and risk stratification of coronary artery disease. Therefore, automated machine learning and computer vision systems are being adopted and becoming popular for clinical use in cardiovascular imaging laboratories, leading to more precise diagnosis and image-guided intervention and, hence, a much higher quality of clinical care.

In summary, this collection of studies gives an overview of different research on vascular and intravascular analysis, discusses different scientific and clinical questions in detail, and proposes advances in clinical treatment and the automatic analysis of medical imaging. We aim to give an overview of the active topics and problems in this field and encourage the community to continue in their search for scientific and clinical answers as to which are the most precise, objective, effective and efficient strategies for atherosclerotic diagnosis, treatment and follow-up, as CVD remains one of the most important health problems of humanity.

Petia Radeva
Jasjit S Suri

Editor biographies

Petia Radeva

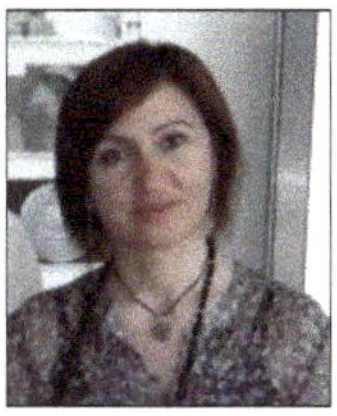

Dr Petia Radeva (PhD 1993, Universitat Autònoma de Barcelona, Spain) is a senior researcher and full professor at the University of Barcelona. She received her PhD degree from the Universitat Autònoma de Barcelona in 1998. She is the head of the Computer Vision and Machine Learning Consolidated Research Group at the University of Barcelona and the head of MiLab of the Computer Vision Center (www.cvc.uab.es). Her current research interests include the development of learning-based approaches (in particular, deep learning methods) for computer vision and image analysis. Radeva has been an AIPR Fellow since 2015, and became an ICREA Academia researcher in 2014 for her outstanding research achievements. In 2015 she received the Aurora Pons Porrata award for her scientific merits as well as the Antonio Caparros award for the best technology transfer.

Jasjit S Suri

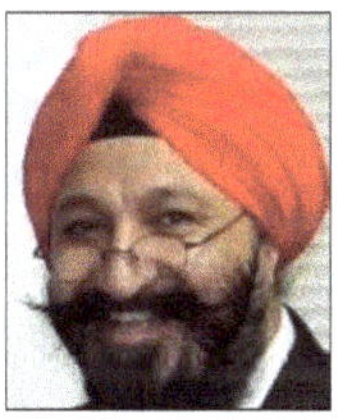

Jasjit S Suri, PhD, MBA, is an innovator, visionary, scientist and an internationally known world leader in the field of biomedical imaging and healthcare management. Dr Suri is a recipient of the Director General's Gold Medal (1980), was named a Fellow of the American Institute of Medical and Biological Engineering by the National Academy of Sciences, Washington, DC (2004), and received a Marquis Life Time Achievement Award (2018). Dr Suri is a board member in several organizations.

List of contributors

Sergio García-Blas
Hospital Clínico Universitario de Valencia, Spain

Santiago Jiménez-Valero
Hospital Clínico Universitario de Valencia, Spain

Clara Bonanad
Hospital Clínico Universitario de Valencia, Spain

Juan Sanchis
Hospital Clínico Universitario de Valencia, Spain

Vicente Bodí
Hospital Clínico Universitario de Valencia, Spain

Joana Delgado Silva
Coimbra's Hospital and University Centre—General Hospital, Portugal

Marco Costa
Coimbra's Hospital and University Centre—General Hospital, Portugal

Lino Gonçalves
Coimbra's Hospital and University Centre—General Hospital, Portugal

Nenad Filipovic
Faculty of Engineering, University of Kragujevac, Serbia

Arindam Bit
National Institute of Technology, Raipur, India

Himadri Chattopadhyay
Jadavpur University, India

Ignacio Labarride
National University of Central Buenos Aires, Argentina

Ehab Essa
Swansea University, UK

Xianghua Xie
Swansea University, UK

Huaizhong Zhang
Edge Hill University, UK

James Cotton
Royal Wolverhampton NHS Trust, UK

Dave Smith
ABMU, UK

Manya V Afonso
Wageningen University and Research, Netherlands

J Miguel Sanches
Institute for Systems and Robotics, Portugal

E Gerardo Mendizabal-Ruiz
University of Guadalajara, Mexico

M'hamed Bentourkia
University of Sherbrooke, Canada

Ioannis A Kakadiaris
University of Houston, TX, USA

Timur Aksoy
Sabanci University, Turkey

Gozde Unal
Istanbul Technical University, Turkey

Franjo Pernus
University of Ljubljana, Slovenia

Ziga Spiclin
University of Ljubljana, Slovenia

Su-Lin Lee
Imperial College London, UK

Angelos Karlas
Technical University of Munich, Germany

Alessio Dore
Imperial College London, UK

Luca Saba
University of Cagliari, Italy

Sumit K Banchhor
National Institute of Technology, India

Harman S Suri
Monitoring and Diagnostic Division, AtheroPoint™, USA

Narendra D Londhe
National Institute of Technology, India

Tadashi Araki
Toho University Medical Center Omori Hospital, Japan

Nobutaka Ikeda
National Center for Global Health and Medicine, Japan

Klaudija Viskovic
University Hospital for Infectious Disease, Croatia

Shoaib Shafique
CorVasc MDs PC, IN, USA

John R Laird
St Helena Hospital, CA, USA

Ajay Gupta
Weill Cornell Medical College, NY, USA

Andrew Nicolaides
Vascular Screening and Diagnostic Centre, UK

Pankaj K Jain
Indian Institute of Technology Varanasi (BHU), India

Ayman El-Baz
University of Louisville, KY, USA

Vimal K Shrivastava
Kalinga Institute of Industrial Technology, India

Shoaib Shafique
CorVasc Vascular Laboratory, IN, USA

Section I

Vascular and intravascular clinical analysis

IOP Publishing

Vascular and Intravascular Imaging Trends, Analysis, and Challenges, Volume 1
Stent applications
Petia Radeva and Jasjit S Suri

Chapter 1

OCT in the evaluation of late stent pathology: restenosis, neoatherosclerosis and late malapposition

Sergio García-Blas, Santiago Jiménez-Valero, Clara Bonanad, Juan Sanchis and Vicent Bodi

1.1 Stent evolution and late stent pathology

Coronary stents were developed to overcome the limitations of percutaneous transluminal coronary angioplasty (PTCA), improving acute success, facilitating the management of complications (mainly coronary dissection and acute vessel closure) and lowering restenosis rates [1, 2]. However, PTCA and subsequent stent deployment are an aggression to the arterial wall and leave a metallic material that must be incorporated into the vascular structure through a complex restoration process called neointimal coverage or re-endothelialization.

The first devices used were bare metal stents (BMSs). Pathological studies have suggested that re-endothelialization occurs with the development of neointimal tissue within the luminal area of stents, reaching an intimal hyperplasia peak from 6 to 12 months after BMS deployment [3]. After BMS deployment, in-stent restenosis (ISR) was still a relevant issue with rates up to 20%–30%, due to excessive neointimal proliferation [1, 2]. Initial reports showed excellent late performance of these stents after the initial phase of higher risk ISR, with clinical stability of the stented site at 8–10 years after BMS implantation [4]. Therefore, ISR is generally considered to be a stable process, with an early peak in intimal hyperplasia followed by a quiescent period. However, there is emerging histological and clinical evidence of late *de novo* in-stent neoatherosclerosis [5–7]. These studies indicate that in some patients there is degenerative evolution of neointima into an unstable atherosclerotic lesion and that ISR should not always be regarded as a benign entity.

doi:10.1088/2053-2563/ab01fach1

Drug-eluting stents (DESs) were designed to inhibit smooth muscle cell proliferation which, together with the extracellular matrix, is the main component of neointimal tissue [8, 9]. A DES comprises a metallic stent frame, antiproliferative drugs and eventually a polymer (although recently polymer-free stents have been developed). They have shown reduced rates of angiographic restenosis and improved clinical outcomes [10, 11] and have become the main agent for treating coronary artery disease. However, some concerns arose some years after the widespread use of DESs was established, mainly due to the emergence of very late stent thrombosis (VLST). First-generation DES-treated patients showed a rate of late stent thrombosis (LST) of 0.53% per year which steadily increased to 3% over 4 years [12, 13]. Proposed mechanisms for this LST include insufficient strut coverage, late-acquired malapposition, or the development of neoatherosclerotic changes within the neointimal layer. New generation stents with other drugs, thinner struts and biocompatible polymers, among other innovations, seem to have overcome the challenge of LST [14]. Despite better outcomes with technological developments, late stent pathology is still an issue and the increasing number of coronary stents being used means that a pathology that affects a small percentage of the population at risk will translate into a significant number of patients. Better understanding is needed of the healing process after stent deployment and the development and evolution of late stent pathology. Furthermore, the clinical manifestations of these entities are frequently severe and have a poor prognosis.

Bioresorbable vascular scaffolds (BVSs) have been developed recently to maintain the initial advantages of stents but disappear after some years, thus leaving no foreign material in the arterial wall. Initial reports of extended follow-up beyond three years suggest a favorable vascular late response after resorption, with late luminal gain due to plaque and vessel remodeling, and potential 'sealing' of plaques by creation of a superficial fibrous tissue layer. This may avoid late complications, however, further evaluation and follow-up of these devices is needed.

1.2 OCT characterization of late stent pathology

Optical coherence tomography (OCT) has a resolution about ten times higher than that of intravascular ultrasound (IVUS)—10–20 μm and 80–120 μm, respectively). It is able to identify stent struts and accurately define and quantify their relationship with the vessel wall. Previous studies have shown the superiority of OCT over IVUS in evaluating strut coverage, apposition and neointimal hyperplasia. OCT can also identify neoatherosclerotic changes. The second generation of OCT imaging systems, i.e. optical frequency domain imaging (OFDI), has provided a substantial advance due to a markedly increased speed of image acquisition, improving the feasibility of this technique and reducing complications and patient discomfort during image acquisition. All these features make OCT a unique tool for the evaluation of acute and late stent performance.

1.2.1 Stent coverage: re-endothelialization

The high spatial resolution of OCT (10–20 μm axial) enables detailed *in vivo* assessment of individual stent strut coverage. Preclinical studies have established the accuracy and reproducibility of OCT in detecting DES endothelialization. Suzuki *et al* analyzed the performance of OCT and IVUS to evaluate neointimal coverage compared to histology in a swine model. They found that OCT had a high correlation with histology measurements (r = 0.980, p < 0.001, for the lumen area; r = 0.978, p < 0.001, for the stent area; and r = 0.961, p < 0.001, for the neointimal area) and a good diagnostic accuracy for detecting a small degree of neointima (AUC = 0.967, 95% CI 0.914–1.019). Conversely, IVUS showed a poorer correlation with histology (AUC = 0.781, 95% CI 0.621–838) [15]. Also, in a pathological study in a porcine coronary model, Murata *et al* demonstrated a high correlation between OCT and histology regarding neointimal thickness, and neointimal and luminal area. Interestingly, OCT and histology detected a similar proportion (1.16% and 1.84%) of uncovered struts. OCT seems to correlate appropriately with histology in either the absence (<20 μm) or the presence (>100 μm) of robust neointima; however, the correlation does not seem to be very linear between these values (the proportions of struts displaying neointimal thicknesses ranging from 20–80 μm differed significantly) [16]. Prati *et al* proved an adequate linear correlation between neointimal measurements obtained by OCT and histological measures, with a correlation coefficient of 0.726 (p <0.0001), in a rabbit model. Furthermore, intra- and inter-observer reproducibility were 0.9 and 0.8, respectively [17]. Initial reports also correlated neointima visualized by OCT with histopathological findings in humans [18]. Nakano *et al* found a good correlation between OCT and histological analysis for strut coverage in 14 human stented coronary segments from autopsy specimens, with a sensitivity of 79%, a specificity of 97% and good inter-observer reproducibility [19].

The second generation of OCT imaging systems, i.e. OFDI, have also shown excellent agreement with histological analysis regarding neointimal thickness (r = 0.90, p < 0.01) and strut coverage (r = 0.96, p < 0.01). Moreover, optical density measurements revealed a significant difference between fibrin- and neointima-covered coronary stent struts, suggesting that differences in optical density provide information on the type of stent strut coverage (see figure 1.1). Namely, the pixel intensity (optical density) of stent strut coverage in OFDI images, normalized

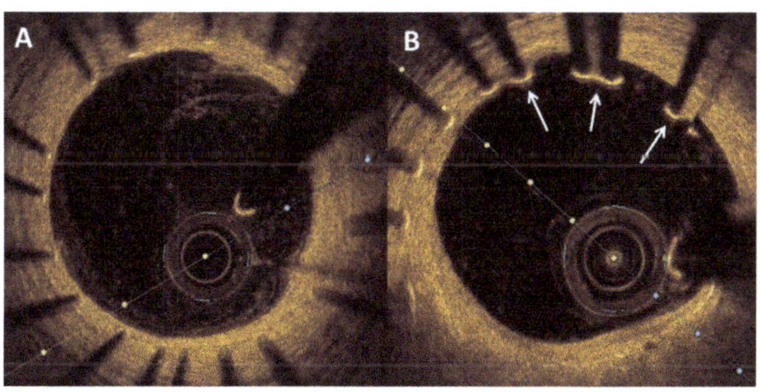

Figure 1.1. Complete versus incomplete strut coverage. (A) A complete homogeneous layer of neoendothelium. (B) Incomplete coverage, struts from 11 to 3 (arrows) are not covered, probably due to slight incomplete apposition.

for optical density of the stent struts, revealed an excellent diagnostic accuracy (AUC = 0.859) for differentiating fibrin versus neointimal stent strut coverage. Therefore, densitometric analysis may represent a promising tool to obtain further information on the type of stent strut coverage [20].

Its accuracy in detecting and quantifying neointima makes OCT a unique technique to evaluate the process of endothelialization *in vivo*. OCT assessment of stent strut coverage is not standardized, and a quantitative or qualitative approach can be used. In the first methodology, strut coverage is evaluated through quantification of tissue coverage area: the operator manually traces the stent and lumen area, deriving the tissue coverage area. Using this type of approach, good intra- and inter-observer agreement has been reported for neointima thickness measurements [17, 21, 22]. Volume measurements can be performed using Simpson's rule, where the areas of each cross section in a pullback multiplied by the slice thickness (frame–frame spacing) are added over the segmented volume of interest [23, 24]. Data can also be quantified at strut-level, measuring the thickness of the covering tissue in each strut, namely the distance between the luminal surface of the covering tissue and the luminal surface of the strut [23, 24]. The second and most used approach to evaluate strut coverage is a visual qualitative classification of strut coverage as a binary variable (covered or not covered). This qualitative evaluation of strut coverage by OCT has proven to have good inter- and intra-observer agreement. The zoom setting is an important bias and the range of intra-observer agreement according to the zoom used is very broad—the same strut can have a 0%–25% probability of being considered as uncovered depending on the zoom used [25]. Qualitative analysis is generally expressed as the percentage of uncovered struts, and other measurements have been proposed, such as the linear distribution of strut coverage [24]. OCT assessment of strut coverage is limited by its axial resolution and by blooming artifacts (intense signal generated by the reflection of light against the metallic struts) which may cause one to overestimate the number of uncovered struts.

Different studies have employed different arbitrary cut-off values for the ratio of uncovered struts which might be considered clinically relevant. For example a rate of >10% uncovered struts was used in the optical coherence tomography in acute myocardial infarction (OCTAMI) trial 28, whereas rates of >5% and >10% uncovered struts were employed in the LEADERS trial. However, histological data showed a higher prevalence of thrombus in stents with a ratio of uncovered struts >30% [26]. Won *et al* analyzed OCT imaging at a median of 851 days after DES implantation in 535 lesions treated with DESs, and found that the best cut-off value for the percentage of uncovered struts for predicting major events was 5.9% [27]. However, to date there is not enough evidence to establish a definitive cut-off value of the percentage of uncovered struts or malapposed struts that is clinically relevant. Thus, a larger OCT study is warranted to evaluate the reliability of the degree of incomplete coverage for identifying patients at a clinically relevant increased risk of LST.

1.2.1.1 Stent coverage according to clinical presentation

Pathological observations suggest that the ratio of uncovered to total stent struts is increased in patients with acute coronary syndrome after DES implantation [28].

OCT evaluation of DES implanted in patients with ST-elevation myocardial infarction (STEMI) revealed a higher frequency of uncovered stent struts at a median follow-up of 9 months when compared with patients with stable coronary disease (93.8% versus 67.7%, $p = 0.048$). Data from the same study showed that DES implantation in STEMI was the only independent predictor for both the presence of uncovered struts and incomplete stent apposition (ISA) at follow-up [29]. This may be one of the underlying factors that make acute coronary syndrome a patient-related factor for stent thrombosis (see further in section 1.2.5).

1.2.1.2 Stent coverage depending on the stent type

Analysis of coverage at strut-level using OCT is the most common surrogate endpoint in OCT studies, providing a measurable variable for comparison between different stents and also being an important parameter for the approval of new drug-eluting stents by regulatory agencies.

- *First-generation DES*s. These include the sirolimus-eluting stent (SES) and paclitaxel-eluting stent (PES).

  Takano *et al* compared 3 month and 2 year OCT findings in patients who had received a first-generation SES. The neointimal coverage had advanced during the follow-up, as shown by a greater thickness of neointima, a lower frequency of uncovered struts and a lower prevalence of patients with a cross section of uncovered strut ratio >0.3 in the 2 year evaluation. However, the prevalence of patients who had any cross-sections with an uncovered strut ratio >0.3 was still significant (38%). Therefore, despite the evolving neointimal coverage, a few stent struts might persist as uncovered struts long-term [30]. Other OCT studies agreed with the conclusion that first-generation SESs showed a higher frequency of incomplete strut coverage compared to BMSs [31, 32].

  Ishigami *et al* evaluated 60 patients classified into three groups according to the time elapsed since SES implantation. The follow-up time was associated with a significant increase in mean neointimal area and neointimal thickness, and a significant decrease in the number of uncovered stent struts. However, even at the later follow-up, only 17.6% of implanted SESs were completely covered by neointima [33].

  In a comparative study between two first-generation stents, OCT examination at 6 months showed that compared to SESs, PESs have a non-uniform and larger neointimal thickness with fewer uncovered struts, and more peri-strut low-density areas, probably related to inflammatory areas and fibrin deposits [34]
- *Second-generation DESs.*

  Second-generation stents have demonstrated a better clinical and angiographic performance compared to first-generation stents [35], and a lower rate of stent thrombosis [14, 36–38]. OCT evaluation of strut coverage has provided insight into the possible mechanisms underlying these better outcomes.

Everolimus-eluting stent (EES): OCT evaluation 8 months after EES implantation showed that most struts were covered with uniform and thin neointima. The frequency of low-intensity neointima was very low, suggesting a good vessel healing pattern [39]. These findings are in concordance with the good clinical outcome data associated with this stent platform, showing a reduction of stent thrombosis compared to first-generation stents [40, 41]. Toledano *et al* reported OCT follow-up (at least one year) of 66 DESs: 21 EESs, 23 SESs and 22 PESs. The average tissue coverage thickness of the struts per stent was greater in EESs than in SESs and PESs, while the percentage of uncovered and malapposed struts was much lower in EESs, with no significant differences between SESs and PESs [42].

Zotarolimus-eluting stent (ZES): OCT imaging studies revealed a higher mean neointimal thickness and a lower prevalence of uncovered struts as well as malapposed struts in ZESs than in SESs [43]. The OCTAMI trial (optical coherence tomography in acute myocardial infarction) found no differences in 6 month follow-up strut coverage and a similar vessel response to ZESs, when compared to identical BMSs, implanted during primary percutaneous coronary intervention (PCI) in STEMI patients [44].

- *Drug-eluting balloons (DEBs).*

  OCT has been established as the reference technique to evaluate stent performance regarding neointimal coverage *in vivo*. Therefore, randomized OCT studies are the cornerstone for the evaluation of newer stents or alternative techniques. A recent 'hybrid' approach tries to combine the advantages of BMSs in terms of strut coverage while reducing the ISR rate, using a BMS and DEB simultaneously, and studies have focused on OCT follow-up to determine its safety.

  The OCTOPUS trial compared strut coverage and neointimal proliferation of a therapy using a BMS postdilated with a paclitaxel DEB to everolimus DESs at 6 month follow-up using OCT, showing comparable results for the percentage of uncovered struts, but more neointimal proliferation in the BMS + DEB group (although there was no difference in the rate of ISR) [45]. Other ongoing studies are also comparing the use of BMSs alone or associated with DEBs in terms of OCT findings at follow-up [46]. OCT studies are thus a valuable tool as a first step in evaluating *in vivo* stent performance, but these data must be supported by clinical outcomes.

- *Biodegradable polymers.*

  Recently published long-term follow-up studies combining data from three large randomized trials showed a reduction in the incidence of LST with biodegradable polymer DESs compared to durable polymer SESs [47–49].

  It has been hypothesized that the lower rates of late adverse events associated with biodegradable polymer stents are related to improved vascular healing as assessed by intravascular imaging. An OCT substudy of the LEADERS trial reported that a biodegradable polymer biolimus-eluting stent (BES) showed superior stent strut coverage at 9 months, despite an overall comparable degree of neointimal suppression compared to a durable polymer SES [50]. However, further data showed that subsequent improvement of SES coverage between 9–24 months resulted in similar strut coverage for the BES and SES at 24 months [51]. On the other hand, the OCTDESI pilot trial compared biodegradable polymer PESs with durable polymer PESs and found no difference in the proportion of uncovered struts at 6 months [52]. Also, a novel rapid-breakdown biodegradable polymer SES compared to a durable polymer EES showed a similar degree of early stent strut coverage as assessed by OCT at 4 months, although coverage patterns were more homogeneous for the biodegradable polymer SES [24].

1.2.1.3 Clinical applications

It has already been stated that OCT assessment of strut coverage is widely used for the evaluation of newer stents and techniques. In the same way, OCT evaluation of this re-endothelialization process may help to define the optimal duration of dual antiplatelet therapy after stent implantation, both to define general strategies and to individualize treatment.

1.2.1.4 Limitations

Current OCT resolution is insufficient to detect thicknesses <20 μm, which prevents accurate distinction between the absence of endothelialization and the presence of a very thin layer of 3–5 endothelial cells.

The vascular healing process involves the participation of the coagulation system and many types of cells in different phases, all of them covering the stent struts. Optical coherence tomography is unable to distinguish between fibrin, giant cells, granulomatous reaction and degree of endothelialization [16]. There are promising findings with optical density analysis that claim to be able to distinguish between neointima and fibrin/thrombus, but further investigation is warranted to confirm them [20].

As previously remarked, there is no clinically validated cut-off value for the percentage of uncovered struts associated with stent thrombosis, and there is a need for a homogeneous definition in order to compare different clinical studies.

1.2.2 Restenosis

ISR is defined as a luminal renarrowing after stent deployment. Binary angiographic restenosis is defined as ⩾50% luminal narrowing at follow-up angiography (see figure 1.2). Complete evaluation must include both an assessment of luminal narrowing and the patient's clinical context [53]. In case of an intermediate lesion, the use of fractional flow reserve or intracoronary imaging can guide the clinical decision.

OCT allows both quantitative and qualitative analysis of ISR (table 1.1). Neointima is defined as the tissue layer between the inner border of stent struts and the luminal border. Therefore, quantification of neointimal tissue is the key to differentiate between the normal process of re-endothelialization and ISR. OCT

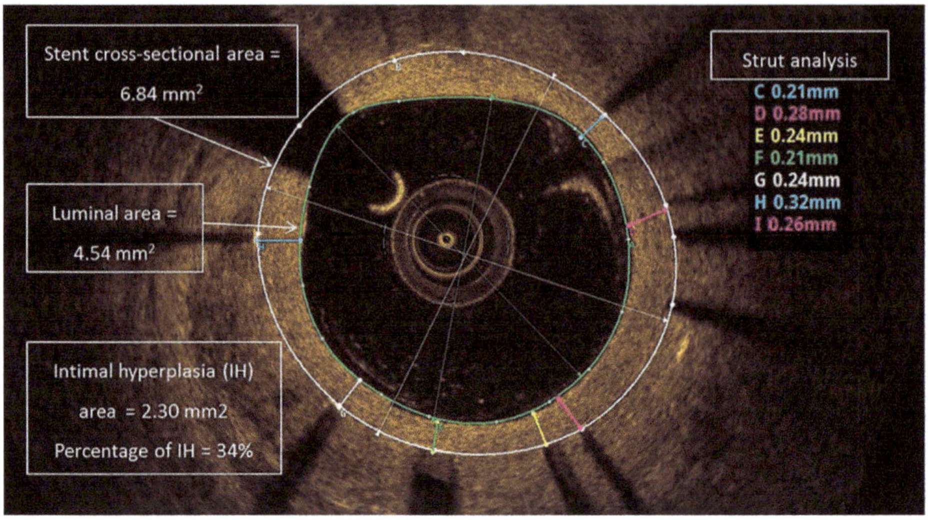

Figure 1.2. Example of ISR measurements.

Table 1.1. OCT assessment of ISR.

Quantitative assessment	Qualitative assessment
Stent area measurements	Structural characteristics
• Stent cross-sectional area	• Homogeneous
• Minimum and maximum stent diameter	• Heterogeneous
• Luminal area	• Layered
• Intimal hyperplasia area	
• Percentage of intimal hyperplasia	
Strut measurements	Intensity
• Mean strut coverage thickness	• Hyperintense
	• Hypointense
Length measurements	Luminal border
	• Regular
	• Irregular
Volume measurements	Microvessels; intraluminal material

allows the accurate measurement of stent cross-sectional area (CSA), minimum and maximum stent diameter, intimal hyperplasia (IH) area (calculated as stent area minus luminal area), and percentage of intimal hyperplasia (IH area divided by stent area) [23].

However, considering ISR as a mere problem of diameters and areas is an oversimplification. ISR is a complex process that is not completely understood, which may reflect different underlying mechanisms (or different stages of the same mechanism). Experimental and clinical studies have identified excessive neointimal hyperplasia as the leading cause of stent restenosis, at least in BMSs [3, 54]. This intimal hyperplasia reaches a peak between 6 and 12 months after BMS deployment, and it was considered to be followed by a quiescent period with no further growth of this layer [3]. Clinical and histological evidence of very late restenosis of BMSs (occasionally observed beyond 4 years), showing late neointimal progression and neoatherosclerosis development, has now turned the paradigm of ISR into an evolving process [5–7, 55]. In DESs, it may be an even more complex process, initially inhibited by antiproliferative drugs, involving different mechanisms and progression.

OCT qualitative studies have provided evidence regarding the nature and evolution of ISR. Its high-resolution images have shown variation in structure, backscatter and composition of the hyperplastic tissue that could not be identified using IVUS. Gonzalo *et al* described three OCT patterns (see figure 1.3) of ISR in a sample of 148 cases (both BMS and DES from first and second generation) [56]:

- *Homogeneous neointima*: uniform signal-rich band without focal variation or attenuation.
- *Heterogeneous neointima*: Focally changing optical properties and various backscattering patterns.
- *Layered neointima*: layers with different optical properties.

Other differential characteristics between restenotic tissue include: high or low backscattering, the presence of microvessels, luminal shape and the presence of intraluminal material [56].

The observation of ISR with different optical properties suggests that it may have different compositions. It has been argued that non-homogeneous patterns may represent an artifact related to the progressive attenuation of the light, but there is no difference in the maximal tissue coverage thickness between the different patterns and sometimes there is a clearly visible border between layers, which support that these images are related to the presence of a different tissue [56]. Pathological studies have shown that restenosis in DESs can consist of heterogeneous components, including proteoglycan-rich tissue, organized thrombus, atheroma, inflammation and fibrinoids, and also the density and orientation of smooth muscle cells vary within restenotic tissue [57, 58]. It can be hypothesized that OCT patterns may translate these tissue differences, although current data regarding correlation of histopathology and OCT appearance is scarce and remains poorly understood [23]. Anecdotal reports have related heterogeneous tissue to the presence of fibrinoids or proteoglycans [59, 60]. Nakano *et al* demonstrated OCT signal (peak intensity and attenuation rate) differences over time in neointima after $\leqslant$6 months and >1 year, thus signal analysis of OCT may also be useful to unveil the components or processes of neointimal growth and ISR [19]. Recently, Itoh *et al* used the normalized standard deviation of OCT signal intensity to assess homogeneity in ISR tissue, finding that high values were a useful predictor for non-homogeneous images, and in some histological samples taken from these patients chronic inflammation and fibrin thrombi were observed [61].

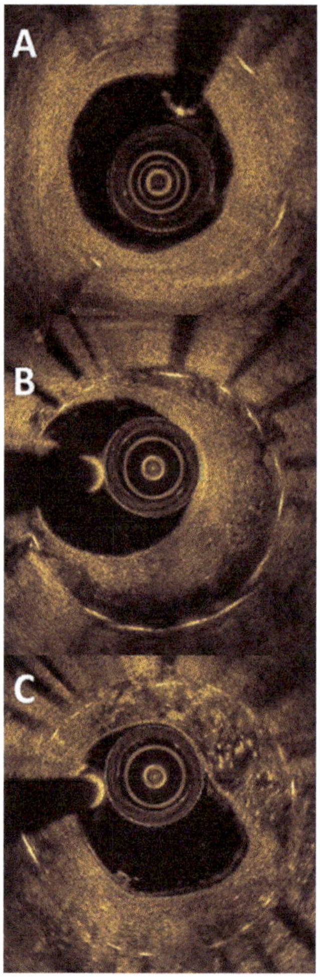

Figure 1.3. Examples of three different restenotic patterns. (A) Homogeneous, showing uniform optical properties. (B) Layered, with two concentric separate areas of different signal intensity. (C) Heterogeneous, several focal changes in optical intensity.

The assessment of ISR patterns by OCT showed low inter- and intra-observer variability. However, low reproducibility has been reported for the evaluation of other parameters such as tissue backscatter, which highlights the need for objective methods for the analysis of image properties to improve the accuracy [56, 62]. Moreover, there are still some limitations of OCT imaging that should be taken into account, such as the relatively low-penetration power of the light source, the influence of catheter position in the tissue backscatter and other possible artifacts.

Further analyses have tried to correlate OCT ISR features and clinical and angiographic characteristics. Heterogeneous neointima is more frequently present in focal restenosis (rather than diffuse) and at minimum lumen area [56, 62]. The time from stent implantation also seems to influence OCT appearance, the layered pattern being more frequent in stents implanted ⩽12 months before the OCT examination, while the heterogeneous pattern has been found in a higher proportion in very late ISR (>5 years) [56, 62]. The homogeneous pattern is more common in the early stages. Yamaguchi *et al* found, in a group of 25 patients with late ISR, that the heterogeneous pattern was more prevalent in patients with late ISR who had more abrupt neointimal growth in serial OCT evaluation, while the homogeneous pattern was associated with a more gradual decrease of luminal area [63].

Acute coronary syndrome is associated with irregular luminal shape, the presence of intraluminal material, or more asymmetric ISR [56]. Both findings suggest that it translates to an active process with potential clinical implications. Following this line of thought, Kim *et al* studied the correlation between in-stent neointimal tissue patterns and major cardiovascular events (MACEs) at follow-up, excluding patients with significant restenosis and definite OCT evidence of neoatherosclerosis. They found that age and initial clinical presentation of acute coronary syndrome were the main independent predictors of heterogeneous neointima, and this pattern was independently associated with MACEs at follow-up [64]. There is also initial observational data suggesting that ISR patterns may have a distinct response to the different treatment modalities (i.e. plain balloon angioplasty, paclitaxel-coated balloon dilatation or DES implantation) [65].

Most of these data are preliminary and need to be confirmed, but they constitute a promising line of investigation where OCT may play a major role.

1.2.3 Neoatherosclerosis

Neoatherosclerosis refers to an atherosclerotic change in neointimal tissue, which is histologically defined as clusters of lipid-laden foamy macrophages within the neointima with or without necrotic core formation [66] (see figure 1.4). In recent years, growing evidence has suggested that neointima is subject to atherosclerotic changes similar to native vessels that may lead to late clinical events. The paradigm that considers neointimal development a quiescent process after the first year of BMS implantation has been widely disproved by clinical, angiographic and histopathological data. Histological studies have found that in the first 2–3 years after stenting, endothelial coverage is formed by smooth muscle and collagen rich neointima, but also chronic inflammation elements can be found (macrophages, T cells and giant cell infiltration); after that (more than 3–4 years) smooth muscle cells are sparse, with abundant collagen toward the lumen and evidence of neoatherosclerosis, namely foamy macrophages around stent struts, with an increasing incidence over time [66, 67]. These neoatherosclerotic changes have been related to very late BMS thrombosis both in autopsy findings and thrombectomy specimen analysis [68, 69].

Moreover, DESs, which were designed to avoid excessive neointimal growth, have proved to also be affected by this neoatherosclerotic process. Clinical and histologic studies of DESs have demonstrated evidence of continuous neointimal growth during long-term follow-up, which is designated as the 'late catch-up' phenomenon [70, 71]. Furthermore, pathological studies suggest that this

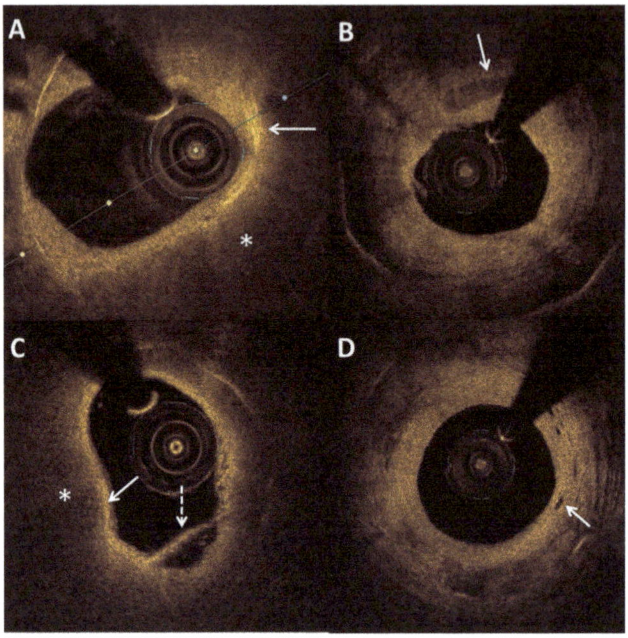

Figure 1.4. OCT findings suggestive of neoatherosclerosis. (A) ISR showing a hypointense area similar to lipidic plaque (asterisk), and linear images with high intensity (arrow) compatible with cholesterol crystals. (B) Heterogeneous restenosis with microcalcifications (arrow). (C) Thin-cap fibroatheroma inside a stent composed of a predominant lipidic component (asterisk), and a thin fibrous cap (solid arrow), with an area of rupture (dashed arrow). (D) Microvessels (arrow).

atherosclerotic change occurs more quickly in DESs than in BMSs [66]. This phenomenon is poorly understood, and it has been speculated to be related to the incomplete maturation of the regenerated endothelium [72].

OCT is recognized as a valuable tool for atherosclerotic plaque quantitative and qualitative evaluation, and some of the plaque characteristics can be identified and quantified with good correlation with pathological findings [23, 73]. Therefore, OCT imaging is a unique tool to determine the presence of these atherosclerotic features within the intrastent lumen and to analyze the evolution and clinical implications of neoatherosclerosis *in vivo*.

Atherosclerotic findings that can be visualized inside the stent neointima include:

- *Calcific intima*: well-delineated, signal-poor region with sharp borders.
- *Lipidic intima*: signal-poor region with diffuse borders [74].
- *Macrophage infiltration*: increased signal intensity accompanied by heterogeneous back shadows [75].
- *Cholesterol crystals*: bright spikes inside a lipidic plaque.
- *Thin-cap fibroatheroma* (TCFA): fibrous cap thickness at the thinnest part $\leqslant 65$ μm and an angle of lipidic tissue $\geqslant 180°$.
- *Neointimal rupture*: break in the fibrous cap that connected the lumen with the underlying lipid pool.

- *Microvessel:* evidence of neovascularization; a small vesicular or tubular dark or hypointense structure with a diameter $\leqslant 200$ μm. In-stent microvasculature is divided into two categories: intraintimal, located within the most superficial 50% of the neointimal thickness, and persistent, within the deepest 50% [7].

Several studies have used OCT to evaluate the presence of neoatherosclerosis and assess its temporal development and clinical implications. Habara *et al* found a high incidence (90.7%) of possible neoatherosclerotic change [35] in restenotic lesions 5 years after BMS implantation, while it was scarce (17.9%) in 1 year ISR. Neointimal disruption, which has an analogous morphology to ruptured fibroatheroma in a native coronary artery, occurred more frequently in $\geqslant 5$ year lesions (18.6%) than in 1 year lesions (0%) [6]. Similarly, Takano *et al* demonstrated that neointima exhibited a homogeneous OCT appearance, and there was a lack of lipid-laden intima in the early phase (6 months). Conversely, lipid-laden intima, intimal disruption and luminal thrombus formation were more frequently observed in the late phase (5 years) when compared to the early phase. Furthermore, although microvasculature was present in both stages, the appearance of intraintimal neovascularization was more prevalent in the late phase and in segments with lipid-laden intima, suggesting that the expansion of neovascularization from persistent to intraintima may contribute to neoatherosclerotic progression [7].

OCT analysis in 50 patients with DES-ISR (median follow-up period 32.2 months) demonstrated a high incidence of TCFA-containing neointima (52%), in-stent neointimal rupture (58%) and intraluminal thrombi. The presence of TCFA was significantly higher in ISR >20 months post-implantation. Interestingly, patients presenting with unstable (versus stable) angina showed a thinner fibrous cap and an increasing number of unstable OCT findings, including TCFA-containing neointima, neointima rupture and thrombus, suggesting a clinical implication for these neoatherosclerotic findings [76]. Current data show that first-generation DESs have a constant rate of VLST (0.26%–0.4%/yr), with little evidence of a plateau up to 5 years [77], and neoatherosclerosis may be a relevant cause that warrants further investigation.

The progression of neoatherosclerosis in the same patient was evaluated by Kim *et al* with serial OCT imaging at 9 months and 2 years after DES implantation. On qualitative evaluation of neointimal morphology, lipid-laden neointima (27.6% versus 14.5%, $p = 0.009$) and thin-cap neoatheroma (13.2% versus 3.9%, $p = 0.07$) were more frequently detected at the 2 year follow-up compared to at 9 months. In matched cross-sectional evaluation, the change of neointimal morphology from a homogeneous to heterogeneous or lipid-laden pattern was observed in 23 (30.3%) of 76 lesions [78].

Neoatherosclerosis has been described in both BMSs and DESs, but they seem to present a different temporal pattern as supported by histological data [66]. OCT has provided further evidence on this aspect. Yonetsu *et al* demonstrated a greater incidence of lipid-laden intima inside DESs than in BMSs at $\leqslant 4$ years post-implantation, although no significant difference was observed afterward, suggesting an earlier onset of neoatherosclerosis in DESs [79]. There was more neovascularization in BMSs than in DESs in the early phase, showing again a different response and vascular healing that may influence the development of neoatherosclerosis [79].

The presence of atherosclerotic features in the neointima can also be objectively quantified by measurements of the attenuation, backscatter, intensity and normalized standard deviation (NSD) of the OCT signal, showing a good correlation with visual assessment [79]. However, there is a lack of consensus regarding cut-off values and further investigation is needed to standardize this quantitative assessment.

Evidence regarding underlying mechanisms and risk factors of neoatherosclerosis is scarce. OCT evaluation of 179 stents with significant neointimal growth (⩾100 μm) found that for a stent age ⩾48 months, all subtypes of drug-eluting stent, current smoking, chronic kidney disease and angiotensin-converting enzyme inhibitors/angiotensin II receptor blockade use were independent predictors for neoatherosclerosis [80]. However, these observational data provide a low level of evidence, and the mechanism of neoatherosclerotic change needs to be investigated in the future, as well as possible therapeutic strategies to avoid its development.

1.2.4 Incomplete stent apposition (malapposition)

1.2.4.1 Definition and quantification

Apposition is defined as contact of the stent struts with the vessel wall. A strut is considered to be malapposed (see figure 1.5) if it is separated abluminally from the luminal contour of the vessel [23]. Evaluation of apposition requires an adequate visualization of both elements, which can only be achieved with intracoronary imaging techniques. OCT is the most precise and sensitive technique to evaluate apposition due to his high spatial resolution and imaging quality. With OCT,

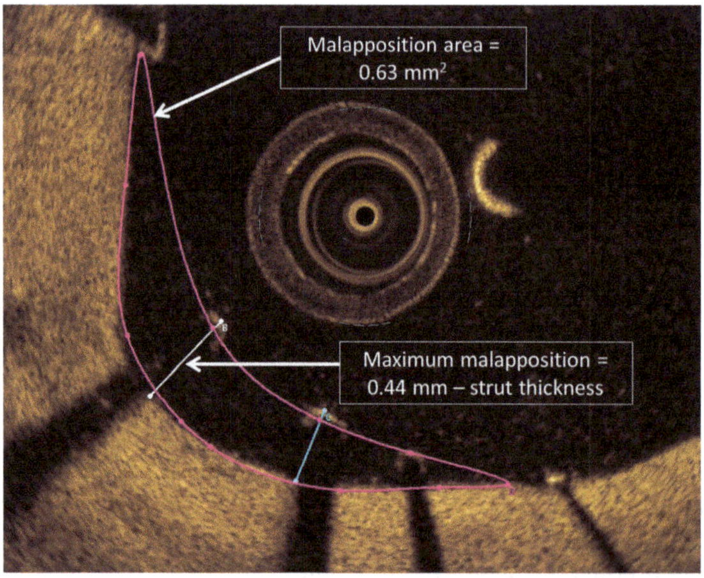

Figure 1.5. Example of measurement of incomplete stent apposition.

metallic stent struts appear as highly reflective surfaces and cast shadows on the vessel wall behind and we can only visualize the adluminal reflection of the strut (while the optical shadow hides the body of the strut and its abluminal side), thus the contact between the strut and the vessel wall cannot be directly assessed by OCT. Apposition must be indirectly assessed by measuring the distance between the adluminal border of the stent and the vessel wall and then subtracting the strut thickness (strut and polymer thickness in DESs). To enhance accuracy, the measurement line should be as perpendicular to the strut and vessel wall as possible [81].

The use of two kinds of correction factors for apposition assessment is recommended. The first one consists of adding an empirical margin between 10–20 μm to take into account the OCT axial resolution. The second approach tries to correct the intense signal generated by the reflection of light against the metallic struts (so-called strut blooming). The true edge of the strut lies somewhere in the middle of that blooming. The correction for blooming consists of measuring its thickness in a random sample of study struts and then adding to the analysis of apposition a correction factor equal to half of the blooming thickness. The use of one or another correction is more of a theoretical methodological issue than a relevant practical matter [82, 83]. To obtain a global estimation of ISA, a thorough cross-sectional analysis is required (at least at 1 mm intervals, choosing the best images with clearly identifiable vessel wall and struts within two frames distal or proximal) and for a certain cross section (or the global stent assessment) measurements can refer to the distance of ISA (maximum, median, average), ISA volume, or percentage of malapposed struts [81, 84].

When analyzing bioresorbable intracoronary devices, the abluminal side of the strut and its contact with or detachment from the vessel wall can be directly evaluated by OCT [85].

Considering apposition, the following classification may be applied [81]:

- *Malapposition* (or ISA): defined as a strut–vessel distance greater than the corrected strut–polymer thickness.
- *Protruding*: a strut–vessel distance more than half of the corrected strut–polymer thickness.
- *Embedded*: a strut–vessel distance less than half of the corrected strut–polymer thickness.

Both protruding and embedded struts are well-apposed. This discrimination might be of interest because of the flow disruption and potential increased thrombogenicity caused by protruding struts. However, recent data suggest that protruding struts and struts malapposed with moderate detachment (ISA distance <100 μm) pose minimal disturbance to blood flow compared to floating struts [86]. Moreover, to the best of current knowledge, there is no evidence of a clinical impact related to protruding struts, and the criterion for optimal stent deployment is to avoid ISA [82].

The evaluation of apposition is not possible in the strut's 'jailed' side branches, and they may be considered as an independent category. There is evidence that coverage of non-apposed side-branch struts is delayed with respect to well-apposed struts in DESs, as assessed by OCT, and similar to ISA struts [87, 88].

Imaging and pathological studies have shown that ISA is correlated with thrombus detection (visualized by OCT in more than 20% of struts with ISA at follow-up compared to 2% of struts with a good apposition ($P < 0.001$)) and LST/VLST [89, 90]. Acute malapposition reflects a procedural failure and is mainly associated with early stent thrombosis. However, it may produce LST after dual antiplatelet treatment discontinuation. ISA is closely associated with delayed neo-intimal healing and incomplete endothelialization [90, 91]. This is probably the ultimate mechanism that triggers stent thrombosis in ISA. Acute stent malapposition can be observed with OCT in more than 60% of lesions, even with angiographic optimization with high pressures and adequately sized balloons, being more frequent within the edges of the stents. Severe diameter stenosis, calcified lesions and stent characteristics (strut thickness and length) have been identified as independent predictors of acute stent malapposition [84, 92].

1.2.4.2 ISA evolution: neointimal healing versus persistent ISA

After acute ISA, the neointimal healing process might spontaneously correct it to some extent, integrating the malapposed regions into the vessel wall, as suggested by sequential quantitative studies with OCT, which reported ISA volumes and percentage of ISA struts decreasing over time [90, 93]. ISA should be considered as a quantitative, rather than binary phenomenon (present or absent), because the quantify influences the evolution regarding strut coverage and flow profile. OCT studies have tried to establish a threshold for ISA that poses a higher risk of incomplete coverage at follow-up. Foin *et al* analyzed 72 stents at baseline and at a 6 month follow-up, finding that segments with an ISA detachment <100 μm at baseline showed complete strut coverage at follow-up, whereas segments with a maximal ISA detachment distance of 100–300 μm and >300 μm had 6.1% and 15.7% of their struts still uncovered, respectively ($P < 0.001$) [86]. Shimamura *et al* evaluated ISA at a 1 year follow-up in EESs and SESs, finding that both stents showed a significant decrease in ISA distance, but with EESs showing better performance. Receiver-operating curve analysis identified that the best cut-off value of OCT-estimated ISA distance at post-stenting for predicting late-persistent ISA at 8–12 month follow-up in EESs and SESs was >355 μm and >285 μm, respectively [94]. This is concordant with the strut–vessel distance threshold of $\leqslant$260 μm in post-stenting OCT images identified as the best cut-off point for resolved malapposed struts in another study [95]. Im *et al* analyzed the OCT images from 351 patients with 356 lesions who received post-stent and follow-up (175 ± 60 days) OCT examinations. 31% of lesions with acute stent malapposition remained malapposed (late-persistent stent malapposition), and they found that an ISA volume >2.56 mm^3 and the location within the stent edges were independent predictors of late-persistent stent malapposition [84]. Another study found a similar predictive value when ISA size was estimated by ISA volume as when it was estimated by the maximum ISA distance per strut, observing that maximum ISA distances <270 μm after stent implantation appeared covered and spontaneously reapposed in 100% of cases at follow-up (distances <400 μm, in 93% of the cases), whereas maximum ISA distances ⩾850 μm resulted in persistent ISA and grossly delayed coverage in 100% of cases [91]. It is not clearly determined how long this healing process is maintained. Serial OCT follow-up examination of DESs 9 months and 2 years after implantation showed that the percentage of malapposed struts was similar (0.6% versus 0.9%, $p = 0.24$), although the percentage of uncovered stent struts significantly decreased [78].

These studies suggest a threshold of ISA detachment estimated by OCT that is associated with persistent ISA and therefore might benefit from optimization during stent implantation. However, to date, no prospective trial has tested this hypothesis and the question of what degree of acute ISA is worth correcting remains unanswered for the interventional cardiologist. Moreover, factors other than ISA measurements can influence this process. OCT studies have identified that DES implantation during primary PCI in STEMI is an independent predictor of ISA at follow-up [29]. Other data suggest that persistent ISA is more frequent over lipid or calcified plaques than over fibrous plaques [96].

OCT analysis can identify different patterns of ISA evolution. Radu *et al* observed four patterns of strut apposition at least 2 months after stent deployment based on the stent area (SA) and vessel wall area (VWA) and morphology: (i) apposed struts, in frames where SA = VWA; (ii) struts overlying the ostium of a side branch (SA = VWA); (iii) malapposed struts, that are clearly separated from the vessel wall where SA < VWA; and (iv) 'pseudo-apposed' struts, struts that are not clearly separated from the vessel wall, but where SA < VWA, creating a sort of 'flower shape'. The authors hypothesized that these different patterns may translate to different tissue coverage, in particular in the pseudo-apposed pattern, where struts often display lower signal brightness than the rest of the vessel wall, which might indicate the presence of fibrin [97]. Histological confirmation and clinical implications of this hypothesis have not yet been established.

Gutierrez-Chico *et al* described six possible OCT morphological patterns at follow-up (see figure 1.6):

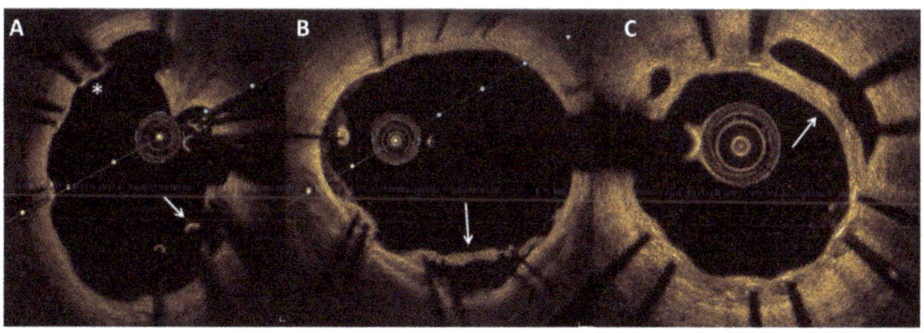

Figure 1.6. Two different coverages of incomplete stent apposition. (A) Strut re-endothelialization of well-apposed struts (asterisk), while non-apposed struts appear uncovered (arrow). (B) Partial coverage (partial bridging) of incomplete apposed struts. (C) Bridged: persisting incomplete stent apposition, entirely covered by a rim of tissue linking the vessel intima with the malapposed struts.

1. *Homogeneous*: ISA integrated into the vessel wall, covered with a homogeneous density, and retaining a smooth lumen contour.
2. *Layered*: ISA integrated into the vessel wall, covered with a double or triple density, often with a layered appearance, and retaining a smooth lumen contour.
3. *Crenellated*: ISA integrated into the vessel wall and grossly covered, but presenting indentations that give the lumen contour a scalloped appearance.
4. *Bridged*: persisting ISA, entirely covered by a rim of tissue linking the vessel intima with the malapposed struts.
5. *Partially bridged*: persisting ISA; a rim of tissue linking the vessel intima with the malapposed struts can be seen but does not cover all the ISA struts.
6. *Bare*: ISA uncovered struts, with little tissue reaction.

Delayed healing was defined by patterns 3–6, while persistent ISA was defined by patterns 4–6. As previously stated, initial ISA size was the only independent predictor for ISA patterns at follow-up. The vascular tissue reaction ends in the complete integration of the ISA into the vessel wall in most cases (71.5%), but two out of three cases of acute ISA have a morphological healing pattern that is not homogeneous. These different OCT patterns may reflect the healing process of acute ISA. The authors argue that the bridged pattern might represent an earlier state in the maturation of neointimal coverage. Small ISA volumes could induce a conformal bridging pattern of healing that ends up connecting the ISA struts with the vessel wall (homogeneous pattern) or that creates a false lumen that undergoes subsequent low-flow and thrombosis phenomena (layered pattern). The layered pattern might also be caused by the cytotoxicity of specific drugs or stents, or by the increased presence of fibrinoids or proteoglycans. The partially bridged and bare patterns might represent the failure of neointima to cover large ISA regions before the vascular healing response ceases [91]. Once more, further investigation is warranted to confirm this hypothesis and its possible clinical relevance. In any case, OCT has been confirmed to be a powerful investigational tool with potential use in *in situ* clinical decision making.

1.2.4.3 Late-acquired ISA

Vessel remodeling and strut coverage after stent deployment is a complex process, and as shown, the evolving result is a mix of different possibilities. Previously reported data describe the possible evolution and determinants after acute malapposition (i.e. immediate ISA after stent deployment), which can be grossly classified at follow-up as 'resolved acute malapposition' or 'late-persistent stent malapposition'. However, there is another important situation at follow-up, 'late-acquired stent malapposition' (LA-ISA), namely, a newly developed stent malapposition that is identified at the follow-up examination despite complete stent apposition during the initial procedure. Acute and late-acquired malapposition can coexist in the same patient. Therefore, OCT studies have shown four possible situations at follow-up regarding stent apposition:

- Resolved acute malapposition, i.e. immediate ISA after stent deployment not persistent in the follow-up.
- Late-persistent stent malapposition, i.e. acute ISA not resolved in the follow-up.
- LA-ISA in a completely well-apposed stent at initial evaluation.
- Resolved acute malapposition with development of LA-ISA in another stent segment.
- Late-persistent stent malapposition with LA-ISA.

In an analysis of 351 patients with 356 lesions treated with DESs (70% second-generation DESs) with post-stent and follow-up OCT examinations, Im *et al* detected LA-ISA in 15% of all lesions (accounting for 3.8% ± 4.5% of the struts) and it was usually (61%) located within the stent body. It was more frequently associated with plaque/thrombus prolapse in post-stent OCT images (70% versus 42%; $P < 0.001$). Lesions classified as late-persistent stent malapposition with LA-ISA had the smallest neointimal hyperplasia thicknesses. In this series, LA-ISA was not related to clinical events, including cardiovascular death, nonfatal myocardial infarction and stent thrombosis, during the follow-up period of 28.6 ± 10.3 months [84].

In a meta-analysis of 17 trials, Hassan *et al* found a higher risk of LA-ISA in DESs compared to BMSs [98]. Also, an OCT follow-up substudy of the HORIZONS-AMI trial showed a higher proportion of malapposed struts in DESs (paclitaxel) [83]. This difference could be attributable to the adverse effect of the drug on the vessel wall, resulting in positive remodeling [99]. Hypersensitivity to the metallic stent, the polymer, or the drug has been associated with positive remodeling and excessive inflammation in the vessel wall [100]. Further studies suggested that the vessel response is different depending of the drug used [101, 102]. Nakano *et al* found that OCT identified histologically confirmed hypersensitivity as luminal surface irregularities and cavity formation around struts, or dark tissue with a moderate signal attenuation rate in the areas adjacent to the stent struts [19].

Coronary imaging studies have suggested two possible mechanisms underlying late-acquired malapposition: regional positive remodeling of the vessel wall (as previously exposed) and decrease of the plaque volume behind the stent (including clot lysis or plaque regression) [99, 103, 104]. In OCT studies, the presence of a plaque/thrombus protrusion has been reported to be a predictor of LA-ISA. Thus, it was suggested that plaque/thrombus dissolution plays an important role in the pathogenesis of late-acquired stent malapposition [84].

Evidence regarding the clinical implications of stent malapposition is controversial and non-conclusive [89, 98, 102, 103]. In a meta-analysis of five studies, Hassan *et al* found a higher risk of LST in patients with LA-ISA [98]. However, other studies have shown no relationship between them [89, 105]. This discordance may be attributable to a different extent of ISA, time of follow-up or other factors, such as length of dual antiplatelet therapy or the use of newer generation stents [106]. Moreover, the relatively low incidence of stent thrombosis makes a large sample size necessary, and follow-up to establish any relationship with certainty is required.

To the best of current knowledge, it is not clear whether the presence of LA-ISA should be treated and how. It is evident that it may persist for years without leading to VLST, and there is no evidence thus far that the optimization of the subtle degrees of ISA detected by OCT is associated with any clinical advantage. We need further investigation to clarify the underlying relationship between LA-ISA and stent thrombosis and its optimal management.

1.2.5 Stent thrombosis

1.2.5.1 Definition and epidemiology

Stent thrombosis is an uncommon, but serious complication of PCI (see figure 1.7). Its cause is total or subtotal thrombotic occlusion of a coronary artery by a thrombus that originates in or close to an intracoronary stent.

There Academic Research Consortium (ARC) established standardized definitions for stent thrombosis according to the diagnostic evidence [53]:

- *Definite stent thrombosis*: angiographic or histopathologic evidence of stent thrombosis at the site of the PCI.
- *Probable stent thrombosis*: unexplained death within 30 days of the procedure or myocardial infarction at any time in the territory of PCI.
- *Possible stent thrombosis*: unexplained death 30 days after the procedure [8].

A classification of the timing of stent thrombosis was also established:

- *Acute stent thrombosis*: occurring within 24 h of the procedure,
- *Early stent thrombosis*: between 24 h and 30 days,
- *LST*: between 31 days and 1 year.
- *VLST*: occurring more than 1 year after the procedure.

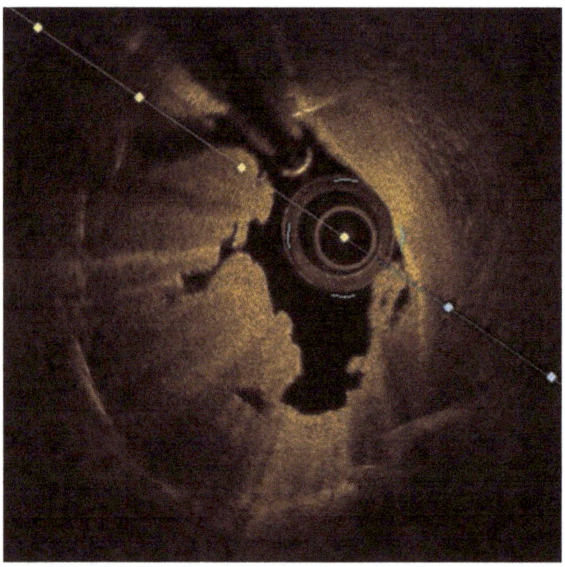

Figure 1.7. Example of stent thrombosis, a high burden of white thrombus is visualized, characterized by high backscatter with low attenuation.

The use of DESs improved PCI outcomes by reducing ISR due to neointimal hyperplasia inhibition. However, after DES use became common, the first reports of VLST pointed out an unexpected safety issue. In 2007, a meta-analysis of clinical trials confirmed an excess of VLST for DESs compared to BMSs [107]. Long-term follow-up data have shown that stent thrombosis is a rare event, and the rate of VLST is between 0.25% and 0.6% per year depending on the study [77, 108, 109]. However, it may have a growing impact because some first-generation DES studies showed that there is a steady increase in incidence, at least at 5 year follow-up [77]. Second-generation DESs have been shown to be associated with reduced rates of VLST compared to first-generation paclitaxel- and sirolimus-eluting stents [14, 36–38].

Regardless of its incidence, VLST is a relevant issue due to the severe clinical manifestations and poor prognosis. Most patients with stent thrombosis present with an acute coronary syndrome, mainly STEMI which accounts for up to 75% [110]. Mortality during hospitalization ranges from 7% to 18%, and reaches up to 25% at one year follow-up [77, 110, 111].

Although initial concerns about VLST have been declining in recent years due to the better performance of new generation stents, it is still a clinical issue in daily practice [112]. Therefore, further investigation is warranted to improve our understanding of this topic. OCT provides a useful tool for this purpose. Its application in experimental and clinical studies has expanded our knowledge regarding the underlying mechanisms of VLST, as described below. Beyond its research applications, OCT can identify stent-related causes in certain individuals with stent thrombosis, making it an essential technique for the evaluation of this issue.

1.2.5.2 Diagnosis

As stated in the definition, diagnosis relies on angiographic evidence of thrombus at the site of a previously implanted stent. The clinical scenario supports the differentiation between stent thrombosis and restenosis. However, sometimes the angiography does not clearly differentiate between them, and both can also coexist. OCT is a reliable tool to confirm diagnosis of stent thrombosis as well as to point out possible underlying mechanisms.

The accuracy of OCT in detecting acute thrombus formation is comparable to that of angioscopy [113], and OCT may reliably differentiate between red and white thrombi. A thrombus in OCT appears as a mass attached to the luminal surface or floating within the lumen. Red thrombi (which are cell-rich structures and consist mainly of red blood cells) are identified as high-backscattering protrusions inside the lumen of the artery, and have a high attenuation with signal-free shadowing. White thrombi (consisted mainly of platelets, fibrin and white blood cells) are less backscattering, homogeneous, and have low attenuation in the OCT image [23]. The ability of OCT to visualize different types of thrombi has been compared to histological diagnosis, which served as the 'gold standard'. Quantitative analysis of OCT images showed no significant differences in peak intensity of OCT signal between red and white thrombi. However, the 1/2 attenuation width of the signal intensity curve (i.e. distance from peak intensity to its 1/2 intensity) was significantly different between red and white thrombi (324 ± 50 versus 183 ± 42 μm, $p < 0.0001$).

A cut-off value of 250 μm in the 1/2 width of signal intensity attenuation can differentiate white from red thrombi with a sensitivity of 90% and specificity of 88% [114]. The distinction between a fibrin clot (a signal-rich structure without back-scattering) and minimal neointimal hyperplasia or other tissue types covering DESs or protruding in the lumen may be more challenging [115] and has yet to be validated in comparative experimental studies. The appearance of an organized thrombus in OCT is hypothesized to be heterogeneous, but the image characteristics of organized thrombi are not well understood or validated.

1.2.5.3 Mechanisms

The mechanisms underlying stent thrombosis can be classified into three types: patient, lesion and stent-related [112]. Patient-related mechanisms are clinical features such as clinical presentation (STEMI), diabetes or chronic kidney disease. These factors cannot be identified as the sole mechanism underlying stent thrombosis in a certain patient, but their presence has been associated with a higher risk of stent thrombosis, mainly early and late. Also premature clopidogrel discontinuation or clopidogrel resistance are patient-related stent thrombosis mechanisms [116, 117]. Lesion characteristics account mainly for a higher risk of early stent thrombosis and include length and the presence of thrombus [112].

Stent-related mechanisms include: underexpansion, incomplete re-endothelialization, malapposition (acute or acquired), inflammation (hypersensitivity) and neo-atherosclerosis [112] (see figure 1.8). OCT provides a unique technique for the

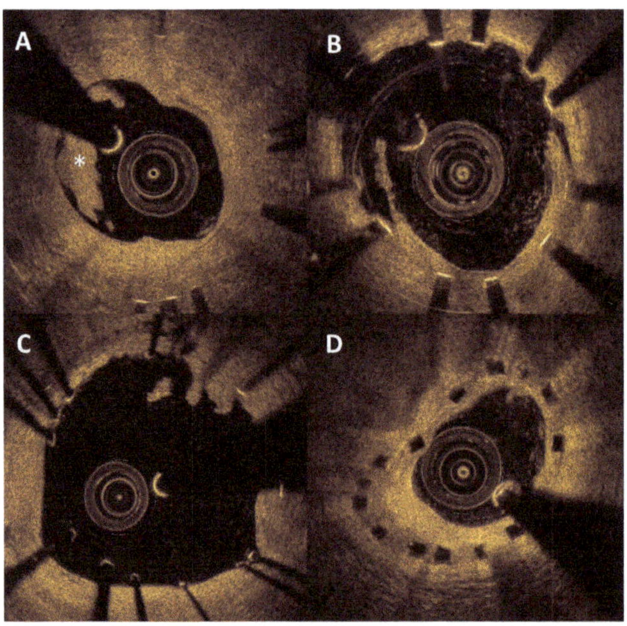

Figure 1.8. Different possible underlying mechanisms of stent thrombosis. (A) ISR. (B) Incomplete strut coverage. (C) Incomplete stent apposition. (D) Stent (BVS) underexpansion.

identification of these factors in a particular patient, and subsequently can guide therapeutic decisions.

- *Underexpansion* is mainly related to early stent thrombosis. It is defined as a minimum stent area (MSA) lower than both the nominal stent and reference vessel areas. Both for IVUS and OCT evaluation, the threshold for an underexpanded stent is a MSA less than 90% of the average reference lumen area (1–5 mm on either side of the stented segment) [73]. OCT can measure the MSA and lumen area of the reference vessel with a higher precision than angiography, thus giving a quick and accurate estimation of the expansion and sizing of the stent [82]. Moreover, OCT may provide information about the underlying causes of stent underexpansion, such as calcified nodules. When diagnosis of underexpansion as the possible mechanism of stent thrombosis is made, postdilatation alone could be the therapeutic approach chosen, avoiding the deployment of an additional stent (stent intrastent) if optimal expansion is achieved.
- *Restenosis* can present as stent thrombosis. If restenosis is identified in a patient with stent thrombosis, the use of DESs is warranted to decrease the probability of recurrence, also a drug-eluting balloon may have a role in this setting. Further insight into IRS and its OCT features has been provided earlier in this chapter.
- *Malapposition* or incomplete stent apposition (ISA) is frequently found in all types of stent thrombosis, but it plays a major role in LST and VLST, mainly driven by its association with incomplete re-endothelialization. Earlier in this chapter, we explained the definition, epidemiology, mechanisms and clinical implications of ISA. Its management may vary depending on its mechanism, but in many cases simple angioplasty to oversize the stent may be sufficient.
- *Incomplete re-endothelialization.* Pathological studies have shown that endothelialization is the best predictor of stent thrombosis in autopsies performed >30 days after DES implantation [26], and first-generation DESs (the sirolimus-eluting stent Cypher and the paclitaxel-eluting stent Taxus) are associated with delayed healing and poorer endothelialization compared with BMSs [118]. The number of uncovered stent struts in histological assessment was associated with a markedly increased risk of LST [26, 118, 119]. OCT evaluation of stent coverage has found a similar relationship with stent thrombosis [106]. The ratio of uncovered to total stent struts has been identified as the OCT parameter that best correlates with the degree of stent endothelialization, and the odds ratio for thrombus in a stent with a ratio of uncovered to total stent struts per section >30% is 9.0 (95% CI, 3.5 to 22) [26]. The relationship between incomplete re-endothelialization and ISA has been described in detail earlier in this chapter.
- *Neoatherosclerosis* can lead to plaque rupture that triggers stent thrombosis. Further insight into neoatherosclerosis is provided earlier in this chapter.

1.2.5.4 Limitations

It is necessary to note that OCT evaluation of stent thrombosis is not always feasible. The thrombus burden may impair adequate contrast clearance of the artery, thus precluding the acquisition of images of sufficient quality for a correct interpretation. Even when an optimal contrast flush is achieved, the intraluminal thrombus may have high attenuation and prevent the visualization of the underlying stent struts and other components of the vessel wall. Thrombus aspiration or balloon angioplasty may decrease the thrombus burden and improve OCT imaging.

1.3 OCT evaluation of bioresorbable vascular scaffolds

In the last few years, bioresorbable vascular scaffolds (BVSs) have been developed and introduced into clinical practice (see figure 1.9). The latest-generation DESs offer excellent short- and long-term results, and their thinner struts and biodegradable polymers have considerably improved their safety profile [40, 48]. However, these stents still leave a permanent metal implant inside the vessel wall, and it may interfere with complete vascular healing and the full recovery of vessel properties.

The rationale for BVS development is to maintain the acute advantages of stents, but to disappear in the long-term, avoiding late complications. Therefore, BVSs offer multiple theoretical advantages over traditional BMSs and DESs [120]:

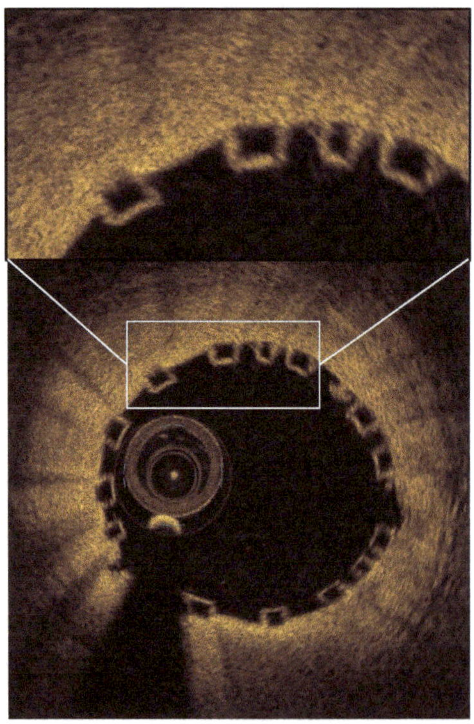

Figure 1.9. OCT imaging of a bioresorbable scaffold (Absorb). Struts are apposed to the vessel wall, and have box-shaped appearance with sharp, defined, bright borders; the strut body shows low reflection.

- They feature a scaffold to avoid initial PCI complications (i.e. elastic recoil, acute closure secondary to dissection, constrictive remodeling and neointimal proliferation).
- They include drug-eluting to avoid neointima proliferation and reduce restenosis risk.
- They allow arterial wall healing.
- They completely disappear after vascular healing, avoiding late stent failure and helping in restoration of physiological vasomotion, mechanotransduction, adaptive shear stress, late luminal gain (as opposed to late luminal loss with permanent stents) and late expansive remodeling [121, 122].
- The absence of any residual foreign material and restoration of functional endothelial coverage can also reduce the risk of stent thrombosis and the need for long-term dual antiplatelet therapy.
- They avoid the permanent 'jailing' of the side branches, overhanging at ostial lesions and the inability to graft the stented segment [123].

However, most of these advantages are theoretical and have not been fully assessed, and data are scarce regarding long-term response.

1.3.1 OCT in the evaluation of long-term BVS performance

The characteristics of OCT (namely its spatial resolution) make it the intracoronary imaging technique of choice to assess arterial wall changes after BVS implantation and reabsorption.

To date the first clinically available BVS is the everolimus-eluting Absorb BVS (Abbot Vascular, Santa Clara, CA). It is made from a bioabsorbable polylactic acid backbone which is coated with a more rapidly absorbed polylactic acid layer that contains and controls the release of the antiproliferative drug. Absorb struts imaged by OCT have the appearance of a black box, leaving no optical shadow [23, 124].

OCT can evaluate the apposition, coverage and neointimal proliferation for BVSs in the same manner as for BMSs and DESs. A novel concept arises in BVS evaluation—reabsorption.

This strut reabsorption is a progressive process. Therefore, four OCT categories have been identified regarding the Absorb strut appearance, which may reflect different stages of reabsorption [124]:

- *Preserved box*: Sharply defined, bright reflection borders with a preserved box-shaped appearance; the strut body shows low reflection.
- *Open box*: the luminal and abluminal long-axis borders show thickened bright reflection; the short axis borders are not visible.
- *Dissolved bright box*: partially visible bright spot, contours poorly defined; no box-shaped appearance.
- *Dissolved black box*: black spot, contours poorly defined, often confluent; no box-shaped appearance.

The initial Absorb series showed at 6 month follow-up that 3% of struts had a preserved box, 30% had an open box, 50% had a dissolved bright box and 18% had a dissolved black-box appearance [124].

The largest study of BVS long-term performance was published by Karanasos *et al* and included 14 patients with a follow-up of 5 years after implantation. The BVS evaluated was the first-generation everolimus-eluting Absorb BVS (Abbot Vascular, Santa Clara, CA). At this late stage, the BVSs have been fully reabsorbed and no remaining struts were present. Therefore, it is impossible to distinguish between the strut area, underlying plaque and neointimal area. In these patients, OCT identifies a signal-rich layer between the lumen border and the internal elastic lamina. This signal-rich layer is the result of the addition of a neointimal layer, resorbed struts and pre-existing fibrous tissue, and it is thought that it may separate thrombogenic plaque components from the lumen, creating a sort of thick fibrous cap that may stabilize the underlying plaque [125]. OCT findings at 5 year follow-up can be summarize as follows:

- Complete strut resorbtion—at 5 years scaffold struts were no longer discernible.
- Late lumen enlargement and increase in luminal symmetry.
- A thick signal-rich layer with a mean minimum thickness of 150 μm.
- Side-branch ostia patency with struts being replaced by thin tissue bridges.

Once again, evidence is scarce and further investigation will clarify if it correlates with better clinical outcomes.

1.3.2 Current pitfalls of BVSs

The aim of this chapter is to describe OCT applications in BVS evaluation, and the current knowledge of OCT findings in this setting. The described findings support a promising perspective for the long-term results of BVSs. However, we want to state that at the moment there are several pitfalls facing this technology that warrant further investigation and development. Moreover, long-term clinical evaluation of a wide spectrum of patients treated with BVSs is needed in order to correlate OCT findings with a real clinical 'vascular healing'.

1.4 Future perspectives

OCT is a promising tool with huge potential both in the research and clinical fields. In our opinion, the future of this technique must address three main issues:

1. *Technological development.*

   OCT imaging systems have improved considerably in recent years, providing better images, faster acquisition and new utilities such as 3D imaging. Current efforts are targeted at enhancing tissular characterization using objective quantitative approaches with dedicated software [126], new technologies such as polarization-sensitive OCT (used to measure the polarization properties of backscattered light) or micro-OCT [127, 128], and cellular targeting agents combined with hybrid OCT systems [129].

2. *Validation.*

   Since it has come into widespread clinical use, OCT has accounted for an increasing number of published papers. However, most of these data come from observational studies. Future investigation must provide histological validation of OCT findings, search for underlying mechanisms and design randomized studies that further support clinical evidence.
3. *Clinical implementation.*

   OCT evaluation is a common tool in many cath laboratories, but there is a lack of evidence-based recommendations for clinical practice. In the near future, consensus and guidelines must take a step forward to establish the usefulness of OCT in guiding clinical decisions.

References

[1] Serruys P W *et al* 1994 A comparison of balloon-expandable-stent implantation with balloon angioplasty in patients with coronary artery disease *N. Engl. J. Med.* **331** 489–95
[2] Fischman D L *et al* 1994 Stent restenosis study investigators. a randomized comparison of coronary-stent placement and balloon angioplasty in the treatment of coronary artery disease *N. Engl. J. Med.* **331** 496–501
[3] Farb A *et al* 1999 Pathology of acute and chronic stenting in humans *Circulation* **99** 44–52
[4] Chousssat R *et al* 2001 Long term outcome after Palmaz–Schatz stent implantation *Am. J. Cardiol.* **88** 10–6
[5] Hasegawa K *et al* 2006 Histopathological findings of new in-stent lesions developed beyond five years *Catheter Cardiovasc. Interv.* **68** 554–8
[6] Habara M, Terashima M and Suzuki T 2009 Detection of atherosclerotic progression with rupture of degenerated in-stent intima five years after bare-metal stent implantation using optical coherence tomography *J. Invasive Cardiol.* **21** 552–3
[7] Takano M *et al* 2009 Appearance of lipid-laden intima and neovascularization after implantation of bare-metal stents extended late-phase observation by intracoronary optical coherence tomography *J. Am. Coll. Cardiol.* **55** 26–32
[8] Forrester J S *et al* 1991 A paradigm for restenosis based on cell biology: clues for the development of new preventive therapies *J. Am. Coll. Cardiol.* **17** 758–69
[9] Virmani R and Farb A 1999 Pathology of in-stent restenosis *Curr. Opin. Lipidol.* **10** 499–506
[10] Moses J W *et al* 2003 Sirolimus-eluting stents versus standard stents in patients with stenosis in a native coronary artery *N. Engl. J. Med.* **349** 1315–23
[11] Stone G W *et al* 2004 A polymer-based, paclitaxel-eluting stent in patients with coronary artery disease *N. Engl. J. Med.* **350** 221–31
[12] Daemen J *et al* 2007 Early and late coronary stent thrombosis of sirolimus-eluting and paclitaxel-eluting stents in routine clinical practice: data from a large two-institutional cohort study *Lancet* **369** 667–78
[13] Wenaweser P *et al* 2008 Incidence and correlates of drug-eluting stent thrombosis in routine clinical practice. 4-year results from a large 2-institutional cohort study *J. Am. Coll. Cardiol.* **52** 1134–40
[14] Raber L *et al* 2011 Long-term comparison of everolimus-eluting and sirolimus-eluting stents for coronary revascularization *J. Am. Coll. Cardiol.* **57** 2143–51

[15] Suzuki Y *et al* 2008 *In vivo* comparison between optical coherence tomography and intravascular ultrasound for detecting small degrees of in-stent neointima after stent implantation *JACC Cardiovasc. Interv.* **1** 168–73
[16] Murata A *et al* 2010 Accuracy of optical coherence tomography in the evaluation of neointimal coverage after stent implantation *JACC Cardiovasc. Imaging* **3** 76–84
[17] Prati F *et al* 2008 Does optical coherence tomography identify arterial healing after stenting? An *in vivo* comparison with histology, in a rabbit carotid model *Heart* **94** 217–21
[18] Kume T *et al* 2005 Visualization of neointima formation by optical coherence tomography *Int. Heart J.* **46** 1133–6
[19] Nakano M *et al* 2012 *Ex vivo* assessment of vascular response to coronary stents by optical frequency domain imaging *JACC Cardiovasc. Imaging* **5** 71–82
[20] Templin C *et al* 2010 Coronary optical frequency domain imaging (OFDI) for *in vivo* evaluation of stent healing: comparison with light and electron microscopy *Eur. Heart J.* **31** 1792–801
[21] Gonzalo N *et al* 2009 Reproducibility of quantitative optical coherence tomography for stent analysis *EuroIntervention* **5** 224–32
[22] Xie Y *et al* 2008 Comparison of neointimal coverage by optical coherence tomography of a sirolimus-eluting stent versus a bare-metal stent three months after implantation *Am. J. Cardiol.* **102** 27–31
[23] Tearney G J *et al* 2012 Consensus standards for acquisition, measurement, and reporting of intravascular optical coherence tomography studies: a report from the International Working Group for Intravascular Optical Coherence Tomography Standardization and Validation *J. Am. Coll. Cardiol.* **59** 1058–72
[24] Tada T *et al* 2013 Early vascular healing with rapid breakdown biodegradable polymer sirolimus-eluting versus durable polymer everolimus-eluting stents assessed by optical coherence tomography *Cardiovasc. Revasc. Med.* **14** 84
[25] Brugaletta S *et al* 2013 Reproducibility of qualitative assessment of stent struts coverage by optical coherence tomography *Int. J. Cardiovasc. Imaging* **29** 5–11
[26] Finn A V *et al* 2007 Pathological correlates of late drug-eluting stent thrombosis: strut coverage as a marker of endothelialization *Circulation* **115** 2435–41
[27] Won H *et al* 2013 Optical coherence tomography derived cut-off value of uncovered stent struts to predict adverse clinical outcomes after drug-eluting stent implantation *Int. J. Cardiovasc. Imaging* **29** 1255–63
[28] Nakazawa G *et al* 2008 Delayed arterial healing and increased late stent thrombosis at culprit sites after drug-eluting stent placement for acute myocardial infarction patients: an autopsy study *Circulation* **118** 1138–45
[29] Gonzalo N *et al* 2009 Incomplete stent apposition and delayed tissue coverage are more frequent in drug-eluting stents implanted during primary percutaneous coronary intervention for ST-segment elevation myocardial infarction than in drug-eluting stents implanted for stable/unstable angina: insights from optical coherence tomography *JACC Cardiovasc. Interv.* **2** 445–52
[30] Takano M *et al* 2008 Long-term follow-up evaluation after sirolimus-eluting stent implantation by optical coherence tomography: do uncovered struts persist? *J. Am. Coll. Cardiol.* **51** 968–9
[31] Chen B X *et al* 2008 Neointimal coverage of bare-metal and sirolimus-eluting stents evaluated with optical coherence tomography *Heart* **94** 566–70

[32] Matsumoto D *et al* 2007 Neointimal coverage of sirolimus-eluting stents at 6-month follow-up: evaluated by optical coherence tomography *Eur. Heart J.* **28** 961–7
[33] Ishigami K *et al* 2009 Long-term follow-up of neointimal coverage of sirolimus-eluting stents--evaluation with optical coherence tomography *Circ. J.* **73** 2300–7
[34] Miyoshi N *et al* 2010 Comparison by optical coherence tomography of paclitaxel-eluting stents with sirolimus-eluting stents implanted in one coronary artery in one procedure. 6-month follow-up *Circ. J.* **74** 903–8
[35] Kandzari D E *et al* 2006 Comparison of zotarolimus-eluting and sirolimus-eluting stents in patients with native coronary artery disease: a randomized controlled trial *J. Am. Coll. Cardiol.* **48** 2440–7
[36] Smits P C *et al* 2011 2-year follow-up of a randomized controlled trial of everolimus- and paclitaxel-eluting stents for coronary revascularization in daily practice. COMPARE *J. Am. Coll. Cardiol.* **58** 11–8
[37] Stone G W *et al* 2011 Randomized comparison of everolimus and paclitaxel-eluting stents. 2-year follow-up from the SPIRIT IV trial *J. Am. Coll. Cardiol.* **58** 19–25
[38] Kandzari D *et al* 2011 Late-term clinical outcomes with zotarolimus- and sirolimus-eluting stents. 5-year follow-up of the ENDEAVOR III *J. Am. Coll. Cardiol. Cardiovasc. Interv.* **4** 543–50
[39] Inoue T *et al* 2011 Optical coherence evaluation of everolimus-eluting stents 8 months after implantation *Heart* **97** 1379–84
[40] Stone G W *et al* 2010 Everolimus-eluting versus paclitaxel-eluting stents in coronary artery disease *N. Engl. J. Med.* **362** 1663–74
[41] Kedhi E *et al* 2010 s-generation everolimus-eluting and paclitaxel-eluting stents in real-life practice (COMPARE): a randomised trial *Lancet* **375** 201–9
[42] Toledano Delgado F J *et al* 2014 Optical coherence tomography evaluation of late strut coverage patterns between first-generation drug-eluting stents and everolimus-eluting stent *Catheter Cardiovasc. Interv.* **84** 720–6
[43] Kim J-S *et al* 2009 Optical coherence tomography evaluation of zotarolimus-eluting stents at 9-month follow-up: comparison with sirolimus-eluting stents *Heart* **95** 1907–12
[44] Guagliumi G *et al* 2010 Strut coverage and vessel wall response to zotarolimus-eluting and bare-metal stents implanted in patients with ST-segment elevation myocardial infarction: the OCTAMI (Optical Coherence Tomography in Acute Myocardial Infarction) Study *JACC Cardiovasc. Interv.* **3** 680–7
[45] Poerner T C *et al* 2014 Stent coverage and neointimal proliferation in bare metal stents postdilated with a paclitaxel-eluting balloon versus everolimus-eluting stents: prospective randomized study using optical coherence tomography at 6-month follow-up *Circ. Cardiovasc. Interv.* **7** 760–7
[46] Burzotta F *et al* 2012 Intimal hyperplasia evaluated by OCT in *de novo* coronary lesions treated by drug-eluting balloon and bare-metal stent (IN-PACT CORO): study protocol for a randomized controlled trial *Trials* **13** 55
[47] Byrne R A *et al* 2011 Biodegradable polymer versus permanent polymer drug-eluting stents and everolimus- versus sirolimus-eluting stents in patients with coronary artery disease: 3-year outcomes from a randomized clinical trial *J. Am. Coll. Cardiol.* **58** 1325–31
[48] Stefanini G G *et al* 2011 Long-term clinical outcomes of biodegradable polymer biolimus-eluting stents versus durable polymer sirolimus-eluting stents in patients with coronary

artery disease (LEADERS): 4 year follow-up of a randomised non-inferiority trial *Lancet* **378** 1940–8
[49] Stefanini G G *et al* 2012 Biodegradable polymer drug-eluting stents reduce the risk of stent thrombosis at 4 years in patients undergoing percutaneous coronary intervention: a pooled analysis of individual patient data from the ISAR-TEST 3, ISAR-TEST 4, and leaders randomized tria *Eur. Heart J.* **33** 1214–22
[50] Barlis P *et al* 2010 An optical coherence tomography study of a biodegradable vs durable polymer-coated limus-eluting stent: a LEADERS trial sub-study *Eur. Heart J.* **31** 165–76
[51] Gutierrez-Chico J L *et al* 2011 Long-term tissue coverage of a biodegradable polylactide polymer-coated biolimus-eluting stent: comparative sequential assessment with optical coherence tomography until complete resorption of the polymer *Am. Heart J.* **162** 922–31
[52] Guagliumi G *et al* 2010 Strut coverage and vessel wall response to a new-generation paclitaxel-eluting stent with an ultrathin biodegradable abluminal polymer: optical coherence tomography drug-eluting stent investigation (OCTDESI) *Circ. Cardiovasc. Interv.* **3** 367–75
[53] Cutlip D E *et al* 2007 Clinical end points in coronary stent trials: a case for standardized definitions *Circulation* **115** 2344–51
[54] Nakatani M *et al* 2003 Mechanisms of restenosis after coronary intervention: difference between plain old balloon angioplasty and stenting *Cardiovasc. Pathol.* **12** 40–8
[55] Kimura T *et al* 2002 Long-term clinical and angiographic follow-up after coronary stent placement in native coronary arteries *Circulation* **105** 2986–91
[56] Gonzalo N *et al* 2009 Optical coherence tomography patterns of stent restenosis *Am. Heart J.* **158** 284–93
[57] van Beusekom H M *et al* 1993 Histology after stenting of human saphenous vein bypass grafts: observations from surgically excised grafts 3 to 320 days after stent implantation *J. Am. Coll. Cardiol.* **21** 45–54
[58] van Beusekom H M *et al* 2007 Drug-eluting stents show delayed healing: paclitaxel more pronounced than sirolimus *Eur. Heart J.* **28** 974–79
[59] Teramoto T *et al* 2010 Intriguing peri-strut low-intensity area detected by optical coherence tomography after coronary stent deployment *Circ. J.* **74** 1257–9
[60] Nagai H, Ishibashi-Ueda H and Fujii K 2010 Histology of highly echolucent regions inoptical coherence tomography images from two patients with sirolimus-eluting stent restenosis *Catheter Cardiovasc. Interv.* **75** 961–3
[61] Itoh T *et al* 2015 Clinical and pathological characteristics of homogeneous and non-homogeneous tissue of in-stent restenosis visualized by optical coherence tomography *Coron. Artery Dis.* **26** 201–11
[62] Habara M *et al* 2011 Difference of tissue characteristics between early and very late restenosis lesions after bare-metal stent implantation *Circ. Cardiovasc. Interv.* **4** 232–8
[63] Yamaguchi H *et al* 2015 Association of morphologic characteristics on optical coherence tomography and angiographic progression patterns of late restenosis after drug-eluting stent implantation *Cardiovasc. Revasc. Med.* **16** 3
[64] Kim J S *et al* 2014 Long-term outcomes of neointimal hyperplasia without neoatherosclerosis after drug-eluting stent implantation *J. Am. Coll. Cardiol. Imaging* **7** 788–95
[65] Tada T *et al* 2015 Association between tissue characteristics assessed with optical coherence tomography and mid-term results after percutaneous coronary intervention for in-stent

restenosis lesions: a comparison between balloon angioplasty, paclitaxel-coated balloon dilatation and drug-eluting stent implantation *Eur. Heart J. Cardiovasc. Imaging* **16** 1101–11
[66] Nakazawa G *et al* 2011 The pathology of neoatherosclerosis in human coronary implants bare-metal and drug-eluting stents *J. Am. Coll. Cardiol.* **57** 14–1322
[67] Inoue K *et al* 2004 Pathological analyses of long-term intracoronary Palmaz–Schatz stenting; is its efficacy permanent? *Cardiovasc. Pathol.* **13** 109–15
[68] Yamaji K *et al* 2012 Bare-metal stent thrombosis and in-stent neoatherosclerosis *Circ. Cardiovasc. Interv.* **5** 47–54
[69] Farb A *et al* 2003 Pathological mechanisms of fatal late coronary stent thrombosis in humans *Circulation* **108** 1701–6
[70] Grube E *et al* 2009 TAXUS VI final 5-year results: a multicentre, randomised trial comparing polymer-based moderate-release paclitaxel-eluting stent with a bare metal stent for treatment of long, complex coronary artery lesions *EuroIntervention* **4** 572–7
[71] Nakazawa G *et al* 2011 Coronary responses and differential mechanisms of late stent thrombosis attributed to first-generation sirolimus- and paclitaxel-eluting stents *J. Am. Coll. Cardiol.* **57** 390–8
[72] Finn A V and Otsuka F 2012 Neoatherosclerosis: a culprit in very late stent thrombosis *Circ. Cardiovasc. Interv.* **5** 6–9
[73] Di Vito L *et al* 2014 Comprehensive overview of definitions for optical coherence tomography-based plaque and stent analyses *Coron. Artery Dis.* **25** 172–85
[74] Yabushita H *et al* 2002 Characterization of human atherosclerosis by optical coherence tomography *Circulation* **106** 1640–5
[75] Tearney G J *et al* 2003 Quantification of macrophage content in atherosclerotic plaques by optical coherence tomography *Circulation* **107** 113–9
[76] Kang S J *et al* 2011 Optical coherent tomographic analysis of in-stent neo-atherosclerosis after drug– eluting stent implantation *Circulation* **123** 2913–5
[77] Kimura T *et al* 2012 Very late stent thrombosis and late target lesion revascularization after sirolimus-eluting stent implantation: five year outcome of the j-Cypher Registry *Circulation* **125** 584–91
[78] Kim J S *et al* 2012 Quantitative and qualitative changes in DES-related neointimal tissue based on serial OCT *J. Am. Coll. Cardiol. Cardiovasc. Imaging* **5** 1147–55
[79] Yonetsu T *et al* 2012 Comparison of incidence and time course of neoatherosclerosis between bare metal stents and drug-eluting stents using optical coherence tomography *Am. J. Cardiol.* **110** 933–9
[80] Yonetsu T *et al* 2012 Predictors for neoatherosclerosis: a retrospective observational study from the optical coherence tomography registry *Circ. Cardiovasc. Imaging* **5** 660–6
[81] Tanigawa J *et al* 2007 Intravascular optical coherence tomography: optimisation of image acquisition and quantitative assessment of stent strut apposition *EuroIntervention* **3** 128 36
[82] Gutiérrez-Chico J L *et al* 2012 Optical coherence tomography: from research to practice *Eur. Heart J. Cardiovasc. Imaging* **13** 370–84
[83] Guagliumi G *et al* 2011 Strut coverage and late malapposition with paclitaxel-eluting stents compared with bare metal stents in acute myocardial infarction: optical coherence tomography substudy of the HORIZONS-AMI Trial *Circulation* **123** 274–81
[84] Im E *et al* 2014 Incidences, predictors, and clinical outcomes of acute and late stent malapposition detected by optical coherence tomography after drug-eluting stent implantation *Circ. Cardiovasc. Interv.* **7** 88–96

[85] Serruys P W *et al* 2010 Evaluation of the second generation of a bioresorbable everolimus drug-eluting vascular scaffold for treatment of *de novo* coronary artery stenosis: 6-month clinical and imaging outcomes *Circulation* **122** 2301–12
[86] Foin N *et al* 2014 Incomplete stent apposition causes high shear flow disturbances and delay in neointimal coverage as a function of strut to wall detachment distance: implications for the management of incomplete stent apposition *Circ. Cardiovasc. Interv.* **7** 180–9
[87] Gutiérrez-Chico J L *et al* 2011 Delayed coverage in malapposed and side-branch struts with respect to well-apposed struts in drug-eluting stents: *in vivo* assessment with optical coherence tomography *Circulation* **124** 612–23
[88] Liu Y *et al* 2011 Assessment by optical coherence tomography of stent struts across side branch—comparison of bare-metal stents and drug-elution stents *Circ. J.* **75** 106–12
[89] Cook S *et al* 2007 Incomplete stent apposition and very late stent thrombosis after drug-eluting stent implantation *Circulation* **115** 2426–34
[90] Ozaki Y *et al* 2010 The fate of incomplete stent apposition with drug-eluting stents: an optical coherence tomography-based natural history study *Eur. Heart J.* **31** 1470–6
[91] Gutiérrez-Chico J *et al* 2012 Vascular tissue reaction to acute malapposition in human coronary arteries: sequential assessment with optical coherence tomography *Circ. Cardiovasc. Interv.* **5** 20–9
[92] Tanigawa J *et al* 2009 The influence of strut thickness and cell design on immediate apposition of drug-eluting stents assessed by optical coherence tomography *Int. J. Cardiol.* **134** 180–8
[93] Kim W H *et al* 2010 Serial changes of minimal stent malapposition not detected by intravascular ultrasound: follow-up optical coherence tomography study *Clin. Res. Cardiol.* **99** 639–44
[94] Shimamura K *et al* 2015 Outcomes of everolimus-eluting stent incomplete stent apposition: a serial optical coherence tomography analysis *Eur. Heart J. Cardiovasc. Imaging* **16** 23–8
[95] Kawamori H *et al* 2013 Natural consequence of post-intervention stent malapposition, thrombus, tissue prolapse, and dissection assessed by optical coherence tomography at mid-term follow-up *Eur. Heart J. Cardiovasc. Imaging* **14** 865–75
[96] Inoue T *et al* 2014 Impact of strut–vessel distance and underlying plaque type on the resolution of acute strut malapposition: serial optimal coherence tomography analysis after everolimus-eluting stent implantation *Int. J. Cardiovasc. Imaging* **30** 857–65
[97] Radu M *et al* 2010 Strut apposition after coronary stent implantation visualised with optical coherence tomography *EuroIntervention* **6** 86–93
[98] Hassan A K *et al* 2010 Late stent malapposition risk is higher after drug-eluting stent compared with bare-metal stent implantation and associates with late stent thrombosis *Eur. Heart J.* **31** 1172–80
[99] van der Hoeven B L *et al* 2008 Stent malapposition after sirolimus-eluting and bare-metal stent implantation in patients with ST-segment elevation myocardial infarction: acute and 9-month intravascular ultrasound results of the MISSION! Intervention Study *J. Am. Coll. Cardiol. Interv.* **1** 192–201
[100] Virmani R, Farb A, Guagliumi G and Kolodgie F D 2004 Drug-eluting stents: caution and concerns for long-term outcome *Coron. Artery Dis.* **15** 313–8
[101] Pires N M *et al* 2007 Sirolimus and paclitaxel provoke different vascular pathological responses after local delivery in a murine model for restenosis on underlying atherosclerotic arteries *Heart* **93** 922–7

[102] Hong M K *et al* 2006 Late stent malapposition after drug-eluting stent implantation: an intravascular ultrasound analysis with long-term follow-up *Circulation* **113** 414–9
[103] Hong M K *et al* 2004 Incidence, mechanism, predictors, and long-term prognosis of late stent malapposition after bare-metal stent implantation *Circulation* **109** 881–6
[104] Mintz G S, Shah V M and Weissman N J 2003 Regional remodeling as the cause of late stent malapposition *Circulation* **107** 2660–3
[105] Tanabe K *et al* 2005 Incomplete stent apposition after implantation of paclitaxel-eluting stents or bare metal stents: insights from the randomized TAXUS II trial *Circulation* **111** 900–5
[106] Parodi G *et al* 2013 Stent-related defects in patients presenting with stent thrombosis: differences at optical coherence tomography between subacute and late/very late thrombosis in the Mechanism Of Stent Thrombosis (MOST) study *EuroIntervention* **9** 936–44
[107] Stettler C *et al* 2007 Outcomes associated with drug eluting and bare-metal stents: a collaborative network meta-analysis *Lancet* **370** 937–48
[108] De la Torre-Hernandez J M *et al* 2008 Drug-eluting stent thrombosis: results from the multicenter Spanish registry ESTROFA (Estudio ESpañol sobre TROmbosis de stents FArmacoactivos) *J. Am. Coll. Cardiol.* **51** 986–90
[109] Roukoz H *et al* 2009 Comprehensive meta-analysis on drug-eluting stents versus bare-metal stents during extended follow-up *Am. J. Med.* **122** 581e1–10
[110] Buchanan G L, Basavarajaiah S and Chieffo A 2012 Stent thrombosis: incidence, predictors and new technologies *Thrombosis* **2012** 956–62
[111] van Werkum J W *et al* 2009 Long-term clinical outcome after a first angiographically confirmed coronary stent thrombosis: an analysis of 431 cases *Circulation* **119** 828–34
[112] Siddiqi O K and Faxon D P 2012 Very late stent thrombosis: current concepts *Curr. Opin. Cardiol.* **27** 634–41
[113] Kubo T *et al* 2007 Assessment of culprit lesion morphology in acute myocardial infarction: ability of optical coherence tomography compared with intravascular ultrasound and coronary angioscopy *J. Am. Coll. Cardiol.* **50** 933–9
[114] Kume T *et al* 2006 Assessment of coronary arterial thrombus by optical coherence tomography *Am. J. Cardiol.* **97** 1713–7
[115] Kume T, Okura H, Kawamoto T, Akasaka T, Toyota E, Watanabe N, Neishi Y, Sadahira Y and Yoshida K 2008 Fibrin clot visualized by optical coherence tomography *Circulation* **118** 426–7
[116] D'Ascenzo F *et al* 2013 Incidence and predictors of coronary stent thrombosis: evidence from an international collaborative meta-analysis including 30 studies, 221,066 patients, and 4276 thromboses *Int. J. Cardiol.* **167** 575–8
[117] Sambu N *et al* 2012 Personalised antiplatelet therapy in stent thrombosis: observations from the Clopidogrel Resistance in Stent Thrombosis (CREST) registry *Heart* **98** 706–11
[118] Joner M *et al* 2006 Pathology of drug-eluting stents in humans: delayed healing and late thrombotic risk *J. Am. Coll. Cardiol.* **48** 193–202
[119] Luscher T F *et al* 2007 Drug-eluting stent and coronary thrombosis: biological mechanisms and clinical implications *Circulation* **115** 1051–8
[120] Iqbal J *et al* 2014 Bioresorbable scaffolds: rationale, current status, challenges, and future *Eur. Heart J.* **35** 765–76
[121] Waksman R 2006 Biodegradable stents: they do their job and disappear *J. Invasive Cardiol.* **18** 70–4

[122] Wykrzykowska J J 2009 Vascular restoration therapy: the fourth revolution in interventional cardiology and the ultimate 'rosy' prophecy *EuroIntervention* **5** F7–8
[123] Okamura T, Serruys P W and Regar E 2010 Cardiovascular flashlight. The fate of bioresorbable struts located at a side branch ostium: serial three-dimensional optical coherence tomography assessment *Eur. Heart J.* **31** 2179
[124] Ormiston J A *et al* 2008 A bioabsorbable everolimus-eluting coronary stent system for patients with single *de-novo* coronary artery lesions (ABSORB): a prospective open-label trial *Lancet* **371** 899–907
[125] Karanasos A *et al* 2014 OCT assessment of the long-term vascular healing response 5 years after everolimus-eluting bioresorbable vascular scaffold *J. Am. Coll. Cardiol.* **64** 2343–56
[126] Soest G *et al* 2010 Atherosclerotic tissue characterization *in vivo* by optical coherence tomography attenuation imaging *J. Biomed. Opt.* **15** 011105
[127] Giattina S D *et al* 2006 Assessment of coronary plaque collagen with polarization sensitive optical coherence tomography (PS-OCT) *Int. J. Cardiol.* **107** 400–9
[128] Liu L *et al* 2011 Imaging the subcellular structure of human coronary atherosclerosis using micro-optical coherence tomography *Nat. Med.* **17** 1010–4
[129] Tahara N, Imaizumi T, Virmani R and Narula J 2009 Clinical feasibility of molecular imaging of plaque inflammation in atherosclerosis *J. Nucl. Med.* **50** 331–4

Chapter 2

Bioresorbable eluting scaffolds in the era of optical coherence tomography: real-world clinical practice

Joana Delgado Silva, Luís Paiva, Marco Costa and Lino Gonçalves

Percutaneous coronary intervention (PCI) is constantly evolving, with cutting-edge technology being developed on a regular basis. Nearly four decades after the first coronary angioplasty was performed, new material and techniques have been adopted in order to progressively improve the outcomes for treated patients and avoid potential complications, such as restenosis and stent thrombosis. Bioresorbable vascular scaffolds (BRSs), considered by experts as the fourth breakthrough in interventional cardiology (after plain old balloon angioplasty, bare metal stents and drug-eluting stents), offer several potential advantages over standard metallic stents. These include the restoration of normal endothelium and hence vessel function after polymeric strut disappearance, the feasibility of a future need for re-PCI or coronary artery bypass grafts, improved non-invasive coronary imaging, late luminal gain, and reduction of late and very-late scaffold thrombosis. Absorb was the first bioresorbable everolimus-eluting scaffold and is the best documented so far. It consists of four main components (a poly-L-lactic acid polymer, a poly-DL-lactide coating, the anti-proliferative drug everolimus and the XIENCE V® delivery system). Although the initial study results were promising, the three-year outcomes showed a two-fold increase in device-oriented clinical events, mostly due to excessive scaffold thrombosis. Consequently, Absorb was discontinued for use in routine clinical practice and its use was limited to clinical registries and studies. Magmaris is a newly redesigned second-generation drug-eluting absorbable metal scaffold, with a shorter resorption time and high radial strength. Twelve-month clinical and safety outcomes are encouraging but a longer follow-up is crucial for the evaluation of device-oriented events. BRS implantation can be

doi:10.1088/2053-2563/ab01fach2

challenging, and proper lesion preparation, optimal scaffold optimization, and the early detection and correction of peri-procedural complications are pivotal for achieving favorable results. Optical coherence tomography (OCT) is a catheter-based imaging system that uses near-infrared light to produce high resolution cross-sectional images of the coronary arteries. It is a state-of-the-art technique, which can precisely measure the vessel lumen and assess scaffold apposition, coverage and the appearance of struts over time. OCT plays an important role in decision making for the best treatment strategy, through accurate plaque characterization, selection of proper landing sites, and avoidance of scaffold malapposition and underexpansion. This chapter aims to review current bioresorbable technology and provide insight into the potential advantages of using OCT for BRS optimization, through a series of real-world clinical cases.

2.1 Introduction

BRSs are considered to be cutting-edge technology and have generated great interest among interventional cardiologists worldwide. Since the introduction of drug-eluting stents (DESs) which release, locally and predictably, anti-proliferative agents, the risk of restenosis and therefore repeat revascularization has been reduced significantly when compared to bare metal stents (BMSs) [1, 2]. It is well known that stents can improve immediate outcomes by sealing any possible intimal tissue flaps, preventing acute vessel closure and optimizing final vessel caliber [3]. DESs, by blocking negative remodeling and limiting neointimal hyperplasia, potentially allow physiological arterial healing. However, early generation sirolimus and paclitaxel-eluting stents have been associated with delayed arterial healing, incomplete endothelization of stent struts, premature neoatherosclerosis [4] and very-late stent thrombosis (ST) [5]. Neoatherosclerosis is a term usually used to characterize the growth of an atherosclerotic plaque inside an implanted coronary stent. The process includes three important stages: macrophage infiltration, detectable atherosclerotic plaque development and necrotic core plaque formation [6]. New generation DESs emerged as a possible solution to prevent delayed re-endothelization and include devices with several features, such as thinner struts, more biocompatible polymers and different anti-proliferative agents, such as zotarolimus and everolimus [7]. A wide range of DESs is now available and they may lower thrombotic risk as they are less prone to hypersensitivity reactions and cause less arterial injury. On the other hand, the permanent caging of the coronary vessel may be associated with suppressed wall motility, altered vasodilation properties, chronic inflammation and very-late ST. Although a fully bioresorbable device has been investigated for over 20 years, the development of a scaffold with sufficient and durable radial strength, without exaggerated thick struts, which allows controlled delivery of an anti-proliferative agent and that can degrade progressively without generating an overwhelming inflammatory response, has been rather challenging.

Importantly, BRSs are associated with potential advantages over standard metallic stents. These include the restoration of vasomotion after the disappearance of struts, late luminal gain, reduction of ST, restoration of functional endothelium, improved lesion imaging with computed tomography, facilitation for grafting the stented segment, and freedom from side-branch obstruction from scaffold struts, struts overhanging on ostial lesions or restenosis induced by stent fracture [8, 9].

This chapter overviews BRS technology and discusses the advantages of performing intracoronary imaging with OCT in real-world clinical practice.

2.2 Historical background and the search for the ideal bioresorbable scaffold

Interventional cardiology has undergone several breakthroughs in the past 40 years, since Andreas Gruentzig, using a manufactured expandable balloon, performed the first coronary angioplasty in an awake patient in 1977, and changed the future of cardiovascular medicine [10]. This technique, now referred to as plain old balloon angioplasty (POBA), although providing an immediate reasonable angiographic result, was associated with compromised outcomes, mainly as a result of acute vessel closure due to coronary dissection, restenosis due to elastic recoil, or accelerated neointimal proliferation. In 1986, Jacques Puel and Ulrich Sigwart implanted the first coronary Wallstent® (Boston Scientific, Natick, MA, USA), a self-expanding device composed of a cobalt-based stainless steel alloy [11]. In 1987 Julio Palmaz, an Argentinian interventional vascular radiologist, and Richard Schatz, an American cardiologist, implanted the first coronary Palmaz–Schatz stent® (Cordis, Warren, NJ, USA), a self-expanding, stainless steel device [12]. This newer technology provided a solution for the early complications surrounding POBA by sealing any dissection flaps and preventing vessel recoil. Restenosis rates were reduced but still remained unacceptably high, with many patients needing repeated revascularizations after BMS index implantation [13]. During the late 1980s and early 1990s, a large number of interventional tools were developed, including rotational atherectomy devices, intravascular ultrasound and improvements in stent design. In 1997, over one million angioplasties had been performed worldwide, positioning this technique as one of the most commonly performed medical interventions. DESs were specifically developed to address the problems encountered with BMSs, namely restenosis and ST. The first DES to be launched was the Cypher® stent (Cordis Corporation, Warren, NJ, USA) in 2003, a sirolimus-eluting, expandable, stainless steel device, which was shortly followed by the Taxus® stent (Boston Scientific Corp., Natick, MA, USA) in 2004, a paclitaxel-eluting, expandable, stainless steel device. Over the following years, several stents followed, with differences focusing on the employed anti-proliferative agent and the design of the stent itself—the type of metal, strut thickness, mechanical properties and polymer specificities.

After POBA, BMSs and DESs, bioresorbable devices are considered the fourth landmark in the history of interventional cardiology. The search for an optimal absorbable device started over two decades ago, but the initial developed scaffolds failed to reach the market as they were associated with marked inflammatory responses, leading to neointimal hyperplasia and/or thrombus formation [14]. The major reason for the delay in expanding this technology was the inability to develop an ideal polymer, which could limit inflammation and restenosis and, at the same time, fully reabsorb, leaving the vessel completely healed over time. The most frequently used polymer in BRSs is poly-L-lactic acid (PLLA), which is a semi-crystalline polymer—regions with high concentration of polymer with a crystalline structure interconnected by amorphous chains binding the crystallites—since an amorphous polymer is more susceptible to hydration than a crystalline one. It is a biodegradable and thermoplastic polyester that undergoes self-catalyzed hydrolytic degradation to lactic acid, with the final products being carbon dioxide and water [15]. The reabsorption process includes several stages that can overlap: hydration of the polymer (absorption of water from the surrounding tissue), depolymerization by hydrolysis, loss of mass (fragmentation into segments of low-weight polymer and reduction of radial strength), assimilation/dissolution of the monomer (phagocytosis of small particles) and, finally, changing of the soluble monomer (L-lactate) into pyruvate, which subsequently enters the Krebs cycle and is converted into carbon dioxide and water. The final products are excreted through the kidneys and lungs, leading to a complete absorption of the device. Semi-crystalline polymers are used predominantly for mechanical support, while amorphous polymers allow for a more uniform drug delivery and structure loss at a predicted time. The duration of the degradation process depends on the crystallization of the polymer and varies between 2 and 4 years [16]. More recently, a metallic scaffold with a backbone made of absorbable magnesium alloy, sirolimus-eluting and with an open cell design, has also been used in clinical practice. The device resorption process has two stages: first, ions and water from the surrounding tissues reach the metallic backbone, creating magnesium hydroxide and beginning corrosion. In the second stage, magnesium phosphate is slowly converted into an amorphous calcium phosphate, cracks appear in the core and the material is resorbed and, within a 12 month period, 95% of the magnesium is resorbed [17].

2.3 Bioresorbable scaffolds: current clinical evidence

Absorbable devices are more accurately called *scaffolds*, due to their transient vessel support and absence of a permanent metallic implant. Several PLLA-based/polymeric absorbable scaffolds have been clinically evaluated for the treatment of coronary artery disease. These include the Absorb® BRS (Abbott Vascular, Santa Clara, CA, USA), the DESolve® myolimus-eluting bioresorbable coronary scaffold system (Elixir Medical Corporation, Sunnyvale, CA, USA) and a tyrosine-derived polycarbonate polymer stent (Reva Medical, San Diego, CA, USA).

The Igaki-Tamai® (Igaki Medical Planning Company, Kyoto, Japan) was the first BRS implanted in humans. It was constructed with PLLA, being both self-expandable and balloon expandable; its zigzag helical coil pattern resulted in less vessel trauma at implantation and also reduced thrombus formation or intimal hyperplasia. Its strut thickness was larger (0.17 mm) and the vessel coverage by struts was greater than for standard metallic stents. Self-expansion was achieved by the use of heated contrast (up to 70°) and expansion was further optimized by inflation of the delivery balloon up to 14 atm. Continued self-expansion of the stent at 37° in the 20–30 min following deployment would optimize the final result.

The first-in-humans study was reported in 2000 by Tamai *et al* [18], comprising 15 patients (25 scaffolds implanted) and revealed no safety concerns. Major adverse cardiovascular events (MACEs), including scaffold thrombosis (ScT), were reported at 6 months follow-up and the neointimal growth was comparable to that of BMSs (0.48 mm). A second study, which randomized 50 patients, had promising outcomes, with intravascular ultrasound (IVUS) demonstrating complete absence of stent struts at 3 years. The MACE-free survival was 82% at 4 years and freedom from cardiac death and MACE at 10 years were 98% and 47%, respectively [19, 20]. Despite the favorable results, the failure of the scaffold to reach the clinical arena was primarily related to the need for high temperatures to induce self-expansion, which is cumbersome to accomplish in routine daily practice, and is associated with concerns related to the potential induction of arterial wall necrosis, which may lead to excessive intimal hyperplasia, increased platelet adhesion and, subsequently, ScT [21]. The device is now used in Europe for peripheral intervention and has no drug elution.

2.3.1 The Absorb® scaffold

The Absorb® (figure 2.1) was the first everolimus-eluting BRS and is the best documented so far. It consists of four components: a bioabsorbable PLLA scaffold based on a proven MULTI-LINK BMS pattern, a poly-DL-lactide (PDLLA) coating that contains and controls the release of the anti-proliferative drug everolimus, and the XIENCE V (Abbott Vascular, Santa Clara, CA, USA) delivery system. Both PLLA and PDLLA are fully resorbable with complete absorption expected at 24–36 months, with minimal inflammatory response [22]. The first-generation device (BVS 1.0) was tested in the ABSORB Cohort A, a single-arm, prospective, open-label study which enrolled 30 patients with a single, *de novo*,

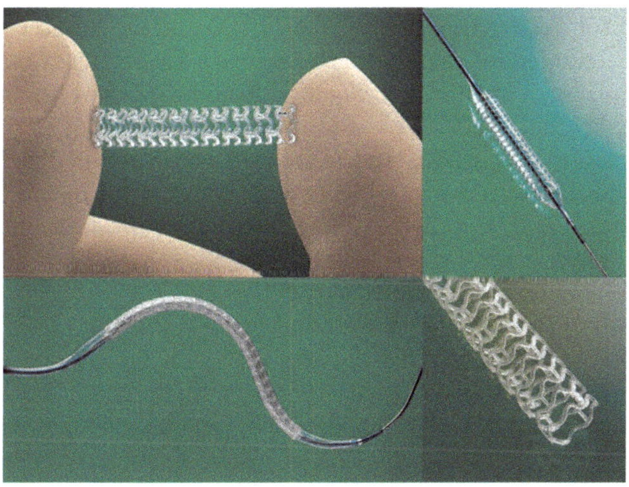

Figure 2.1. The Absorb everolimus-eluting bioresorbable scaffold. Reprinted with permission from Abbott Vascular.

coronary artery lesion [23–25]. At 5 years of follow-up, the ischemia driven MACE incidence was 3.4% and ScT was not reported. Interestingly, between 6 months and 2 years, an enlargement of the vessel lumen was detected by intravascular imaging (IVUS and OCT), although with no change in the angiographic late loss. Vessel motility tests were performed at 2 years and physiological response to vasoactive stimuli was present, suggesting the return of the vessel's vasomotion in the scaffolding area. A second-generation Absorb (BVS 1.1) was tested in the Absorb Cohort B, as a single-arm, multicenter trial that included 101 patients with a maximum of two *de novo* coronary artery lesions, with a maximum diameter of 3 mm and a length up to 14 mm [26, 27]. The studied population was further divided in two groups: the first 45 patients were randomized to a 6 and 24 months follow-up with invasive imaging (quantitative coronary angiography (QCA), IVUS and OCT) (cohort B1) and the remaining 56 patients were randomized to the same tests at 12 and 36 months (cohort B2). At 2 years, nine clinical events were reported, including six ischemia driven (ID) target lesion revascularizations (TLRs). At the 2 year follow-up, a similar neointimal growth was observed between small and large vessels and only one patient in each group had detectable incomplete stent apposition. In cohort B2, the late lumen loss and neointimal growth were slightly larger than in B1 at 6 months, but similar to other studies at the same time point. Furthermore, the authors reported that the scaffolded segments clearly responded to vasomotion stimuli. Three intravascular imaging techniques (OCT, IVUS gray-scale and IVUS-virtual histology) were used for monitoring the resorption activity and documented several stages of the ongoing process. The Absorb EXTEND, a prospective, open-label clinical study, assessed the safety and performance of the Absorb BRS in a larger and more diverse population, with increased lesion complexity [28]. A report concerning the 12 month follow-up of the first 512 patients was disclosed in 2015 and revealed an ID-MACE and ID-target vessel failure of 4.3% and 4.9%, respectively. Four cases of ScT were recorded, two subacute and the other two occurring as late ScT. A comparison between the Absorb EXTEND and the SPIRIT trial (XIENCE V® EES) in the treatment of *de novo* native coronary lesions, regarding the incidence and clinical sequelae of small side-branch occlusion (SBO)—1209 branches of 435 patients in the Absorb EXTEND versus 682 side branches in 237 patients in the SPIRIT—revealed that the BRS was associated with a higher incidence of SBO when compared to EES, and that patients with SBO had an increased incidence of in-hospital myocardial infarction (MI) (6.5% in SBO group versus 0.5% in non-SBO, $p < 0.01$). A post hoc analysis showed that the BRS was associated with SBO only in vessels with a reference vessel diameter $\leqslant 0.5$ mm [29].

The ABSORB II [30–33] is a single-blind, prospective, multicenter randomized clinical trial (RCT) that compared the Absorb® with the Xience® metallic stent, admitting treatment of *de novo* coronary lesions in different major epicardial vessels, with pre-determined diameters: (i) a maximum lumen diameter between 2.25–3.8 mm (QCA) and (ii) a maximum lesion length of $\leqslant 48$ mm. Primary endpoints were the evaluation of vasomotion through the assessment of both mean and minimum lumen diameters at 3 years. In a cohort of 501 patients, acute lumen gain was lower in the BRS group. However, the 1 year rates of angina were lower in the BRS arm, whereas performance during maximum exercise was similar in both groups. The 2 year analysis of the clinical results showed there were no statistically significant differences between the two devices regarding the composite clinical endpoints: 'patient-oriented composite endpoint' (PoCE), 'device-oriented composite endpoint' (DoCE), target lesion failure (TLF) or MACE. Although the absolute rate of definite or probable ScT was higher in the Absorb® group, it was not statistically significant (1.5% versus 0%, $p = 0.174$). Furthermore, at 3 years the clinical endpoints were not different between the groups. Nonetheless, the DoCE was significantly higher in the Absorb arm, driven by target vessel MI (6.0% versus 1.0%, $p = 0.011$), although 52% of the cases were peri-procedural. Eight definite ScT and one late probable ScT were documented after BRS implantation, against none in the XIENCE group ($p = 0.033$). Potential mechanisms leading to early versus late ScT include protruding or malapposed struts (early ScT) and incomplete lesion coverage, malapposition, strut discontinuity and underexpansion (late and very-late ScT).

Although BRSs may have several advantages over DESs—maintaining normal vessel function, allowing for a future percutaneous or surgical revascularization if necessary, elimination of potential triggers for late ScT, such as chronic inflammatory response and delayed endothelization—the resorbable scaffold experience and outcomes in routine clinical practice were largely unknown. GHOST-EU [34] is a retrospective, non-randomized, multicenter registry comprising 1189 patients with coronary artery lesions suitable for stenting, undergoing single or multivessel PCI with the Absorb device. The inclusion criteria encircled a great number of patients, with complex clinical scenarios (myocardial infarction, chronic kidney disease, depressed left ventricle function) and complex coronary disease (ostial lesions, bifurcations, chronic total occlusions, left main disease). TLF had a cumulative incidence of 2.2% at 30 days and 4.4% at six months, and diabetes was the only predictor of TLF, with a 2.4 fold increase. The cumulative incidence of ScT was higher than expected, 1.5% at 30 days and 2.1% at 6 months, with 70% of the cases occurring subacutely. ScT is known to be a multifactorial event, associated with different causal mechanisms, according to the timing of its occurrence. Early events are usually due to procedural issues—dissection, device malapposition and underexpansion—and late events are usually related to the device's inner characteristics and vessel response. The Absorb scaffold is a thick-strutted platform, and has been described as having 1.5 fold more thrombogenicity than thin-strutted metallic stents [35]. Nonetheless, it is still unknown if any deleterious struts-induced event may outweigh the late benefits, after scaffold biodegradation and vessel healing. The authors concluded that early and midterm outcomes in this cohort of patients with unselected clinical characteristics and lesions were acceptable and comparable to second-generation DESs, with ScT comparable to the first-generation DESs.

ABSORB China [36], ABSORB III [37], ABSORB Japan [38], AIDA [39], EVERBIO II [40] and TROFI II [41] are randomized trials which showed more adverse events, mainly attributable to excessive ScT, in the BRS group when compared to the XIENCE stent. In ABSORB II, the rates of recurrent angina were less frequent in the Absorb arm. ABSORB IV [42] is a prospective RCT, designed to be an extension of ABSORB III, with TLF as the predesignated primary endpoint and angina as the major secondary outcome. The results showed non-inferiority between the scaffold and the metallic DES group regarding TLF, and also similar rates of angina at 1 year.

A significant number of trials and studies regarding the use of BRSs in different clinical settings have been published, potentially expanding the indications and advantages of absorbable scaffolds in specific clinical scenarios: (i) in acute coronary syndromes (POLAR-ACS [43], BVS-EXAMINATION [44] and PRAGUE-19 [45]) BRSs were reported as a safe and feasible device, with a high rate of procedural success; (ii) in chronic total occlusions (CTOs) (CTO-Absorb Pilot Study [46] and Goktekin *et al* [47]), CTO recanalization with a BRS had excellent feasibility and safety, with adequate lesion preparation being fundamental to device success; (iii) and ostial lesions (GHOST-EU registry), where BRSs, with suboptimal technique implantation, were an independent predictor of clinical events.

The excessive ScT seen for resorbable scaffolds in recent clinical trials, particuarly in the ABSORB III, led to Absorb being pulled off the market in September 2017. The poor device results may be accounted for by the thicker struts, the limited ability to over-expand, poor outcomes in smaller vessels and the need for precise sizing and optimal implantation techniques.

2.3.2 Metallic magnesium BRSs

The first magnesium-based metallic scaffold to be implanted in humans was AMS-1® (Biotronik AG, Bülach, Switzerland), a balloon expandable device with a strut thickness of 165 μm, which was evaluated in the PROGRESS-AMS trial [48]. Magnesium was the chosen metal as it is one of the major intracellular cations in the body. It is an important cofactor not only for numerous enzymes, transporters and nucleic acids, but also for several functions such asneuromuscular activity [49]. In the former trial, immediate angiographic results were similar to those of other metallic stents but the radial support was lost in the short term, due to an almost complete degradation of the scaffold only after 4 months, resulting in early neointimal growth and negative remodeling. Additionally, the device had no anti-proliferative drug and, hence, high rates of late loss and TLR. Yet, no myocardial infarction, ScT or death occurred. These findings suggested that the scaffold lacked sufficient mechanical strength or support. A few years later, an improved drug-eluting version emerged, DREAMS 1G® (magnesium-based, paclitaxel-eluting), which was evaluated in the prospective, multicenter, first-in-man trial Biosolve I. The scaffold was associated with good safety and efficacy at 12 months (7% of TLR) [50] and no cardiac death or ScT. The newer DREAMS 2G® is an absorbable scaffold made of a refined magnesium alloy backbone and contains a PLLA-based polymer coated with sirolimus with an absorption period of 12 months. BIOSOLVE-II, a prospective, multicenter, non-randomized trial, revealed low rates of TLR/TLF and no ScT at 6 months follow-up [51]. BIOSOLVE-III was designed to confirm the positive outcomes of the modified metallic scaffold, now being called Magmaris®—sirolimus-eluting, 150 μm strut thickness and width, higher acute radial strength, resorption rate of 95% at 12 months [52]. Although BIOSOLVE-III included more patients with type B2/C lesions and more severe calcification, late lumen loss was nearly identical to BIOSOLVE-II, and TLR was 3.3% at 1 year in comparison to 6.6% for Absorb, 5.2% for EES and 5.7% for DESolve [53], with no ScT observed. Overall, safety device improvement may be due to the shorter resorption rate of the magnesium scaffold in contrast to the polymeric ones, in which the resorption occurs at 3 years. BIOSOLVE-IV, a prospective multicenter registry, reported a 12 month TLF rate of 4.2% and one case of ScT due to double antiplatelet therapy interruption, corroborating the excellent safety profile reported in the previous clinical trials [54].

2.3.3 Other resorbable scaffolds

DESolve® (Elixir Medical, Sunnyvale, CA, USA) is a PLLA-based scaffold coated with the anti-proliferative drug myolimus, with more than 85% of the drug being released in 4 weeks. Features include the potential to maintain adequate mechanical support with bioabsorption at about 1 year, a wide safety margin for postdilation without strut fracture and the ability to self-correct to the vessel wall in cases of minor malapposition. It was evaluated in the prospective, multicenter DESolve First-in-Man Trial which included 15 patients [55]. At 6 months, imaging studies with OCT and IVUS revealed a late lumen loss of 0.19 ± 0.19 mm with no evidence of scaffold recoil or late malapposition. At 12 months there were no reports of ScT or MACEs directly attributable to the device, and assessment with computed tomography showed excellent vessel patency. Currently, the second-generation DESolve CX, with thinner struts (120 μm) is being evaluated in clinical trials.

The REVA® stent (Reva Medical, CA, USA) is made of a tyrosine-derived polycarbonate polymer that is both resorbable and radiopaque, after being chemically modified to incorporate iodine molecules. It metabolizes to aminoacids, ethanol and carbon dioxide, with tyrosine entering the Krebs cycle. Its degradation time can reach 2 years, depending on the molecular weight of the polymer [56]. The REVA has a distinctive feature, a 'slide-and-lock' mechanism, conceived to prevent deformation and weakening of the polymer during stent deployment; the locking system, aside from preventing the stent from going back during deployment, provides additional support in a later stage, during vessel remodeling. RESORB, a first-in-human multicenter study which included 30 patients, began its enrollment in 2007. At 6 months follow-up there was no significant elastic recoil or neointimal hyperplasia. However, TLR was unacceptable with a rate of 66.7%, probably due to focal mechanical failures and the absence of an anti-proliferative substance. The scaffold was redesigned and evaluated in ReZolve®—a more robust polymer, a spiral slide-and-lock mechanism and a coating of sirolimus, with 95% of the drug being eluted at 90 days. In the RESTORE Pilot Study, the technical success rate was only 85% due to the high crossing profile and sheathed delivery system. Twelve-month results showed an excellent acute lumen gain, the occurrence of two cases of TLR and one cardiac death [57]. ReZolve2® is a second-generation sirolimus-eluting scaffold and was designed to overcome ReZolve's failures. It has a lower profile, a sheathless delivery system and a 30% increase in radial strength. In 2014,

REVA transitioned to a new platform, Fantom®, which is sirolimus-eluting and was designed to have an even lower crossing profile, higher visibility, a large expansion range with a high safety margin against strut fracture, increased radial strength and complete reabsorption within 3 years, with potential full restoration of natural vasomotion. Results from the second-generation Fantom BRS, a scaffold with thinner struts (125 μm), enhanced radial strength and minimal recoil, were presented at PCR 2018. Fantom II showed a low MACE and very-late ScT rates (5% and 0.4%, respectively), and no evidence of chronic scaffold recoil [58]. The Fantom clinical trial program is still ongoing.

2.4 The clinical utility of optical coherence tomography in the optimization of bioresorbable scaffolds

In the past 15 years OCT has become an important technology in the evaluation of coronary artery structure, overcoming the limited spatial resolution and drawbacks in the assessment of vulnerable plaques of IVUS. It is a catheter-based imaging system that uses near-infrared light to produce cross-sectional images of the inner vascular wall, with a resolution of 10–20 μm, which is approximately ten-fold higher than that of IVUS, with the caveat of limited depth penetration [59]. It is unable to penetrate red blood cells, so it has to be performed in a blood-free environment, through the injection of a contrast medium, allowing operators to visualize long coronary segments in a matter of seconds. As a result of this exceptional high resolution, deep plaque analysis and more accurate detection of PCI-associated complications is now possible, leading to more favorable clinical outcomes [60], and turning OCT into one of the most useful techniques to assess lumen geometry and guide coronary intervention. In addition to identifying the thickness of the tissue layers that separate the superficial plaque from the lumen, and being capable of accurate plaque characterization—a sensitivity of 96% and a specificity of 97% in detecting calcified nodules [61]—it provides a clear evaluation of the interface between the lumen of the vessel and the stent, allowing for clear detection of malapposition, underexpansion, edge dissection or tissue protrusion. BRSs have important differences when compared to standard metallic stents, which can be depicted by a thorough OCT analysis. For metallic stents, struts are clearly visible and neointimal growth can be measured at any time—the area between the struts and the lumen contour. For BRSs, at an early stage, struts are still visible and neointimal proliferation can still be assessed, with degradation progressing steadily. However, in the long term, as the resorption process subsides with vascular repair, and the polymer is progressively replaced by a provisional matrix of proteoglycan, scaffold struts are no longer visible and distinguishing between the strut area and underlying plaque becomes a challenge. Even though OCT is not capable of differentiating PLLA from proteoglycan, which is one of the first structural changes to occur in vascular repair [62], it is able to precisely measure the lumen and scaffold and assess scaffold apposition, coverage and the appearance of polymeric struts over time. Thus OCT has been one of the favorite techniques for studying BRSs. Serruys *et al* have assessed dynamic vessel changes in the entire population of the Absorb

Cohort B trial using several imaging modalities (QCA, IVUS, radio-frequency backscattering (IVUS-VH) and OCT) at different time points [63]. The overall OCT analysis showed that, after an initial decrease in minimal and mean lumen area, values stabilized. Increase in neointima between one and three years was compensated by a simultaneous enlargement in minimum and mean scaffold area (in cohort B2 the mean scaffold area increase was $0.88 \pm 1.72\ mm^2$, $p < 0.001$, with neointimal formation of $0.93 \pm 0.94\ mm^2$). The number of struts counted in all-frame analysis steadily increased from baseline to 1 and 3 years, a finding interpreted as the dismantling of the scaffold, and 98% of the struts showed coverage, with the mean black core area unchanged up to 3 years. In the discussion, the authors refer to the fact that some preclinical investigation showed that changes in strut appearance in OCT correspond to the appearance of connective tissue which will subsequently shrink and ultimately disappear. As this last process is associated with wall thinning, this change may have an impact on lumen enlargement. In contrast to IVUS, OCT was able to detect the endoluminal interface of the vessel wall behind the polymeric struts with near perfect delineation of the neointimal tissue surrounding them. IVUS mainly detected the lumen boundaries determined by strut brightness. This difference has some impact in the follow-up: no change in mean lumen area with OCT versus an increase with IVUS. Allahwala *et al* aimed to determine if OCT, after successful angiographic BRS implantation, influenced decision making with regard to the need for postdilation, in a small population of patients with predominant type A lesions [64]. The authors observed that 28% of patients with optimal angiographic results required further BRS optimization following OCT, a similar finding to the ABSORB trial, and hypothesized that this number could increase if more complex lesions had been included. Bourantas *et al* evaluated the implications of the Absorb BRS on the morphology of superficial plaques and included 46 patients with BRS versus 20 patients with BMSs who underwent OCT at baseline and follow-up [65]. The study revealed that plaques in native coronary segments maintained the same morphology, in contrast to treated segments in which neointimal formation covered calcific spots and turned thin-capped fibroatheromas into thick-capped ones. Also, there was a significantly higher reduction in lumen dimensions in BMSs than in BVSs. In Absorb BRSs, neointimal tissue continued to develop after short-term follow-up and did not compromise luminal dimensions, as the scaffold was shown to expand. Finally, the distribution of neointimal tissue over thin-capped fibroatheromas and calcific plaques in both BMSs and BRSs revealed a similar pattern. These findings are discrepant when compared to other studies, maybe due to the use of different imaging modalities to measure neointimal thickness, as well as the implantation of two different types of stents in the BMS group.

Nakatani *et al* published a consensus amongst multiple core labs and expert researchers of OCT, and proposed a new standardized and comparative method for quantitative analysis on OCT, that specifically applies to the Absorb BRS and, in general, for metallic stents [66]. These authors focused their attention on the following parameters: tracing of both the luminal and abluminal stent/scaffold contours, measurement of the endoluminal and abluminal incomplete stent apposition (ISA) area—in metallic stents is the area between the endoluminal leading edge of the struts, and in polymeric scaffolds is the area between the abluminal side of the strut and the lumen contour [67]. They also quantified the area occupied by the scaffold/stent struts, with exclusion of the strut and neointimal areas from the flow area and usage of interpolated lumen contour to assess the degree of strut embedment on the vessel wall. The authors emphasize that after the integration of the BRS in the vessel wall, measurements of scaffold area, neointimal area and ISA area can no longer be used and, at long-term follow-up, only the flow area is a comparable parameter, between metallic and bioresorbable devices.

So far, limited data exist in the vascular healing process associated with absorbable metal scaffolds. OCT analysis performed in a subgroup of patients in BIOLSOVE-II showed that the minimal lumen area decreased significantly from post-procedure to 6 months. However, between 6 and 12 months the difference was not significant. In addition, maximum backscattered values also decreased significantly from the post-procedure to 6 months. At baseline, magnesium struts appear as bright structures with shadowing, but over time they are resorbed and only vestiges of struts are visible at 12 months. This process is evident through the changes in the maximum values of backscattering and attenuation values. According to this data, serial imaging of the magnesium scaffold appears to reflect the restoration of the vessel anatomy, with an almost complete reabsorption at 12 months [68].

2.5 Bioresorbable scaffolds in real-world clinical settings

The following cases depict the use of the bioresorbable technology in real-world clinical cases, and the utility of OCT for pre-device assessment, scaffold optimization and evaluation of intravascular complications after scaffold implantation, which are often not visible on coronary angiography.

2.5.1 Case 1—the need for state-of-the-art peri-procedural intravascular imaging

A 57 year old male, obese patient with a past medical history of hypertension, dyslipidemia and past smoking was admitted to the intensive cardiac care unit with a non-ST-elevation acute myocardial infarction. He underwent coronary angiography that revealed three vessel diseases: occluded mid-right coronary artery (RCA) with visible retrograde filling, occluded mid-circumflex artery (LCX) with visible retrograde filling, and left anterior descending artery (LAD) with a subocclusive lesion in its mid portion. Left ventriculography revealed postero-basal hypokinesia. RCA was considered the culprit and PCI was performed using a standard floppy 0.014″ guidewire, a 2.5/14 mm compliant balloon for predilation and an Absorb 3.5/18 mm stent (slowly deflated). Postdilation was not performed due to the optimal angiographic result with apparent good apposition (figures 2.2 and 2.3).

Two days later, the patient was submitted to staged PCI of the LAD. After predilation with a 2.5/20 mm compliant balloon, a second lesion (75% by QCA) was evident in the mid/distal segment of the LAD and predilated with a 2.0/15 mm compliant balloon. Subsequently, two Absorbs were implanted, 2.5/18 mm distally

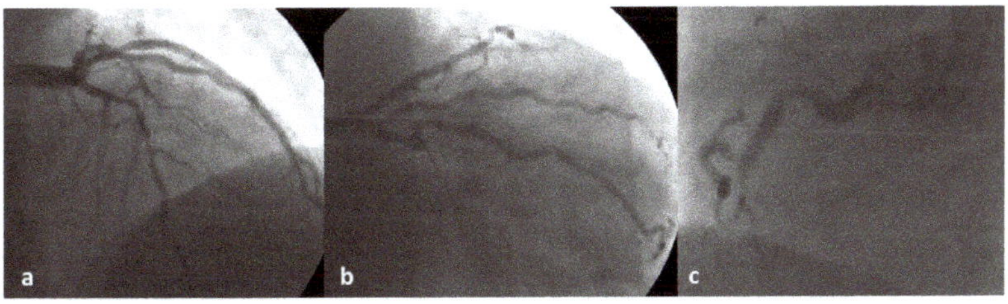

Figure 2.2. (a) LAD with a subocclusive lesion in its mid portion, (b) LCX occluded after the second obtuse marginal branch (OM) and (c) RCA occluded in its mid segment.

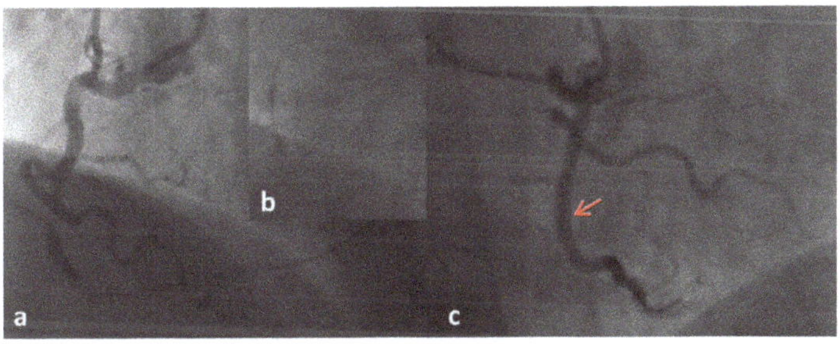

Figure 2.3. (a) RCA after predilation with a 2.5/14 mm compliant balloon, (b) slow deflation of an Absorb 3.5/18 mm stent and (c) final result (arrow pointing at the Absorb site).

and 3.0/23 mm proximally without overlap, followed by postdilation of both scaffolds with a non-compliant 3.0/12 mm balloon. The final angiographic result was good, with no visible complications (figure 2.4).

One month after the procedures, the patient reported mild shortness of breath during moderate effort which worsened throughout the following months, though no chest pain was reported. The patient maintained dual antiplatelet therapy with aspirin (100 mg per day) and ticagrelor (90 mg twice a day). Angiographic revision was scheduled and performed six months after the index event, revealing an occluded mid LAD with retrograde filling by the RCA, before the first implanted BRS. OCT was performed in the RCA, which revealed malapposition in the mid portion of the scaffold (figure 2.5). PCI of the LAD was performed with double cannulation. After the guidewire was advanced into the LAD, dilation with a non-compliant 2.0/20 mm balloon was performed. OCT showed diffuse restenosis of both the distal and proximal BRS and two significant additional lesions, one in the gap between the scaffolds, and the other proximal to the first implanted BRS (edge dissection during the first device implantation? A *de novo* lesion?). Dilation with non-compliant balloons was accomplished, followed by the implantation of a DES in the first lesion, overlapping the proximal scaffold. In the second lesion, a new DES was implanted overlapping both BRS scaffolds. Afterwards, dilation of the distal BRS with a drug-eluting balloon was performed. Final OCT showed no edge dissections and good strut apposition (figures 2.6–2.8). This case illustrates the

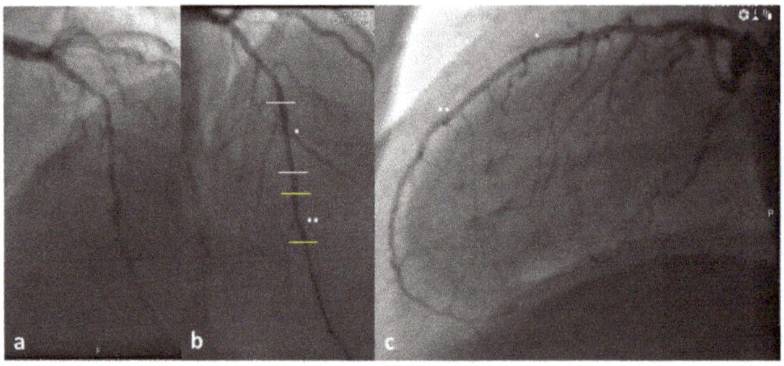

Figure 2.4. (a) LAD predilation with two compliant balloons (2.0/15 mm distally and 2.5/20 mm proximally), (b) LAD after implantation of two Absorbs (one dot: 3.0/23 mm; two dots: 2.5/18 mm) and (c) final result, after postdilation.

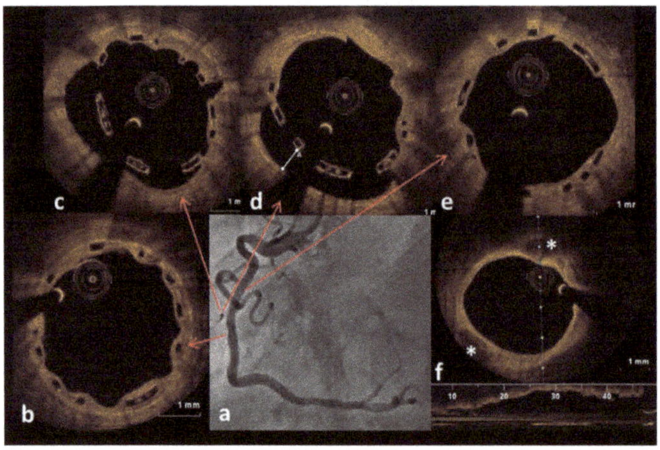

Figure 2.5. (a) RCA at 6 months after the index event with a good angiographic result, (b) distal part of the scaffold, with neointimal growth covering the polymeric struts, (c) and (d) mid portion of the scaffold with malapposition between 5 and 10 o'clock, (e) proximal part of the scaffold with good apposition and luminal area, and (f) proximal RCA with calcified plaques (*).

usefulness of OCT during PCI, both in type A and in more complex lesions. It is unknown whether an edge dissection was present after implantation of the BRS in the LAD or if any other mechanism was responsible for the subsequent proximal vessel occlusion. Restenosis remains an important limitation of current generation DESs, with reported rates of TLR ranging from 5%–10% [69]. Regarding BRS restenosis, current data are very limited and treatment strategies remain to be elucidated.

2.5.2 Case 2—a careful OCT interpretation

A 40-year-old male patient presented to the emergency department with an oppressive and recurrent chest pain, and was diagnosed with a non-ST-elevation

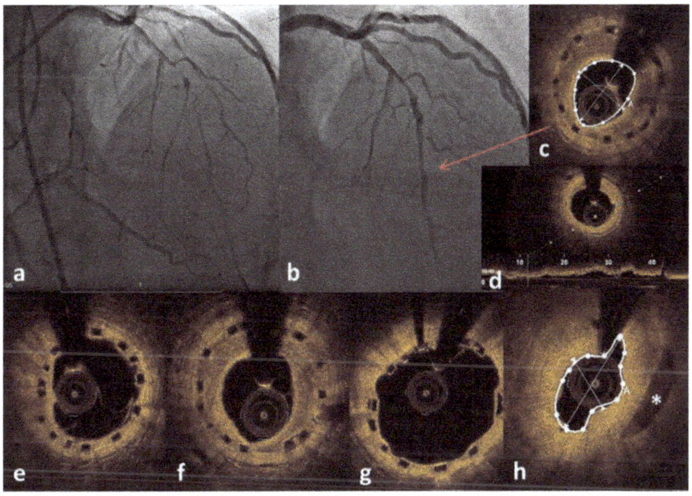

Figure 2.6. (a) Double cannulation of RCA and LAD showing occlusion of the mid segment of the LAD, proximal to the previously implanted BRS, (b) LAD, after dilation with a 2.0/20 mm non-compliant balloon, (c) restenosis of the distal BRS, with a mean luminal area of 1.45 mm^2, (d) a gap between the two scaffolds with a fibrotic plaque, (e) distal part of the proximal scaffold with good apposition and neointimal coverage of the struts, (f) restenosis of the mid portion of the proximal scaffold, (g) proximal segment of the proximal scaffold with good apposition and (h) lesion proximal to the scaffolds, fibrotic and calcified (*), with a mean luminal area of 1.00 mm^2.

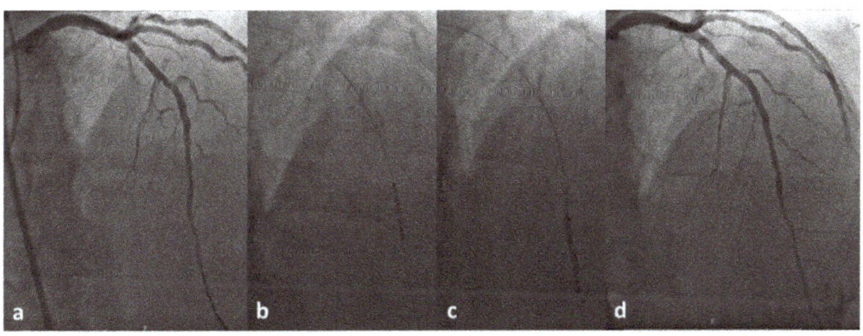

Figure 2.7. (a) LAD after implantation of a DES 3.0/18 mm proximal to the first scaffold, overlapping the proximal BRS, (b) and (c) implantation of a DES 2.75/12 mm in the gap between scaffolds followed by prolonged drug-eluting balloon dilation in the distal scaffold and (d) final result.

acute myocardial infarction. He was a smoker with hypertension and uncontrolled dyslipidemia. Coronary angiography showed a 75% lesion in the mid segment of the LAD and LCX occluded proximally, filling distally by RCA collaterals. OCT was performed in the LAD and revealed a 15 mm fibrolipid lesion, with a mean diameter of 1.2 mm (mean reference diameter of 2.33 mm), absence of calcium and proper plaque free landing zones (figure 2.9). According to these findings, predilation with a 2.0/12 mm compliant balloon was conducted and a BRS 2.5/18 mm was implanted and postdilated with a 3.0/15 mm non-compliant balloon inflated at nominal pressure. The final OCT confirmed good expansion and apposition and revealed

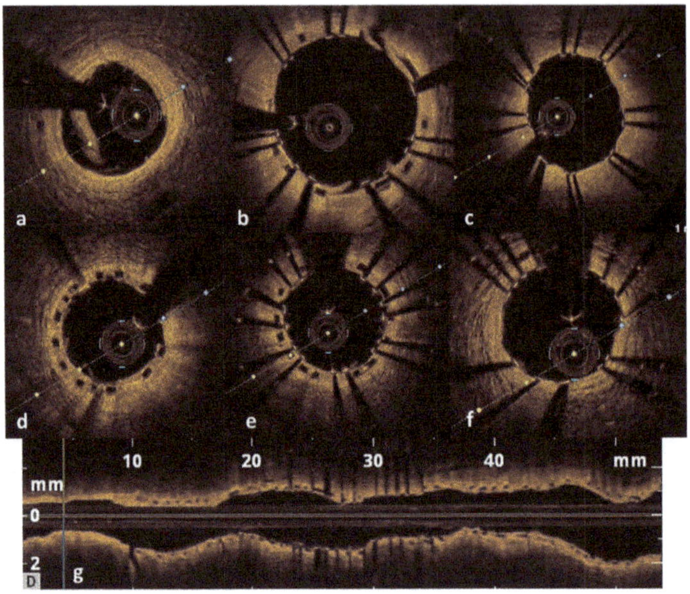

Figure 2.8. (a) Dissection visible in the gap between the scaffolds, pre-DES implantation, (b) and (c) after proximal DES implantation with scaffold overlap and good apposition, (d) distal scaffold after drug-eluting balloon dilation, (e) and (f) after implantation of the second DES, overlapping both scaffolds, showing good apposition and (g) long view, final pullback.

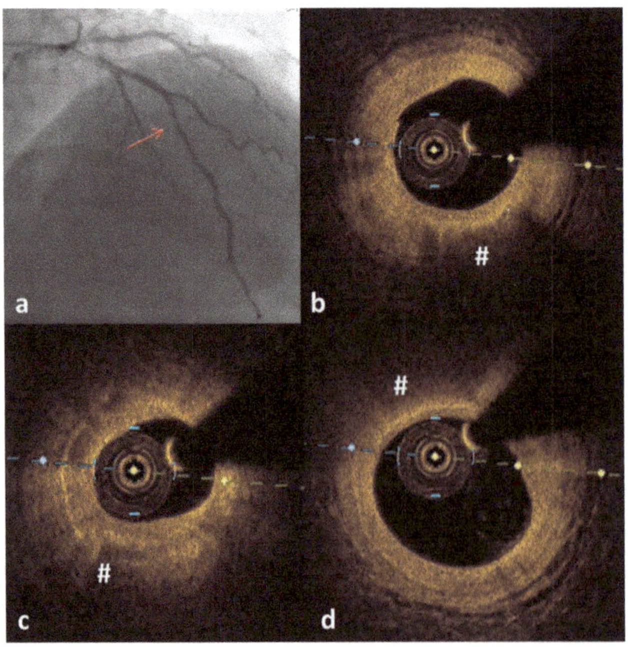

Figure 2.9. (a) LAD with a 75% lesion in its mid segment and (b)–(d) OCT revealing a fibrolipid lesion (# lipid pools).

the presence of a small distal edge dissection (3 mm), without flow compromise and not visible angiographically, so no further measure was taken (figure 2.10).

PCI of the LCX CTO was performed 2 weeks later. After the guidewire progressed to the distal vessel and the lesion was predilated with a 2.0/20 mm compliant balloon, OCT was performed and revealed a long obstructive lesion, with small amounts of calcium and abundant red thrombus (figure 2.11). Two Absorbs were implanted, a 2.5/28 mm distally and a 3.0/18 proximally, with overlap. OCT

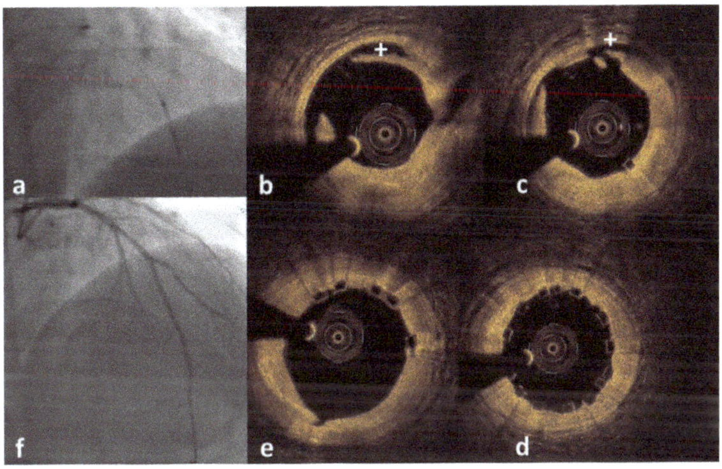

Figure 2.10. (a) A BRS 2.5/18 mm being slowly deflated, (b) and (c) small edge dissection without flow limitation and not angiographically visible, (d) BVS struts ('black box' appearance) with good expansion and apposition, (e) proximal edge of the scaffold, dissection free, and (f) final result.

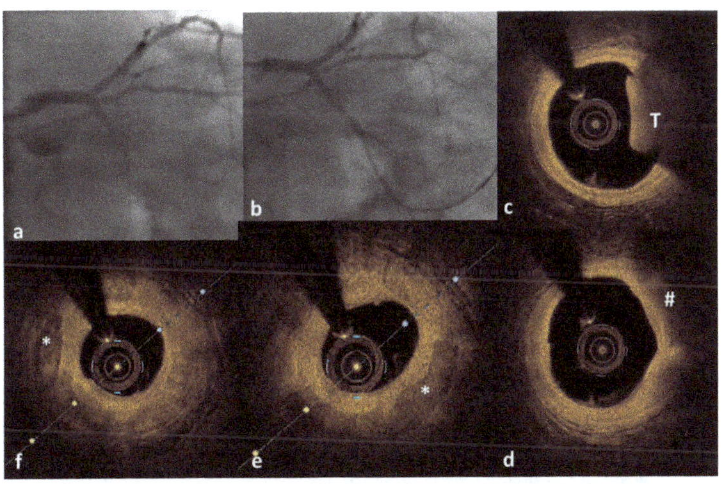

Figure 2.11. (a) CTO of the proximal LCX, (b) progression of the guidewire to the distal vessel and predilation with a compliant 2.0/20 mm balloon, (c) red thrombus (T) visible at the distal part of the lesion, (d) plaque with abundant lipid pools (#) and (e) and (f) severe calcified (*) stenosis.

showed malapposition with plaque/thrombus protrusion (figure 2.12) and postdilation was achieved with non-compliant balloons, 2.5/20 and 3.0/20 mm for the distal and proximal scaffolds, respectively. Final angiography and OCT confirmed a good result (figure 2.13). The 2 week OCT revaluation of the LAD showed a sealed coronary dissection (figure 2.14). Fourteen months later, the patient underwent an angiographic/OCT follow-up showing no scaffold restenosis (figure 2.15).

2.5.3 Case 3—BRS in calcified vessels. Does OCT have a role?

A 50-year-old male patient with hypertension, dyslipidemia and current smoking was referred to invasive risk stratification due to stable angina (class III of the Canadian Cardiovascular Society) and documented myocardial ischemia in a

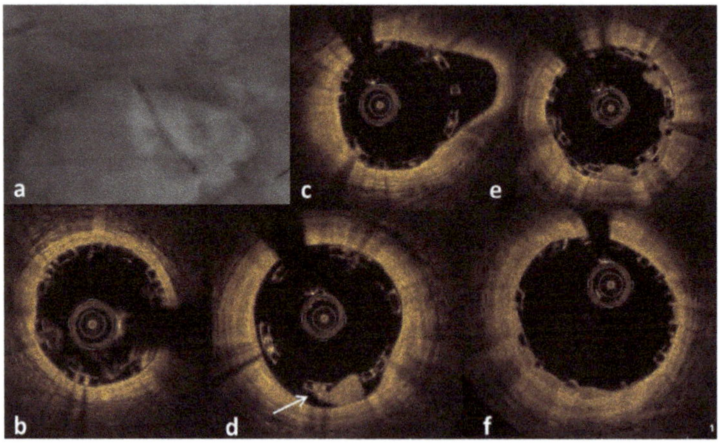

Figure 2.12. (a) Distal BRS 2.5/28 mm implantation, (b) distal edge with no dissection, (c) OM bifurcation, (d) scaffolds struts with malapposition and plaque/thrombus protrusion (arrow), (e) overlap area with plaque protrusion and (f) proximal edge.

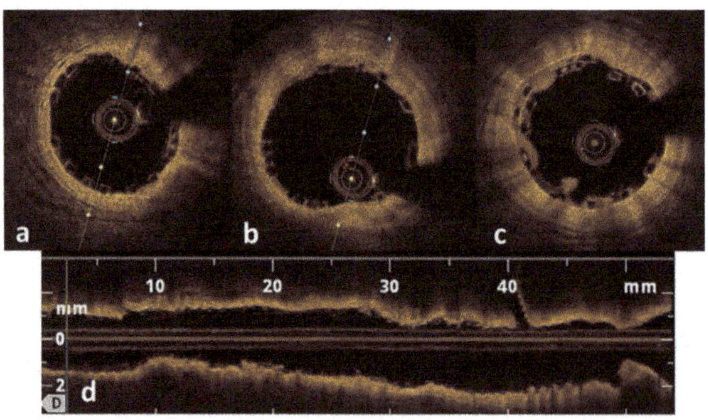

Figure 2.13. (a) Distal edge, (b) previous malapposition area, (c) overlap of the two scaffolds, and (d) long view showing good expansion and apposition.

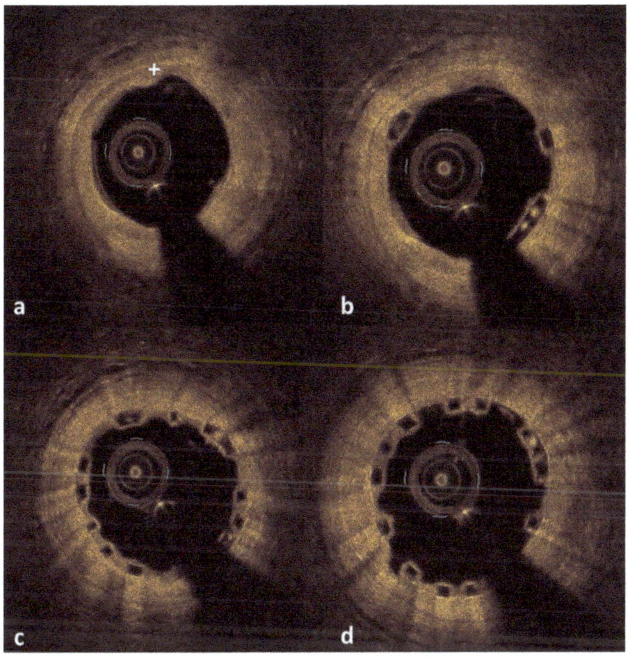

Figure 2.14. LAD follow-up after 2 weeks. (a) Previous dissection area (+) with no visible complications and (b)–(d) good expansion and apposition, with some evident neointimal strut coverage.

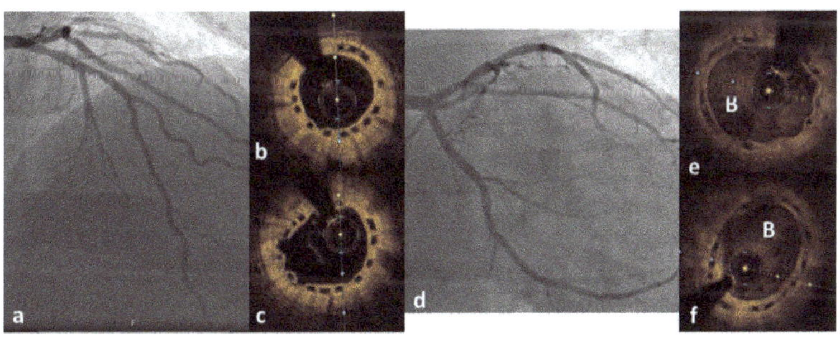

Figure 2.15. LAD and LCX 14 month follow-up. (a) LAD with a patent scaffold, (b) and (c) struts with neointimal coverage, no visible restenosis and maintained vessel architecture, (d) LCX in angiography with patent scaffolds, and (e) and (f) no restenosis, visible neointimal growth, blood in the lumen (B).

non-invasive imaging stress test. Coronary angiography revealed a 75% stenosis in the mid segment of the LAD (diffuse atherosclerosis) and two apparently significant lesions in the RCA (non-dominant, small caliber vessel). OCT guided PCI of the LAD was performed, revealing a long calcified lesion with a mean reference diameter of 3.1 mm (figure 2.16). Predilation was executed with a 3.0/20 mm compliant balloon followed by the implantation of a BRS 3.5/28 mm. OCT disclosed an inadequate expansion on the most severe calcified segment (figure 2.17) and postdilation with a non-compliant 3.5/15 mm balloon was achieved. Final

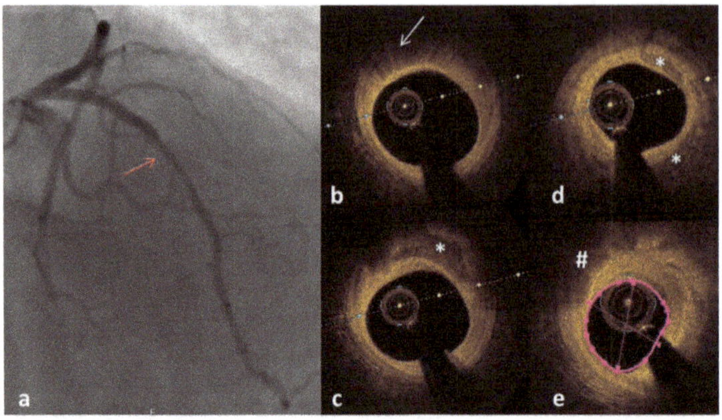

Figure 2.16. (a) LAD with a 75% calcified lesion in its mid segment (red arrow), (b) lipid pool with inflammatory activity and apparent macrophage accumulation (white arrow), (c) and (d) calcified lesion (*), and (e) mixed plaque with fibrotic tissue, lipids (#) and calcium (mean luminal area of 1.49 mm^2).

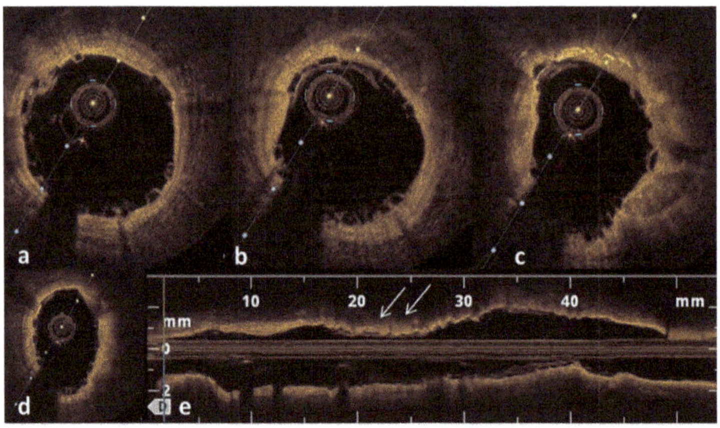

Figure 2.17. (a) Distal scaffold edge, no complications, (b) struts well apposed, over a calcific plaque, (c) and (d) underexpansion of the scaffold due to calcified lesions, and (e) long view showing evident underexpansion (white arrows).

OCT confirmed good scaffold expansion and apposition (figure 2.18). Angiographic follow-up attained 14 months later showed mild intra-scaffold hyperplasia, with no significant restenosis (figure 2.19).

2.5.4 Case 4—BRS in ST-elevation myocardial infarction and long-term evaluation by OCT

A female patient, 66 years of age, presented to a non-primary-PCI-capable center with typical angina symptoms. An anterior ST-elevation acute MI was diagnosed and thrombolytic therapy was administered, with signs of reperfusion. She was transferred to a PCI-capable center to perform coronary angiography which

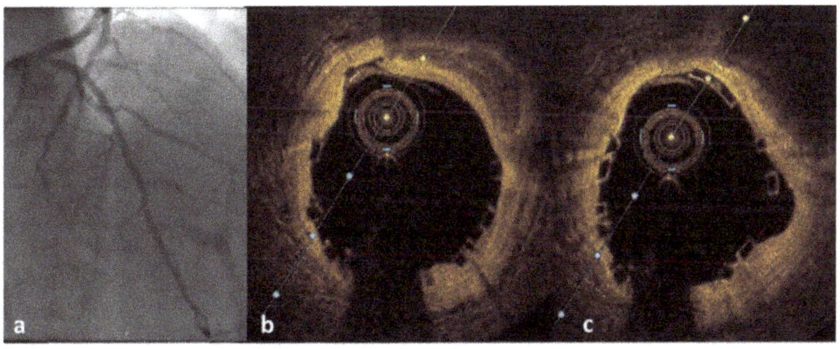

Figure 2.18. (a) Final LAD angiography, (b) and (c) struts well apposed and expanded over calcium.

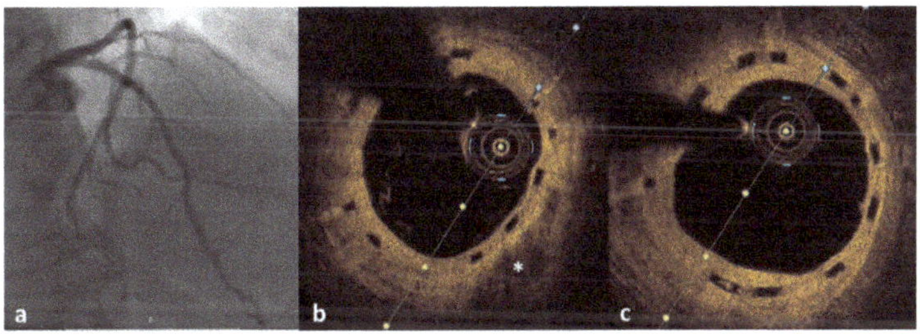

Figure 2.19. (a) LAD follow-up (14 months), (b) and (c) struts with neointimal coverage, 'black boxes' perfectly discernible, calcium (*) visible.

revealed an occluded mid LAD, next to the bifurcation with the first diagonal, and a 75% stenosis in the mid segment of the RCA. Complete revascularization was performed. The LAD and diagonal branch were wired, predilation of the LAD was accomplished with a 2.0/20 mm compliant balloon and a 3.0/28 mm BRS was implanted and postdilated with a 3.0/20 mm non-compliant balloon (figure 2.20). A DES was implanted in the RCA, and no complications were observed. Follow-up with angiography and OCT was performed 25 months later and revealed a patient artery with neointimal growth and a mild degree of neoatherosclerosis. At this time point, scaffold struts could still be identified, although their appearance corresponded mostly to remnants of struts covered by tissue and not exposed to bloodstream (figure 2.21). In the proximal segment, a 50% lesion (QCA) was identified and OCT revealed a mean lumen area of 1.79 mm^2. The patient was asymptomatic and, as such, evaluation with fractional flow reserve was performed and showed a value of 0.84 (figure 2.22).

2.5.5 Case 5—different devices for different lesions

The patient was a 48-year-old male with two-vessel coronary artery disease with repeated TVR. Different devices were implanted with different timings and in different clinical settings, according to lesion characteristics and location (figure 2.23).

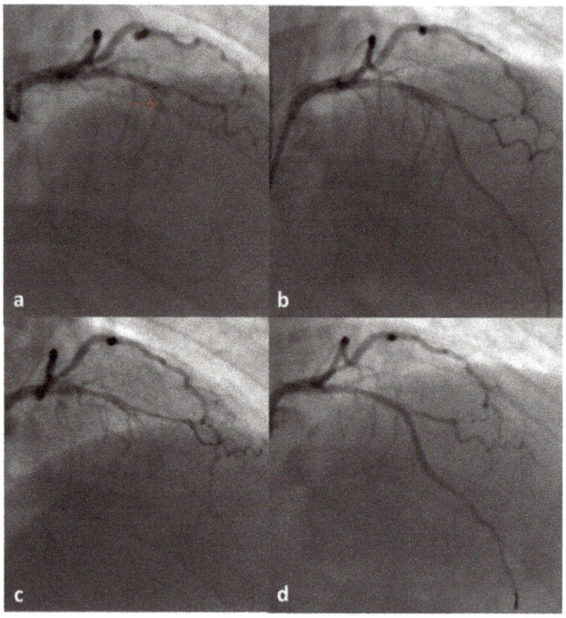

Figure 2.20. (a) LAD occlusion after the first diagonal (arrow), (b) vessel opening after predilation with a 2.0/20 mm compliant balloon, (c) BRS 3.0/28 mm and (d) final result.

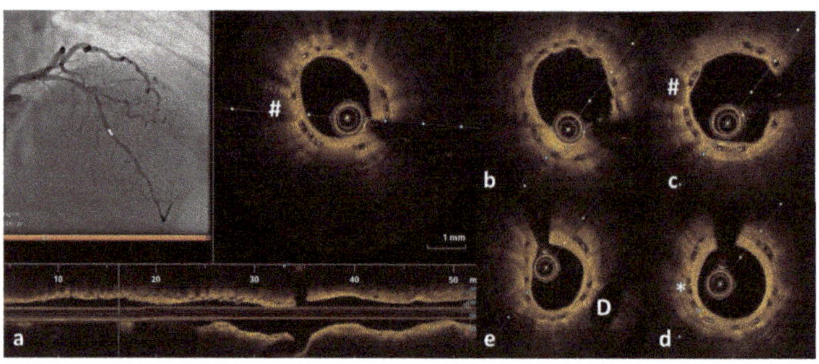

Figure 2.21. LAD OCT with angiographic co-registration, at 25 months of follow-up. (a) Visible struts/strut-like structures with neointimal coverage, (b) neoatherosclerosis, (c) visible strut free zones, and (d) and (e) proximal end of the scaffold. Calcium (*); lipid pool (#); diagonal branch (D).

2.6 Conclusions

Coronary artery lesions selected for percutaneous coronary intervention require more than just plain old balloon angioplasty in order to avoid complications and maintain long-term vessel patency. Drug-eluting stents are the current preferred strategy and have proved their efficacy in preventing stent restenosis. However, they are associated with a permanent caging of the vessel and long-term safety issues such

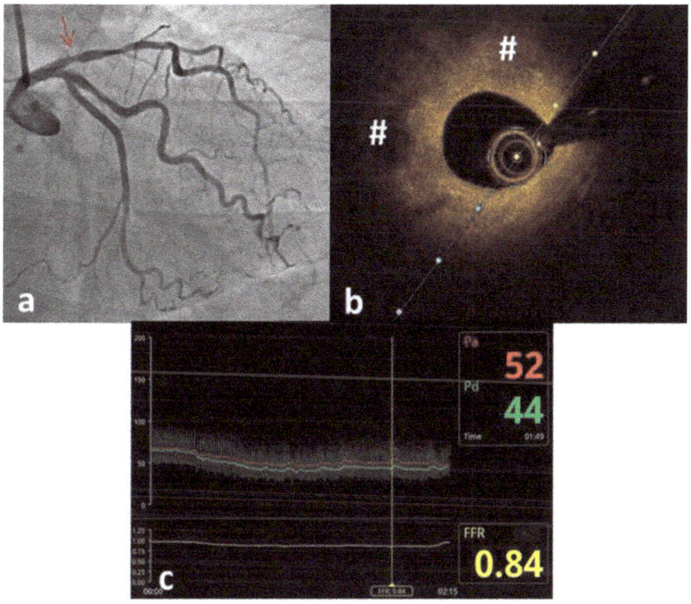

Figure 2.22. (a) LAD with a proximal 50% stenosis (QCA), (b) OCT evaluation showed a fibrolipid plaque with a mean lumen area of 1.79 mm^2 and (c) fractional flow reserve evaluation displayed a value of 0.84 (not significant). Lipid accumulation (#).

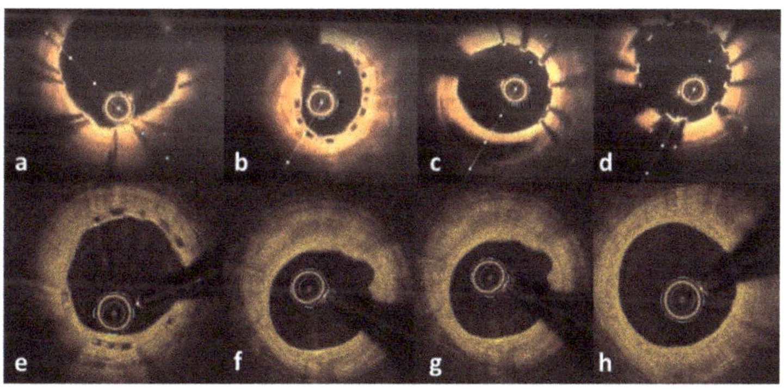

Figure 2.23. (a) DES implanted in proximal LAD, (b) 3-month-old Absorb, (c)–(d) newly implanted 3.0/25 mm Magmaris, (e) 15-month-old Absorb and (f)–(h) Magmaris after one year (shadowing is visible but struts are no longer discernible).

as late and very-late stent thrombosis. Bioresorbable platforms are a more recently developed technology that provide a transient scaffold for the coronary artery, with potential long-term benefits, namely the return of normal vascular function. Optical coherence tomography is an essential intravascular imaging method, giving insight into plaque morphology, optimal landing sites and the need for scaffold optimization.

References

[1] Morice M C *et al* 2002 A randomized comparison of a sirolimus-eluting stent with a standard stent for coronary revascularization *N. Engl. J. Med.* **346** 1773–80

[2] Stettler C *et al* 2007 Outcomes associated with drug-eluting and bare-metal stents: a collaborative network meta-analysis *Lancet* **370** 937–48

[3] Mintz G, Popma J, Pichard A, Kent K, Satler L, Wong C, Hong M, Kovach J and Leon M 1996 Arterial remodeling after coronary angioplasty: a serial intravascular ultrasound study *Circulation* **94** 35–43

[4] Joner M *et al* 2006 Pathology of drug-eluting stents in humans: delayed healing and late thrombotic risk *J. Am. Coll. Cardiol.* **48** 193–202

[5] Silva J, Carrillo X and Salvatella N 2011 Simultaneous two-vessel very-late stent thrombosis and coronary aneurysm formation after sirolimus eluting stent implantation: an intra-vascular ultrasound evaluation *J. Invas. Cardiol.* **23** E128–31

[6] Nakazawa G, Vorpahl M, Finn A V, Narula J and Virmani R 2009 One step forward and two steps back with drug-eluting-stents: from preventing restenosis to causing late thrombosis and nouveau atherosclerosis *JACC Cardiovasc. Imaging* **2** 625–8

[7] Stefanini G G, Taniwaki M and Windecker S 2014 Coronary stents: novel developments *Heart* **100** 1051–61

[8] Serruys P W, Garcia-Garcia H M and Onuma Y 2012 From metallic cages to transient bioresorbable scaffolds: change in paradigm of coronary revascularization in the upcoming decade? *Eur. Heart J.* **33** 16–25b

[9] Okamura T, Serruys P W and Regar E 2010 Cardiovascular flashlight. The fate of bioresorbable struts located at a side branch ostium: serial three-dimensional optical coherence tomography assessment *Eur. Heart J.* **31** 2179

[10] Hurst J W 1986 The first coronary angioplasty as described by Andreas Gruentzig *Am. J. Cardiol.* **57** 185–6

[11] Puel J, Joffre F, Rousseau H, Guermonprez B, Lancelin B, Valeix B, Imbert G and Bounhoure J P 1987 Endo-prothèses coronariennes autoexpansives dans la prévention des resténoses après angioplastie transluminale *Arch. Mal. Coeur.* **8** 1311–2

[12] Schatz R A, Palmaz J C, Tio F O, Garcia F, Garcia O and Reuter S R 1987 Balloon-expandable intracoronary stents in the adult dog *Circulation* **76** 450–7

[13] Serruys P W, de Jaegere P, Kiemeneij F, Macaya C, Rutsch W, Heyndrickx G, Emanuelsson H, Marco J, Legrand V and Materne P 1994 A comparison of balloon-expandable-stent implantation with balloon angioplasty in patients with coronary artery disease: Benestent Study Group *N. Engl. J. Med.* **331** 489–95

[14] van der Giessen W J, Lincoff A M, Schwartz R S, van Beusekom H M, Serruys P W, Holmes D R Jr, Ellis S G and Topol E J 1996 Marked inflammatory sequelae to implantation of biodegradable and nonbiodegradable polymers in porcine coronary arteries *Circulation* **94** 1690–7

[15] Oberhauser J P, Hossainy S and Rapoza R J 2009 Design principles and performance of bioresorbable polymeric vascular scaffolds *EuroIntervention* **5** F15–22

[16] Onuma Y and Serruys P W 2011 Bioresorbable scaffold: the advent of a new era in percutaneous coronary and peripheral revascularization? *Circulation* **123** 779–97

[17] Rapetto C and Leoncini M 2017 Magmaris: a new generation metallic sirolimus-eluting fully bioresorbable scaffold: present status and future perspectives *J. Thorac. Dis.* **9** S903–13

[18] Tamai H, Igaki K, Kyo E, Kosuga K, Kawashima A, Matsui S, Komori H, Tsuji T, Motohara S and Uehata H 2000 Initial and 6-month results of biodegradable poly-l-lactic acid coronary stents in humans *Circulation* **102** 399–404
[19] Tsuji T, Tamai H, Igaki K, Hsu Y-S, Kosuga K, Hata T, Okada M, Nakamura T and Fujita S 2004 Four-year follow-up of the biodegradable stent (Igaki–Tamai stent) *Circ. J.* **68** 135
[20] Nishio S 2010 Long-term (10 years) clinical outcomes of first-in-man biodegradable poly-l-lactic acid coronary stents *Eurointervenion* **6** H44
[21] Post M J, de Graaf-Bos A N, van Zanten H G, de Groot P G, Sixma J J and Borst C 1996 Thrombogenicity of the human arterial wall after interventional thermal injury *J. Vasc. Res.* **33** 156–63
[22] Otsuka F *et al* 2014 Long-term safety of an everolimus-eluting bioresorbable vascular scaffold and the cobalt chromium XIENCE V stent in a porcine coronary artery model *Circ. Cardiovasc. Interv.* **7** 330–42
[23] Serruys P W *et al* 2009 Absorb trial first-in-man evaluation of a bioabsorbable everolimus-eluting coronary stent system: two-year outcomes and results from multiple imaging modalities *Lancet* **373** 897–910
[24] Dudek D, Onuma Y, Ormiston J A, Thuesen L, Miquel-Hebert K and Serruys P W 2012 Four-year clinical follow-up of the ABSORB everolimus-eluting bioresorbable vascular scaffold in patients with *de novo* coronary artery disease: the ABSORB trial *EuroIntervention* **7** 1060–1
[25] Onuma Y, Dudek D, Thuesen L, Webster M, Nieman K, Garcia-Garcia H M, Ormiston J A and Serruys P W 2013 Five-year clinical and functional multislice computed tomography angiographic results after coronary implantation of the fully resorbable polymeric everolimus-eluting scaffold in patients with *de novo* coronary artery disease: the ABSORB cohort A trial *JACC Cardiovasc. Interv.* **6** 999–1009
[26] Diletti R *et al* 2013 Clinical and intravascular imaging outcomes at 1 and 2 years after implantation of absorb everolimus eluting bioresorbable vascular scaffolds in small vessels. Late lumen enlargement: does bioresorption matter with small vessel size? Insight from the ABSORB cohort B trial *Heart* **99** 98–105
[27] Serruys P W *et al* 2011 Evaluation of the second generation of a bioresorbable everolimus-eluting vascular scaffold for the treatment of *de novo* coronary artery stenosis: 12-month clinical and imaging outcomes *J. Am. Coll. Cardiol.* **58** 1578–88
[28] Abizaid A *et al* 2015 The ABSORB EXTEND study: preliminary report of the twelve-month clinical outcomes in the first 512 patients enrolled *EuroIntervention* **10** 1396–401
[29] Muramatsu T *et al* 2013 Incidence and short-term clinical outcomes of small side branch occlusion after implantation of an everolimus-eluting bioresorbable vascular scaffold: an interim report of 435 patients in the ABSORB-EXTEND single-arm trial in comparison with an everolimus-eluting metallic stent in the SPIRIT first and II trials *JACC Cardiovasc. Interv.* **6** 247–57
[30] Serruys P W *et al* 2015 A bioresorbable everolimus-eluting scaffold versus a metallic everolimus-eluting stent for ischaemic heart disease caused by *de-novo* native coronary artery lesions (ABSORB II): an interim 1-year analysis of clinical and procedural secondary outcomes from a randomised controlled trial *Lancet* **385** 43–54
[31] Diletti R *et al* 2012 ABSORB II randomized controlled trial: a clinical evaluation to compare the safety, efficacy, and performance of the Absorb everolimus-eluting bioresorbable vascular scaffold system against the XIENCE everolimus-eluting coronary stent system in

the treatment of subjects with ischemic heart disease caused by *de novo* native coronary artery lesions: rationale and study design *Am. Heart J.* **164** 654–63

[32] Chevalier B *et al* 2016 Randomised comparison of a bioresorbable everolimus-eluting scaffold with a metallic everolimus-eluting stent for ischaemic heart disease caused by de novo native coronary artery lesions: the 2-year clinical outcomes of the ABSORB II trial *EuroIntervention* **12** 1102–7

[33] Serruys P W *et al* 2016 Comparison of an everolimus-eluting bioresorbable scaffold with an everolimus-eluting metallic stent for the treatment of coronary artery stenosis (ABSORB II): a 3 year, randomised, controlled, single-blind, multicentre clinical trial *Lancet* **388** 2479–91

[34] Capodanno D *et al* 2015 Percutaneous coronary intervention with everolimus-eluting bioresorbable vascular scaffolds in routine clinical practice: early and midterm outcomes from the European multicentre GHOST-EU registry *EuroIntervention* **10** 1144–53

[35] Holmes D R Jr, Kereiakes D J, Garg S, Serruys P W, Dehmer G J, Ellis S G, Williams D O, Kimura T and Moliterno D J 2010 Stent thrombosis *J. Am. Coll. Cardiol.* **56** 1357–65

[36] Xu B *et al* 2017 Comparison of everolimus-eluting bioresorbable vascular scaffolds and metallic stents: three-year clinical outcomes from the ABSORB China randomised trial *EuroIntervention* pii: EIJ-D-17-00796

[37] Kereiakes D J *et al* 2017 ABSORB III investigators. 3-year clinical outcomes with everolimus-eluting bioresorbable coronary scaffolds: the ABSORB III trial *J. Am. Coll. Cardiol.* **70** 2852–62

[38] Onuma Y *et al* 2016 Two-year clinical, angiographic, and serial optical coherence tomographic follow-up after implantation of an everolimus-eluting bioresorbable scaffold and an everolimus-eluting metallic stent: insights from the randomised ABSORB Japan trial *EuroIntervention* **12** 1090–101

[39] Shah S R, Fatima M, Dharani A M, Shahnawaz W and Shah S A 2017 Bioresorbable vascular scaffold versus metallic stent in percutaneous coronary intervention: results of the AIDA trial *J. Community Hosp. Intern. Med. Perspect.* **7** 307–8

[40] Arroyo D *et al* 2017 Comparison of everolimus- and biolimus-eluting coronary stents with everolimus-eluting bioresorbable vascular scaffolds: two-year clinical outcomes of the EVERBIO II trial *Int. J. Cardiol.* **243** 121–5

[41] Katagiri Y *et al* 2018 Three-year follow-up of the randomized comparison between everolimus-eluting bioresorbable scaffold and durable polymer everolimus-eluting metallic stent in patients with ST-segment elevation myocardial infarction (TROFI II Trial) *EuroIntervention* **14** e1224–6

[42] Stone G W *et al* 2018 Blinded outcomes and angina assessment of coronary bioresorbable scaffolds: 30-day and 1-year results from the ABSORB IV randomised trial *Lancet* **392** 1530–40

[43] Dudek D *et al* 2014 Bioresorbable vascular scaffolds in patients with acute coronary syndromes: the POLAR ACS study *Pol. Arch. Med. Wewn.* **124** 669–77

[44] Brugaletta S *et al* 2015 Absorb bioresorbable vascular scaffold versus everolimus-eluting metallic stent in ST-segment elevation myocardial infarction: 1-year results of a propensity score matching comparison: the BVS-EXAMINATION Study (bioresorbable vascular scaffold—a clinical evaluation of everolimus eluting coronary stents in the treatment of patients with ST-segment elevation myocardial infarction) *JACC Cardiovasc. Interv.* **8** 189–97

[45] Kočka V, Malý M, Toušek P, Buděšínský T, Lisa L, Prodanov P, Jarkovský J and Widimský P 2014 Bioresorbable vascular scaffolds in acute ST-segment elevation myocardial infarction: a prospective multicentre study 'Prague 19' *Eur. Heart J.* **35** 787–94
[46] Vaquerizo B, Barros A, Pujadas S, Bajo E, Estrada D, Miranda-Guardiola F, Rigla J, Jiménez M, Cinca J and Serra A 2015 Bioresorbable everolimus-eluting vascular scaffold for the treatment of chronic total occlusions: CTO-ABSORB pilot study *EuroIntervention* **11** 555–63
[47] Goktekin O, Yamac A H, Latib A, Tastan A, Panoulas V F, Sato K, Erdogan E, Uyarel H, Shah I and Colombo A 2015 Evaluation of the safety of everolimus-eluting bioresorbable vascular scaffold (BVS) implantation in patients with chronic total coronary occlusions: acute procedural and short-term clinical results *J. Invasive Cardiol.* **27** 461–6
[48] Erbel R *et al* 2007 Temporary scaffolding of coronary arteries with bioabsorbable magnesium stents: a prospective, non-randomised multicentre trial *Lancet* **369** 1869–75
[49] Bringhurst F R, Demay M B, Krane S M and Kronenberg H M 2012 Bone and mineral metabolism in health and disease *Harrison's Principles of Internal Medicine* ed D L Longo, A S Fauci, D L Kasper, S L Hauser, J L Jameson and J Loscalzo 18th edn (New York: McGraw-Hill)
[50] Haude M *et al* 2013 Safety and performance of the drug-eluting absorbable metal scaffold (DREAMS) in patients with *de-novo* coronary lesions: 12 month results of the prospective, multicentre, first-in-man BIOSOLVE-I trial *Lancet* **381** 836–44
[51] Haude M *et al* 2016 Safety and performance of the second-generation drug-eluting absorbable metal scaffold in patients with *de-novo* coronary artery lesions (BIOSOLVE-II): 6 month results of a prospective, multicentre, non-randomised, first-in-man trial *Lancet* **387** 31–9
[52] Haude M *et al* 2018 Safety and clinical performance of a drug eluting absorbable metal scaffold in the treatment of subjects with *de novo* lesions in native coronary arteries: pooled 12-month outcomes of BIOSOLVE-II and BIOSOLVE-III *Catheter Cardiovasc. Interv.* **92** E502–11
[53] Stone G W *et al* 2016 1-year outcomes with the absorb bioresorbable scaffold in patients with coronary artery disease: a patient-level, pooled meta-analysis *Lancet* **387** 1277–89
[54] Lee M K-Y 2018 BIOSOLVE-IV: twelve-month outcomes with a resorbable magnesium scaffold in a real-world setting *TCT 2018*
[55] Verheye S *et al* 2014 A next-generation bioresorbable coronary scaffold system: from bench to first clinical evaluation: 6- and 12-month clinical and multimodality imaging results *JACC Cardiovasc. Interv.* **7** 89–99
[56] Grube E 2009 Bioabsorbable stent. The Boston Scientific and REVA technology *EuroPCR (Barcelona, Spain)*
[57] Anderson J, Abizaid A, Brachmann J, Dudek D, Frey N, Heigert M, Lutz M and Schmermund 2013 REVA RESTORE trial: interim 12-month clinical results of the ReZolve® bioresorbable scaffold and ReZolve2 clinical program update *EuroPCR (Paris, France)*
[58] Abizaid A 2018 New 24-month data from the FANTOM II clinical trial *EuroPCR 2018*
[59] Huang D *et al* 1991 Optical coherence tomography *Science* **254** 1178–81
[60] Prati F *et al* 2012 Angiography alone versus angiography plus optical coherence tomography to guide decision-making during percutaneous coronary intervention: the Centro per la Lotta contro l'Infarto-Optimisation of Percutaneous Coronary Intervention (CLI-OPCI) study *EuroIntervention* **8** 823–9

[61] Yabushita H *et al* 2002 Characterization of human atherosclerosis by optical coherence tomography *Circulation* **106** 1640–5
[62] Onuma Y, Serruys P W, Ormiston J A, Regar E, Webster M, Thuesen L, Dudek D, Veldhof S and Rapoza R 2010 Three-year results of clinical follow-up after a bioresorbable everolimus-eluting scaffold in patients with *de novo* coronary artery disease: the ABSORB trial *EuroIntervention* **6** 447–53
[63] Serruys P W *et al* 2014 Dynamics of vessel wall changes following the implantation of the absorb everolimus-eluting bioresorbable vascular scaffold: a multi-imaging modality study at 6, 12, 24 and 36 months *EuroIntervention* **9** 1271–84
[64] Allahwala U K, Cockburn J A, Shaw E, Figtree G A, Hansen P S and Bhindi R 2015 Clinical utility of optical coherence tomography (OCT) in the optimization of Absorb bioresorbable vascular scaffold deployment during percutaneous coronary intervention *EuroIntervention* **10** 1154–9
[65] Bourantas C V *et al* 2015 Bioresorbable vascular scaffold treatment induces the formation of neointimal cap that seals the underlying plaque without compromising the luminal dimensions: a concept based on serial optical coherence tomography data *EuroIntervention* **11** 746–56
[66] Nakatani S *et al* 2016 Comparative analysis method of permanent metallic stents (XIENCE) and bioresorbable poly-L-lactic (PLLA) scaffolds (Absorb) on optical coherence tomography at baseline and follow-up *EuroIntervention* **12** 1498–509
[67] Gomez-Lara J *et al* 2011 A comparative assessment by optical coherence tomography of the performance of the first and second generation of the everolimus-eluting bioresorbable vascular scaffolds *Eur. Heart J.* **32** 294–304
[68] Karjalainen P, Paana T, Sia J and Nammas W 2017 Neointimal healing evaluated by optical coherence tomography after drug-eluting absorbable metal scaffold implantation in *de novo* native coronary lesions: rationale and design of the Magmaris-OCT study *Cardiology* **137** 225–30
[69] Farooq V, Gogas B D and Serruys P W 2011 Restenosis: delineating the numerous causes of drug-eluting stent restenosis *Circ. Cardiovasc. Interv.* **4** 195–205

Section II

Computer modeling and computational fluid hemodynamics

IOP Publishing

Vascular and Intravascular Imaging Trends, Analysis, and Challenges, Volume 1
Stent applications
Petia Radeva and Jasjit S Suri

Chapter 3

Computer modeling of blood flow and plaque progression in the stented coronary artery

Nenad Filipovic

In this chapter, nonlinear stent deployment modeling with plaque formation and progression for specific patients in the coronary arteries is described. First, the introduction section describes the state-of-the-art in the reported investigations of blood flow in stented arteries. In the methods section, image segmentation methods for arteries with stents are briefly described. Blood flow simulation is described using Navier–Stokes and continuity equations. Blood vessel tissue is modeled with nonlinear viscoelastic material properties. The governing finite element (FE) equations used in modeling wall tissue deformation, with emphasis on the implementation of nonlinear constitutive models, are described. Continuum-based methods for modeling the evolution of plaque are derived. Low-density lipoprotein (LDL) penetration is defined by the convection–diffusion equation, while the endothelial permeability is shear stress dependent. The coupling of fluid dynamics and solute dynamics at the endothelium is achieved using the Kedem–Katchalsky equations. The inflammatory process is modeled using three additional reaction–diffusion partial differential equations. The coupled method is viewed as the motion of the collection of dissipative particle dynamics (DPD) particles inside a finite element mesh. The motion of each DPD particle is described by the corresponding Newton's law. In the results section, examples of rigid and deformable arterial walls with stented and unstented arteries are presented. Effective stress analysis results for stent deployment are shown. It can be seen that stents reduce wall shear stress significantly after deployment, which is caused by opening the artery and reducing the narrowing. Some results are presented for stent a deployment model obtained with a solver developed using the PAK software package.

From the results it may be seen that places marked as risky in the baseline showed varied progression after six months. At the end of the chapter, some results for stent deployment and plaque formation and development are discussed.

doi:10.1088/2053-2563/ab01fach3

3.1 Introduction

Coronary artery disease (CAD) is the leading cause of death worldwide; it is on the rise and has become a true pandemic that respects no borders [1]. CAD has reached enormous proportions striking more and more at younger subjects. It is expected that in coming years CAD linked with atherosclerosis will become the greatest epidemic of mankind. Atherosclerosis involves the gradual development of fatty streaks in arterial walls into atheroma and characteristic plaques. The acute rupture of these atheromatous plaques causes local thrombosis, leading to partial or total occlusion of the affected artery. The clinical consequences of these plaques depend on their site and the degree and speed of vessel occlusion [2]. For atherosclerosis, a major clinical manifestation is ischemic heart disease (IHD). IHD is a major cause of morbidity and mortality; in the UK alone, annual deaths number at 123 000 [3]. The associated direct and indirect costs of IHD are a major cost for healthcare systems. Among the available treatment techniques are percutaneous invasive interventions (PCIs), including percutaneous transluminal coronary angioplasty and stent implantation. In the last decade there has been a steady and significant increase in the rate of stent implantation for IHD.

The advent of coronary stents resulted in a dramatic reduction in procedure-related complications, such as acute closure, and markedly improved long-term outcomes. The development of bare-metal stents (BMSs) was a major advance relative to balloon angioplasty in the management of symptomatic coronary artery disease. Coronary stents have ultimately been the preferred method of performing PCI, replacing unstented balloon angioplasty, due to the observed improvements in angiographic and clinical outcomes [4, 5]. Nowadays, the majority of PCI procedures include the utilization of a coronary stent, and interventional cardiologists are faced with a wide spectrum of coronary stents. This spectrum starts with the conventional BMSs and drug-eluting stents (DESs), which are widely used in clinical practice, followed by newer stents, such as DESs with biodegradable polymers, polymer-free DESs, DESs with novel coatings, and bioresorbable vascular scaffolds (BVS) stents [6–10]. As the advantages of stent implantation saw its evolution from a 'bail out' to a standard treatment strategy [11], three important limitations have been recognized: (i) in-stent restenosis (ISR), (ii) stent thrombosis (ST) and (iii) stent failure.

To reduce or remove obstructions inside arteries, such as plaque formations, which block normal blood flow and reduce oxygen supply to vital organs, angioplasty and stents were introduced to dilate the area of arterial blockage. The plaque is squeezed along the artery wall with the inflation of the balloon and the stent is implanted around the diameter of the artery. Stents can reduce the restenosis rate to 20%–30% compared to balloon angioplasty [12]. Nowadays, coating stents with antiproliferative drugs seems to work well for patients, since the restenosis rate decreases by 85% or more [13]. These drugs act by inhibiting neointimal proliferation. However, the drug can be delivered to the tissue only for a specific period of time, hence the long-term clinical outcome of such stents is still unknown.

While an implanted stent effectively enables a widening of the stenosed part of the blood vessel, it causes local injury to the vascular endothelium and also affects local hemodynamics in a manner conducive to growth of new tissue, which is termed neointimal hyperplasia (NI), and subsequent restenosis [14, 15]. Recent evidence indicates that alterations in wall shear stress (WSS) distributions after stent implantation may represent an important contributing factor in the process of restenosis. Restenosis is the excessive growth of new tissue in the stented segment which can re-block the artery. The success of the stenting procedure depends on the severity of the restenosis. Neointimal hyperplasia has been shown to be dependent on several factors including arterial injury, areas of flow-induced low WSS less than 0.5 N m^2, areas of flow-induced high wall shear stress gradients (WSSG) higher than 200 N m^3, as well as other patient-specific medical factors such as diabetes mellitus [16, 17]. Non-uniform WSS within an arterial segment also affects the establishment of cell density gradients, gene expression, migration and proliferation after vascular injury [18].

The wall injury deriving from stent implantation results in the exposure of underlying atheromatous tissue and the elution of macromolecules. These macrophages transmigrate into the vascular wall and release further cytokines, metalloproteinase and growth factors, which in turn play a significant role in the initiation of the restenosis process. With the increased risk of restenosis being in the range of 20%–30% [19], DESs have been designed to release pharmacological agents after deployment to inhibit the response to injury. As a consequence, DESs have significantly reduced the risk of coronary ISR and the necessity for target lesion revascularization, however, current rates of ISR in clinical practice are high, reaching 10% [20].

ST is characterized by angiographic or post-mortem evidence of a recently formed thrombus in a previously stented segment. ST presents as a mix of thrombotic and inflammatory components including platelet-rich thrombus, fibrin fragments, and leukocytes of both the neutrophil and eosinophil lineages, and can be classified as thrombosis within the first 30 days; late ST is thrombosis occurring beyond 30 days. Early ST is more common than late, accounting for ~50%–70% of all cases, depending on the overall time frame of reference [21]. The risk factors for ST can be classified as patient-, procedure-, or device-specific. Specifically, in early ST among the key factors are those related to the process of stent implantation: stent undersizing, the presence of residual dissection, impaired thrombolysis in myocardial infarction flow, and residual disease proximal or distal to the stented artery. In addition, stent device-specific factors play a significant role in the risk of early ST. ST is a devastating complication that results in high morbidity and mortality in patients who have undergone stent implantation [22]. In-hospital mortalities have been reported to be as high as 7.9% for acute ST (occurring <24 h after stent implantation) and subacute ST (SAST; occurring within 30 days after stent implantation), 3.8% for late ST (occurring within the first year) and 3.6% for very late ST, occurring more than 1 year after stent implantation [23]. The development of a thrombus inside a previously implanted stent can be affected by the geometry, materials and coatings. Optical coherence tomography (OCT) data from patients that had undergone stenting showed that thin-strut DESs were associated with improved rates of stent strut coverage compared to thick-strut DESs at 6–8 months follow-up [24]. The biodegradable polymer-coated stents enhance biocompatibility and permit a more physiological vascular healing response after stenting. These stents have bio-absorbable polymers which dissolve within a specified time period, with a residual metal scaffolding that achieves a similar safety profile to BMSs.

Computational fluid dynamics (CFD) techniques have the advantages of greater flexibility and ease of use with respect to experimental or *in vivo* methods. They can provide detailed information on critical local flow parameters near the stent struts and the arterial wall which are not accessible in biological flows. However, modeling often has its own limitations in the form of simplifications to the real problem.

Many computational studies in the literature have dealt with the influence of stent physical parameters on fluid dynamical changes correlated with the restenosis process [25–30]. The stent strut spacing and thickness and number of struts were found to influence the distribution of low and high shear stress values. However, the unrealistic assumption in the computational models that the stented artery is a simple cylindrical, rigid tube or even flat plane is implicit to most of these investigations. In reality, the coronary vasculature within which stents are commonly deployed exhibits a highly complex geometry with extensive curvature. This vessel curvature can have a significant effect on the skewness of the velocity profile and the general behavior of the flow in the stented segment.

A variety of studies was performed to compare steady-state versus pulsatile flow simulations and investigated the effect of non-Newtonian blood properties on the resulting flow parameters. The pulsatile flow simulations showed in one investigation that the flow separation zones in the region between the stent wires also periodically increase and decrease in size. These results suggest that in pulsatile flow, the character of stent induced flow disturbance is highly dynamic. Some analyses revealed that while the non-Newtonian properties have a very limited impact on the global characteristics of the flow field, they do lead to a modest reduction in the size of the flow separation zone downstream of the stent [30–33].

Failure to deploy a coronary stent not only results in wasted expenditure but also in inadequate myocardial revascularization, which may lead to increased morbidity and mortality rates and the need for additional revascularization procedures [34, 35]. The identification and the analysis of the underlying mechanisms related to stent fracture would allow for more precise delineation of rates of fracture, more focused evaluation and assessment of secondary intervention and allow for primary interventions to minimize and reduce the occurrence of clinically significant outcomes associated with stent fracture [36]. In the last 20 years, stenting has been among the most evolving operative techniques. The introduction of various generations of stents will dramatically improve the outcome of this intervention, however, much effort should be made to reduce the risk of ISR and ST.

The stent biomedical industry and development pipelines for drug-eluting BVSs present significant differences depending on the type of stent (design, material, drug coating, etc), but have the same essential components and serve the same need—to design and develop a medical device which will improve the outcomes for the patient's health, minimize the presence of side effects, have low development costs and achieve a shorter time for being introduced onto the market. Currently, the stent biomedical industry for drug-eluting BVSs includes the following phases: (i) pre-clinical assessment, (ii) clinical assessment for efficacy and (iii) post-market analysis. In the design phase, computer-aided engineering technologies are used, enabling the development of refined biomechanical stent simulations which are sometimes used in pre-clinical assessment. However, the different aspects of stent performance, including the mechanical, deployment, drug-delivery and degradation aspects, have not been studied.

In general, healthcare is based upon a 'one-size-fits-all' approach. However, every patient is different, presenting a different type and progress of atherosclerosis, comorbidities and lifestyle. Current clinical trial designs essentially do not take into account this complexity, with the heterogeneity of the patients in a trial translating in a similar heterogeneity of responses to drug-eluting BVS implantation, forcing in this way doctors to gamble with their patients' health. Due to the differences in patients' arterial cardiovascular physiology and other patient-specific factors, some patients are expected to improve, but some might even become worse due to a scaffold badly fitted to their biological make-up. Patients are provided with drug-delivery BVSs that have been found statistically to be the best option for a similar group of patients. However, this approach does not always mean the majority of patients will recover after this implantation. It is expected that a fraction will respond positively, while others may actually present adverse outcomes effects (ISR, ST) or might even die.

In summary, there are strong limitations to the reported investigations of blood flow in stented arteries, mainly with respect to an idealized geometry of the artery and stent. To the best of the authors' knowledge, no study so far has reported a universally applicable method to perform a blood flow analysis in a patient-specific artery where a stenting intervention to widen the stenosed part of the artery was performed.

3.2 Methods

3.2.1 Geometrical stent modeling

A qualitative description of the integrated bio-anatomical patient-specific model parts which are integrated in ARTool from the ARTreat project (www.artreat.org, www.artreat.kg.ac.rs) is presented in this section.

The clinical user must be able to predict the post-interventional artery shape and possible damage to the endothelium, as well as the effects of the stenting on the vessel wall, the blood flow characteristics and the biological response. To enable such complex predictions, a simulation of the stenting procedure as an integral part of the Patient Specific 3D Modeller consists of the following steps: extracting the region of interest of the stenosed artery segment including plaque identification, the generation of a stent model from CAD data or geometry description, virtual placement/delivery of the stent and balloon into the selected artery segment, simulation of the physical deployment of the stent, generation of a resulting geometry of the stented artery including stent details and output to the blood flow module.

Consequently, a method was developed which enables a virtual stenting intervention in a patient-specific, stenosed artery. To accomplish the simulation of this highly complex physical problem, all system components of this stenting procedure are included, namely the stenosed artery, the stent and the balloon to inflate the stent. These parts have been modeled with different complexity and assumptions.

Voros *et al* [37] presented a study for the evaluation of 3D quantitative measurements of coronary plaque by computed tomography coronary angiography (CTCA) against intravascular ultrasound (IVUS). Another similar approach was introduced by Graaf *et al* [38]. A semi-automated methodology for 3D reconstruction of arteries and their plaque morphology using CTCA was presented by Athanasiou *et al* [39], showing that CTCA can be used for the accurate assessment and reconstruction of coronary arteries. Our method is able to accurately reconstruct a part of the arterial tree including the lumen and outer wall calcified and non-calcified plaques.

The 3D reconstruction and plaque characterization tool will enable the 3D reconstruction of a vessel based on IVUS/OCT and angiography or CT. Fusion of angiography and IVUS as well as OCT is a well-established technique. Bourantas *et al* [40] developed an automated user-friendly system (ANGIOCARE), for rapid 3D coronary reconstruction, integrating angiographic and IVUS data. ANGIOCARE incorporates the method by Plissiti *et al* [41–43] for border extraction. 3D reconstruction and plaque characterization tools will extend this method to also incorporate the reconstruction of plaque lesions that are significant for accurate virtual stent deployment simulation.

The 3D reconstruction and plaque characterization tool will allow the semi-automatic stent reconstruction and evaluation of stent deployment. Deployment evaluation is well established for IVUS and OCT [44, 45] and will be included in the main functionalities of the 3D reconstruction and plaque characterization tool. The 3D reconstruction and plaque characterization tool provides the ability to automatically detect stent struts from OCT or IVUS modalities. Wang *et al* [46–48] presented a robust algorithm to process an entire IVOCT pullback run, which requires neither *a priori* status information, nor lumen or vessel wall contours. Accurate strut detection is the main requirement for extracting stent deployment quantitative measurements. For stent deployment analysis with computed tomography angiography (CTA) imaging studies, the methodology presented for CTA reconstruction by Athanasiou *et al* [49] will be adapted. Our method extracts the interface of the stent (figure 3.1) that will be used to extract the corresponding measures. Moreover, using the stent profile, ISR can be also evaluated.

The 3D reconstruction and plaque characterization tool will also be used to detect scaffold fracture (SF). According to Nakazawa [47] there are five types of SF. The identification of types I and II is rather difficult [48] using any modality. Our method is focused on the semi-automatic detection of type III, IV and V SFs. The method will use the scaffold profiling method and strut detection in order to identify measures indicative of SF. Those measures include the distance between neighboring

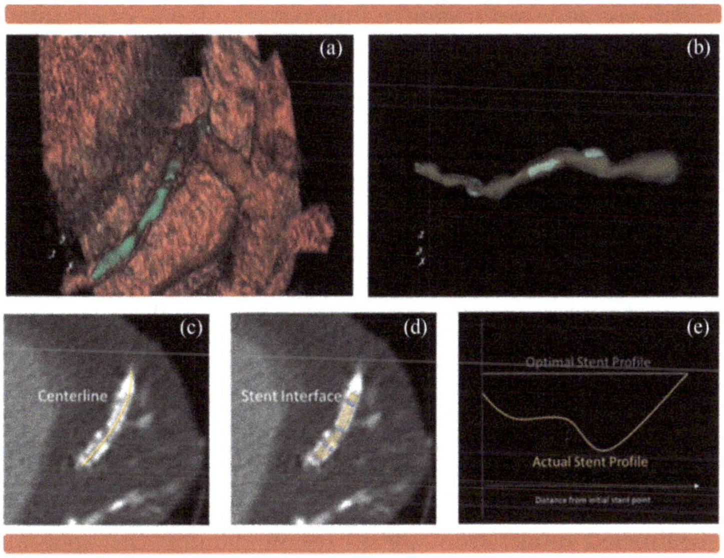

Figure 3.1. (a) Volume rendering of the heart with the vessel (green) superimposed. (b) The 3D vessel with lumen (red), outer wall (green) and calcified plaques (white). (c) Initial stent centerline. (d) Stent interface extraction. (e) Stent profile extraction.

struts, abrupt changes in scaffold centerline and other measures to estimate the probability of different SF types.

Currently, imaging studies (CCTA, IVUS, OCT and angiography) of the same patient, acquired at the same or two separate times, are interpreted separately. Our method will provide the tools to semi-automatically co-register imaging studies from the same or different modalities.

In the CT case, the comparison of two studies is typically performed by individual multiplanar orientation and/or curvilinear displays. This process is time consuming and it is difficult to ensure that identical views of the artery are presented to the clinician in both scans. The 3D reconstruction and plaque characterization tool will provide the ability to co-register two different studies from the same patient. The goal of CT co-registration is to estimate the transformation that aligns coronary arteries in 3D space. The registration tool will rely on the two-step procedure described by Woo *et al* [49] including: (i) a rigid co-registration based on a pre-segmented binary mask and (ii) a final nonlinear co-registration that accounts for local vessel deformation after histogram matching of the intensity distribution in the two scans.

The 3D reconstruction and plaque characterization tool will provide the ability to co-register CT with IVUS or OCT imaging studies. In the literature, CT and IVUS registration has been used in several studies for comparison of atherosclerosis and evaluation of 3D reconstruction. The algorithm for CT and IVUS/OCT co-registration relies on the method presented by Marquering *et al* [50] and has the same principles as the method followed by Athanasiou *et al* [40]. Briefly, the method registers specific vessel segments by initially identifying the vessel segment on both modalities and performing a transversal global orientation based on landmarks (calcifications, side branches and bifurcations). Finally, the registration of the individual cross-sectional slices will be performed.

As a result of a virtual stenting intervention, the clinician is not only provided with comprehensible animations and graphical outputs showing the process and final state of the implanted device, but with a number of indicators which allow a judgment on the performance of the selected stent and of its interactions with the specific artery. Such indicators include the inflation pressure–lumen area relationship, the final dilation of the artery, stress and strain distributions not only for the stent but also for the artery, and the contact stress between the stent struts and vessel wall. These output values also provide clear markers for the assessment of arterial injury sustained during intervention (figure 3.2).

3.2.2 Blood flow simulation

In general, the sequence used to perform blood flow simulations is the acquisition of the 3D reconstructed model from the image modalities, the application of the appropriate input data and, finally, the acquisition of the desired output. Blood flow simulations are performed in three different categories of arteries: (a) in unstented

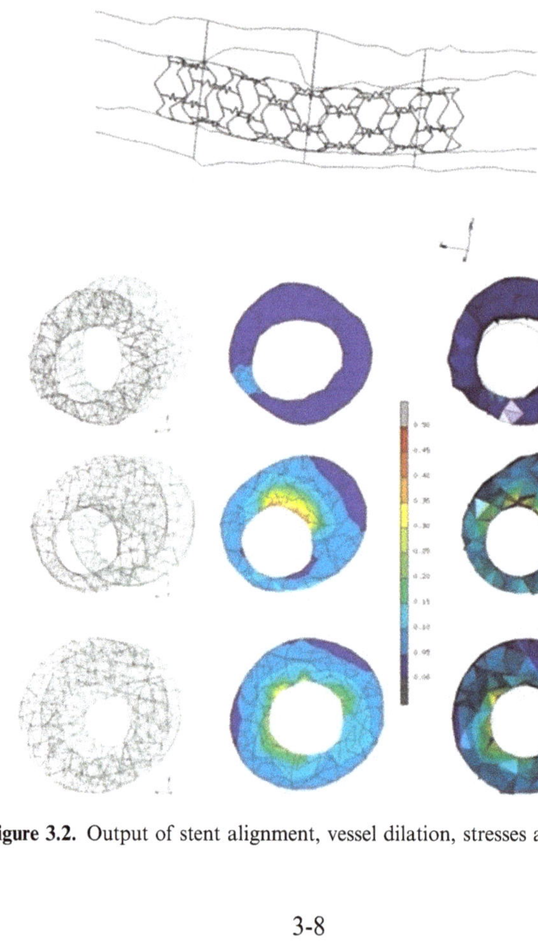

Figure 3.2. Output of stent alignment, vessel dilation, stresses and strains.

arteries assuming the walls to be rigid, (b) in unstented arteries with deformable walls and (c) in stented arteries with rigid walls.

The blood can be considered as an incompressible homogeneous viscous fluid for flow in large blood vessels. Also, laminar flow is dominant in physiological flow environments. Therefore, the fundamental laws of physics which include the balance of mass and balance of linear momentum are applicable here. These laws are expressed by the continuity equation and the Navier–Stokes equations.

Here we present the final form of these equations to emphasize some specifics related to blood flow. The incremental-iterative balance equation of a finite element for a time step n and equilibrium iteration i has the form

$$\begin{bmatrix} \frac{1}{\Delta t}\mathbf{M} + {}^{n+1}\widetilde{\mathbf{K}}_{vv}^{(i-1)} & \mathbf{K}_{vp} \\ \mathbf{K}_{vp}^{T} & \mathbf{0} \end{bmatrix} \begin{Bmatrix} \Delta\mathbf{V}^{(i)} \\ \Delta\mathbf{P}^{(i)} \end{Bmatrix}_{\text{blood}} = \begin{Bmatrix} {}^{n+1}\mathbf{F}_{\text{ext}}^{(i-1)} \\ 0 \end{Bmatrix} - \begin{bmatrix} \frac{1}{\Delta t}\mathbf{M} + {}^{n+1}\mathbf{K}^{(i-1)} & \mathbf{K}_{vp} \\ \mathbf{K}_{vp}^{T} & 0 \end{bmatrix} \begin{Bmatrix} {}^{n+1}\mathbf{V}^{(i-1)} \\ {}^{n+1}\mathbf{P}^{(i-1)} \end{Bmatrix} + \begin{Bmatrix} \frac{1}{\Delta t}\mathbf{M}^{n}\mathbf{V} \\ 0 \end{Bmatrix}, \tag{3.1}$$

where ${}^{n+1}\mathbf{V}^{(i-1)}$ ${}^{n+1}\mathbf{P}^{(i-1)}$ are the nodal vectors of blood velocity and pressure, with the increments in time step $\Delta\mathbf{V}^{(i)}$ and $\Delta\mathbf{P}^{(i)}$ (the index 'blood' is used to emphasize that we are considering blood as the fluid); Δt is the time step size, and the left upper indices n and $n+1$ denote the start and end of the time step; the matrices and vectors are defined in [51]. Note that the vector ${}^{n+1}\mathbf{F}_{\text{ext}}^{(i-1)}$ of external forces includes the volumetric and surface forces. In the assembling of these equations, the system of equations of the form (3.1) is obtained, with the volumetric external forces and the surface forces acting only on the fluid domain boundary (the surface forces among the internal element boundaries cancel).

The specifics for the blood flow are that the matrix ${}^{n+1}\mathbf{K}^{(i-1)}$ may include variability of the viscosity if non-Newtonian behavior of blood is considered. We have that

$$[K_{KJ}^{(i-1)}]_{mk} = \left[\hat{K}_{KJ}^{(i-1)}\right]_{mk} + \int_{V} \mu^{(i-1)} N_{K,j} N_{J,j} dV, \tag{3.2}$$

where $\mu^{(i-1)}$ corresponds to the constitutive law for the last known conditions (at iteration $i-1$). In the case of using the Cason relation (3.2), the second invariant of the strain rate $D_{\text{II}}^{(i-1)}$ is to be evaluated when computing $\mu^{(i-1)}$.

We note here that the penalty method can also be used, as well as the ALE formulation in the case of large displacements of blood vessel walls [52].

In addition to the velocity and pressure fields of the blood, the distribution of stresses within the blood can be evaluated. The stresses ${}^{t}\sigma_{ij}$ at time t follow from

$${}^{t}\sigma_{ij} = -{}^{t}p\delta_{ij} + {}^{t}\sigma_{ij}^{\mu}, \tag{3.3}$$

where

$${}^{t}\sigma_{ij}^{\mu} = {}^{t}\mu\ {}^{t}(v_{i,j} + v_{j,i}) \tag{3.4}$$

is the viscous stress. Here, ${}^t\mu$ is the viscosity corresponding to the velocity vector ${}^t\mathbf{v}$ at a spatial point within the blood domain. The field of the viscous stresses is given by equation (3.4).

Further, the wall shear stress at the blood vessel wall is calculated as

$$ {}^t\tau = {}^t\mu \frac{\partial\, {}^t v_t}{\partial n}, \tag{3.5} $$

where ${}^t v_t$ denotes the tangential velocity and n is the normal direction at the vessel wall. Practically, we first calculate the tangential velocity at the integration points near the wall surface, and then numerically evaluate the velocity gradient $\partial {}^t v_t / \partial n$; finally, we determine the viscosity coefficient ${}^t\mu$ using the average velocity at these integration points. In essence, the wall shear stress is proportional to the shear rate γ at the wall and the blood dynamic viscosity μ.

For a pulsatile flow the mean wall shear stress within a time interval T can be calculated as [53]

$$ {}^T\tau_{\text{mean}} = \left| \frac{1}{T} \int_0^T {}^t\tau_n dt \right|. \tag{3.6} $$

Another scalar quantity is a time-averaged magnitude of the surface traction vector, calculated as

$$ {}^T\tau_{\text{mag}} = \frac{1}{T} \int_0^T |{}^t\mathbf{t}| dt, \tag{3.7} $$

where the vector ${}^t\mathbf{t}$ is given by the Cauchy formula.

3.2.3 Modeling the deformation of blood vessels

Blood vessel tissue has complex mechanical characteristics. The tissue can be modeled by using various material models, from linear elastic to nonlinear viscoelastic. We here summarize the governing finite element equations used in modeling wall tissue deformation with emphasis on implementation of nonlinear constitutive models.

The finite element equation of balance of linear momentum is derived from the fundamental differential equations of balance of forces acting at an elementary material volume. In dynamic analysis we include the inertial forces in this equation. Then, by applying the principle of virtual work

$$ \mathbf{M}\ddot{\mathbf{U}} + \mathbf{B}^w \dot{\mathbf{U}} + \mathbf{K}\mathbf{U} = \mathbf{F}^{\text{ext}}. \tag{3.8} $$

Here the element matrices are as follows: $\mathbf{M}$ is mass matrix; $\mathbf{B}^w$ is the damping matrix, in the case when the material has a viscous resistance; $\mathbf{K}$ is the stiffness matrix; and $\mathbf{F}^{\text{ext}}$ is the external nodal force vector which includes the body and surface forces acting on the element. By the standard assembling procedure, the dynamic differential equations of motion are obtained. These differential equations can further be integrated in the way described, with a selected time step size Δt.

The nodal displacements ${}^{n+1}\mathbf{U}$ at the end of the time step are finally obtained according to

$$\hat{\mathbf{K}}_{\text{tissue}}{}^{n+1}\mathbf{U} = {}^{n+1}\hat{\mathbf{F}}, \tag{3.9}$$

where the tissue stiffness matrix $\hat{\mathbf{K}}_{\text{tissue}}$ and vector ${}^{n+1}\hat{\mathbf{F}}$ are expressed in terms of the matrices and vector in equation (3.8). Note that this equation is obtained under the assumption that the problem is linear: displacements are small, the viscous resistance is constant and the material is linear elastic.

In many circumstances of blood flow the wall displacements can be large, as in the case of aneurysm of the heart, hence the problem becomes geometrically nonlinear. Also, the tissues of blood vessels have nonlinear constitutive laws, leading to a materially nonlinear FE formulation. Therefore, the approximations adopted to obtain equation (3.9) may not be appropriate. For a nonlinear problem, instead of equation (3.9) we have the incremental-iterative equation

$${}^{n+1}\hat{\mathbf{K}}^{(i-1)}_{\text{tissue}}\,\Delta\mathbf{U}^{(i)} = {}^{n+1}\hat{\mathbf{F}}_{(i-1)} - {}^{n+1}\mathbf{F}^{\text{int}(i-1)}, \tag{3.10}$$

where $\Delta\mathbf{U}^{(i)}$ are the nodal displacement increments for the iteration i, and the system matrix ${}^{n+1}\hat{\mathbf{K}}^{(i-1)}_{\text{tissue}}$, the force vector ${}^{n+1}\hat{\mathbf{F}}_{(i-1)}$ and the vector of internal forces ${}^{n+1}\mathbf{F}^{\text{int}(i-1)}$ correspond to the previous iteration.

Here we emphasize the material nonlinearity of blood vessels, which is used in further applications. As presented, the geometrically linear part of the stiffness matrix, $({}^{n+1}\mathbf{K}_L)^{(i-1)}_{\text{tissue}}$, and nodal force vector, ${}^{n+1}\mathbf{F}^{\text{int}(i-1)}$, are defined in

$$({}^{n+1}\mathbf{K}_L)^{(i-1)}_{\text{tissue}} = \int_V \mathbf{B}_L^T\,{}^{n+1}\mathbf{C}^{(i-1)}_{\text{tissue}}\mathbf{B}_L dV,\ ({}^{n+1}\mathbf{F}^{\text{int}})^{(i-1)} = \int_V \mathbf{B}_L^T\,{}^{n+1}\boldsymbol{\sigma}^{(i-1)} dV, \tag{3.11}$$

where the consistent tangent constitutive matrix ${}^{n+1}\mathbf{C}^{(i-1)}_{\text{tissue}}$ of tissue and the stresses at the end of time step ${}^{n+1}\boldsymbol{\sigma}^{(i-1)}$ depend on the material model used. Calculation of the matrix ${}^{n+1}\mathbf{C}^{(i-1)}_{\text{tissue}}$ and the stresses ${}^{n+1}\boldsymbol{\sigma}^{(i-1)}$ for the tissue material models are used in further applications. In each of the subsequent sections we will give the basic data about the models used in the analysis.

3.2.4 Plaque formation and progression modeling—continuum approach

Continuum-based methods are an efficient way to model the evolution of plaque. In our model, LDL concentration is first introduced into the system of partial differential equations as a boundary condition. The model simulates the inflammatory response formed at the initial stages of plaque formation.

Regarding the particle dynamics, the model is based on the involvement of LDL/oxidized LDL, monocytes and macrophages, and foam cells and extracellular matrix. Reaction–diffusion differential equations are used to model these particle dynamics. The adhesion rate of the molecules depends on the local hemodynamics, which is described by solving the Navier–Stokes equations. Intima LDL concentration is a function of the wall shear stress, while the adhesion of monocytes is a function of shear stress and VCAM. Finally, the alterations of the arterial wall are simulated. A finite element solver is used to solve the system of the equations. The lumen is defined as a 2D domain while the intima is simplified as 1D model due to its thin geometry. First, the LDL penetration to the arterial wall as well as the wall shear stress is calculated. Then the concentration of the various components of the model is calculated in order to simulate the intima fattening in the final step.

The LDL penetration is defined by the convection–diffusion equation, while the endothelial permeability is shear stress dependent. This model produces results about the initial stages of the atherosclerotic plaque formation. More specifically, concentration of LDL is calculated on the artery wall and in the next step the oxidized LDL. Furthermore, monocytes and their modified form (macrophages) are also counted. The solution to the system provides the user with the concentration of foam cells created when a threshold LDL concentration is reached.

The previous model describes the initial stages of atherosclerosis. However, atherosclerosis is characterized by the proliferation of smooth muscle cells (SMCs). A medical user needs a prediction for plaque formation, which is based on the concentration of SMCs, the necrotic core and the extracellular matrix. In this respect a new approach to count the concentration of SMCs is being developed. The user is also provided with results regarding the formation of plaque in an overall manner.

The fluid is assumed to be steady, incompressible and laminar. For modeling fluid dynamics in the lumen, the following Navier–Stokes equations are used:

$$-\mu\nabla^2 u_l + \rho(u_l \cdot \nabla)u_l + \nabla p_l = 0 \tag{3.12}$$

$$\nabla u_l = 0, \tag{3.13}$$

where u_l is blood velocity, p_l is pressure, μ is blood dynamic viscosity and ρ is blood density.

Darcy's law were used to model mass transfer across the wall (transmural flow) of the blood vessel:

$$u_w - \nabla\left(\frac{k}{\mu_p} p_w\right) = 0 \tag{3.14}$$

$$\nabla u_w = 0, \tag{3.15}$$

where u_w is transmural velocity, p_w pressure in the arterial wall, μ_p is the viscosity of the blood plasma and k is the Darcian permeability coefficient of the arterial wall (3.14) and (3.15). Convective diffusion equations are used for modeling mass transfer in the lumen:

$$\nabla \cdot (-D_l \nabla c_l + c_l u_l) = 0, \tag{3.16}$$

where c_l represents the blood concentration in the lumen and D_l is the diffusion coefficient of the lumen.

The following convective diffusion reactive equation is used for modeling mass transfer in the wall, related to transmural flow:

$$\nabla \cdot (-D_w \nabla c_w + K c_w u_w) = r_w c_w, \tag{3.17}$$

where c_w is the solute concentration in the arterial wall, D_w is the diffusive coefficient of solution in the wall, K is the solute lag coefficient and r_w is the consumption rate constant.

The coupling of fluid dynamics and solute dynamics at the endothelium was achieved by the Kedem–Katchalsky equations:

$$J_v = L_p(\Delta p - \delta_d \Delta \pi) \tag{3.18}$$

$$J_s = P\Delta c + (1 - \delta_f) J_v \bar{c}, \tag{3.19}$$

where L_p is the hydraulic conductivity of the endothelium, Δc is the solute concentration difference across the endothelium, Δp is the pressure drop across the endothelium, $\Delta \pi$ is the oncotic pressure difference across the endothelium, σ_d is the osmotic reflection coefficient, σ_f is the solvent reflection coefficient, P is the solute endothelial permeability and $\bar{c}$ is the mean endothelial concentration [54].

The inflammatory process is modeled using three additional reaction–diffusion partial differential equations [55]:

$$\begin{aligned} \partial_t O &= d_1 \Delta O - k_1 O \cdot M \\ \partial_t M + \operatorname{div}(v_w M) &= d_2 \Delta M - k_1 O \cdot M + S/(1 + S) \\ \partial_t S &= d_3 \Delta S - \lambda S + k_1 O \cdot M + \gamma(O - O^{\text{thr}}), \end{aligned} \tag{3.20}$$

where O is the oxidized LDL in the wall, M and S are concentrations in the intima of macrophages and cytokines, respectively; d_1, d_2, d_3 are the corresponding diffusion coefficients; λ and γ are the degradation and LDL oxidized detection coefficients; and v_w is the inflammatory velocity of plaque growth [55, 56].

3.2.5 Discrete approach

Blood flow in the small coupled domain within an FE mesh is viewed as a motion of the collection of DPD particles. The motion of each DPD particle is described by the following Newton's law equation:

$$m_i \dot{\mathbf{v}}_i = \sum_j \left(\mathbf{F}_{ij}^C + \mathbf{F}_{ij}^D + \mathbf{F}_{ij}^R\right) + \mathbf{F}_i^{\text{ext}}, \tag{3.21}$$

where m_i is the mass of particle i; $\dot{\mathbf{v}}_i$ is the particle acceleration as the time derivative of velocity; $\mathbf{F}_{ij}^C$, $\mathbf{F}_{ij}^D$ and $\mathbf{F}_{ij}^R$ are the conservative (repulsive), dissipative and random (Brownian) interaction forces that particle j exerts on particle i, respectively, provided particle j is within the radius of influence r_c of particle i; and $\mathbf{F}_i^{\text{ext}}$ is the external force exerted on particle i, which usually represents gradient of pressure or

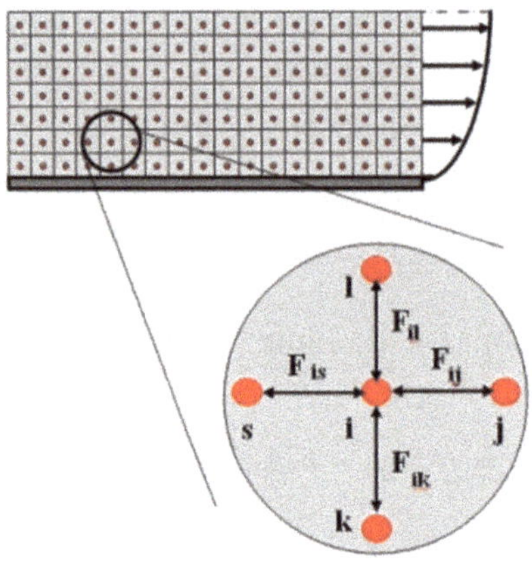

$$\mathbf{F}_{ij} = \mathbf{F}_{ij}^{\text{Conservative}} + \mathbf{F}_{ij}^{\text{Disipative}} + \mathbf{F}_{ij}^{\text{Random}}$$

Figure 3.3. Interaction forces in the DPD approach.

gravity force as a driving force for the fluid domain [57]. Hence, the total interaction force $\mathbf{F}_{ij}$ (figure 3.3) between the two particles is

$$\mathbf{F}_{ij} = \mathbf{F}_{ij}^{C} + \mathbf{F}_{ij}^{D} + \mathbf{F}_{ij}^{R}. \tag{3.22}$$

3.2.6 DPD modeling of oxidized LDL particle adhesion to the wall

When an oxidized LDL comes close to the wall and if the shear rate allows, it binds to the wall. However, when adhered LDL particles are exposed simultaneously to other forces stronger than the binding forces, the bonds break. To incorporate LDL adhesion to vessel walls, we introduce an attractive (bonding) force ($\mathbf{F}_{ij}^{a}$) in addition to the conservative, viscous and random interaction forces. As an approximation, we model the attractive force with a linear spring attached to the LDL's surface. The spring is attached to the vessel wall or to an already adhered LDL particle. The effective spring constant for LDL adhesion on the vessel wall, or to another stationary LDL particle, is denoted by k_{bw}.

The additional parameter involved in the model is the size of the domain from the LDL coated wall ($L_{\text{max}}^{\text{wall}}$) for which the action of attractive force needs to be considered. We take the attractive force as

$$F_{w}^{a} = k_{bw}(1 - L_{w}/L_{\text{max}}^{\text{wall}}) \tag{3.23}$$

where L_w is the distance of the oxidized LDL from the wall.

3.3 Results

3.3.1 Coupled method for modeling of atherosclerosis

Atherosclerosis development for two patients specific in the left and right coronary artery was simulated. Upstream of the bifurcation level there was plaque progression

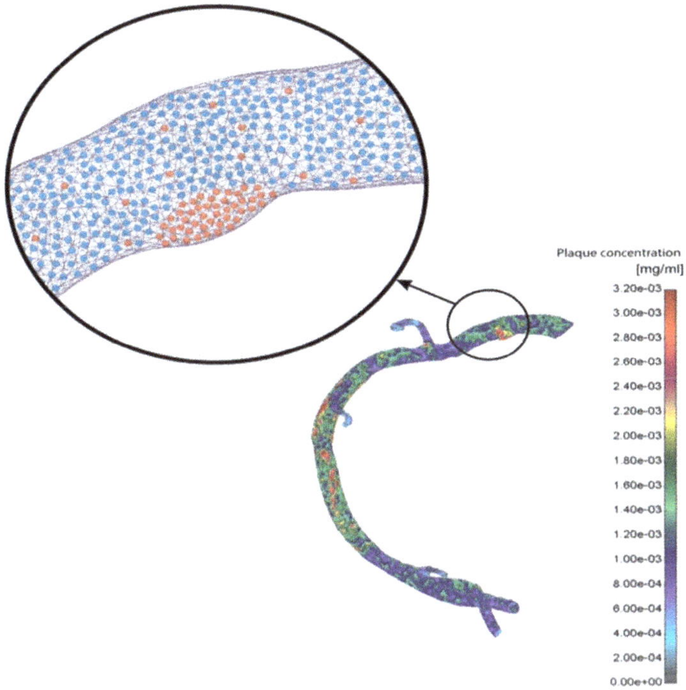

Figure 3.4. The right coronary artery for a specific patient. Coupled simulation FE and DPD method.

(figure 3.4). The biomolecular parameters ICAM1, LDL, high-density lipoprotein (HDL) and triglycerides are used for the computer simulation. The coupled continuum and discrete method were implemented.

3.3.2 Stent deployment modeling

A system of stent deployment is modeled which consists of three parts: the balloon, stent and blood vessel. The first part, the elastic balloon, should be inflated in order to open the stent and blood vessel with stenosis. The second part is the stent, a wired structure that should open and hold the narrowed blood vessel. The third part is the blood vessel with a narrowing caused by plaque progression.

The model consists of eight-node brick linear finite elements. The materials of all three structures are linearly elastic but with large deformations. The boundary conditions applied in this model are fixed nodes at the beginning and at the end of the blood vessel with stenosis, a prescribed pressure in the balloon and symmetry boundary conditions at all three parts of the FE mesh (because we model half of the model based on symmetry assumptions). The value of the pressure is not significant in this case, because it is fitted only to open stenosis. The pressure increases linearly over time. The simulation has 200 time steps of 5 ms. In addition to the mentioned number of 3D finite elements, when the balloon and stent are in contact, or when the stent and blood vessel are in contact, there is a variable number of elastic support elements, which depends on the contact area size between the 3D elements in contact.

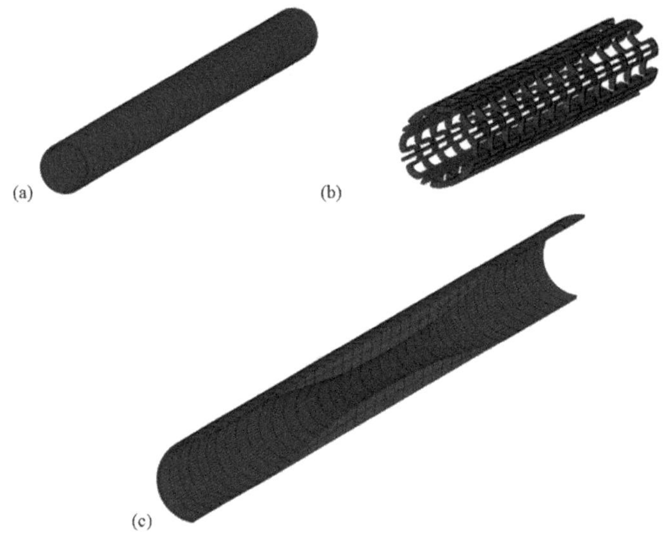

Figure 3.5. FE model of (a) the elastic balloon, (b) the stent and (c) the blood vessel with stenosis.

The three parts of the model are shown separately in figure 3.5. There are (a) the FE mesh of the balloon, (b) the FE mesh of the stent and (c) the FE mesh of the blood vessel with stenosis obtained using parametrized geometry.

The initial results for the stent deployment model obtained with the solver developed using the PAK software package are presented [51]. The PAK software is upgraded with a contact algorithm developed during this study. The initial model is parametric, as explained in the previous section.

The results for a stent opened by an inflated balloon are given in figure 3.6. There are two time steps: time step 10 and 160. These two steps are characteristic because in time step 10 contact appears between the elastic balloon and stent, and in time step 160 the narrowed blood vessel is completely opened by the balloon and stent. As can be seen from the images, at the beginning of the simulation, there is no contact between the elastic balloon and stent, and only the balloon has deformation. At time step 10 the contact appears, and the balloon starts opening the stent and also the blood vessel. At time step 160 the diameter of the narrowed blood vessel is restored to its original dimensions.

3.3.3 Deformable artery wall

In the case of arteries with deformable walls, additional input data are required for blood flow simulations compared to the case of arteries with rigid walls. First, the 3D geometry model of the arterial wall is required (figure 3.7). In addition to the boundary conditions for the fluid domain, the user must also specify the appropriate boundary conditions for the solid domain. The boundary condition for the solid domain is the area that is considered to be fixed, in order for the model to be constrained. This is an issue of great importance since it greatly alters the generated results regarding the displacement of the arterial wall. Furthermore, the interface

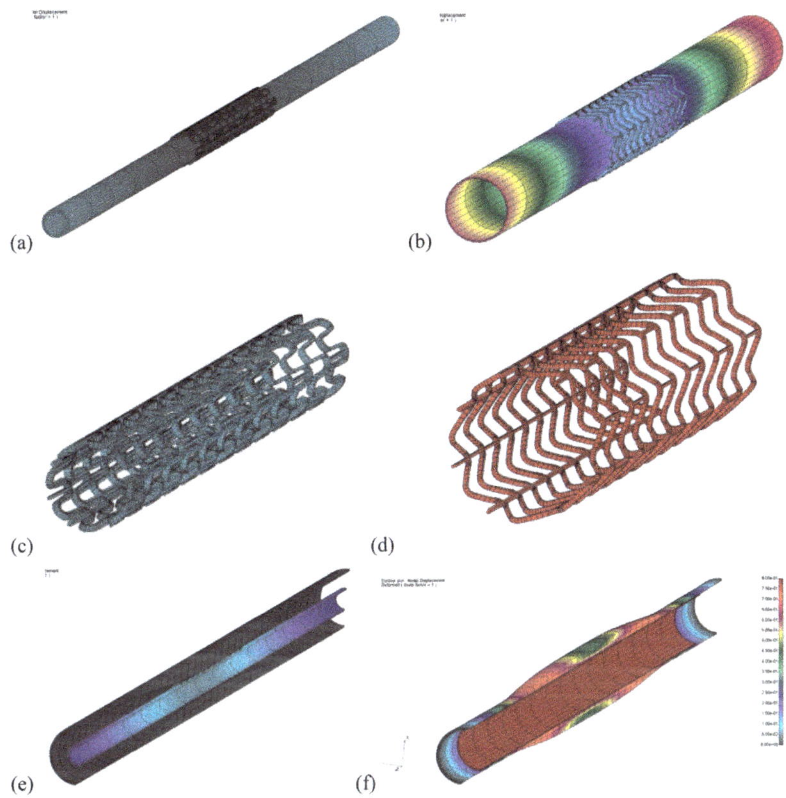

Figure 3.6. Results obtained using the developed parametric model. The displacement fields for: the stent with balloon, (a) time step 10 and (b) time step 160; the stent, (c) time step 10 and (d) time step 160; and the whole model, (e) time step 10 and (f) time step 160.

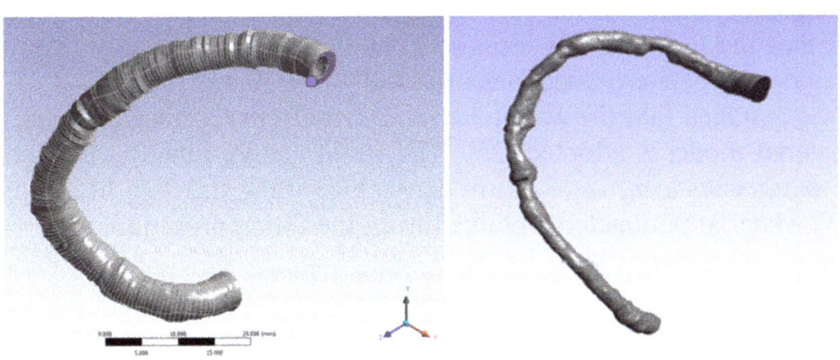

Figure 3.7. 3D reconstructed model for the arterial wall (right) and the lumen (left).

between the arterial wall and the lumen is specified as fluid–structure interface where interaction occurs between the fluid (blood) and the solid (wall). Furthermore, the user must also specify the material of the arterial wall (i.e. linear elastic, hyperelastic, etc). The choice of the wall material can also influence the obtained results on WSS

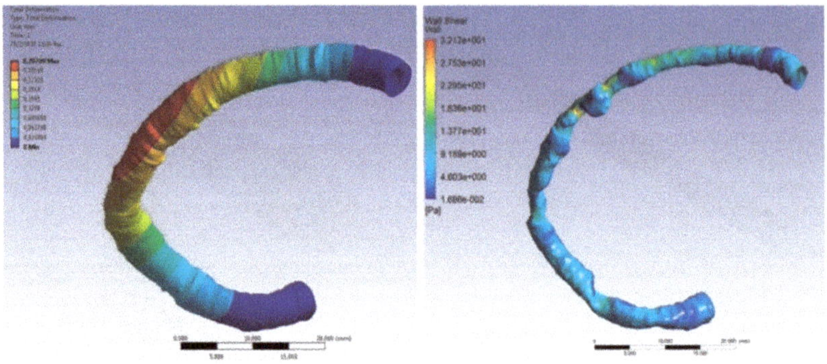

Figure 3.8. Wall deformation (right) and WSS distribution (left).

distribution as well as the wall deformation. However, there is also a great difference regarding computational time. Moreover, the definition of these parameters is of great significance since it is very difficult to acquire exact patient-specific data. The final output data include the areas of low WSS, the WSS distribution within the arterial wall and the wall deformation (figure 3.8), which can provide useful information on plaque generation and progression. The user has the capability to visualize the results in an appropriate environment.

3.3.4 Nitinol material model

In order to perform computer modeling of the combined effects of the surrounding arterial wall and inner forces of blood and stent deployment against the arterial wall, a 3D reconstruction from IVUS and angiography is derived.

The FE model consists of the solid domain and the fluid domain. The solid domain consists of the stent and arterial wall. The fluid and solid domains are modeled using 3D-eight-node FEs.

The boundary conditions for the solid surrounding the artery are as follows. It is assumed that the first and last cross-sections do not move axially, hence all FE element nodes in these cross-sections are axially restrained.

It is also assumed that the wall material is orthotropic nonlinear elastic, and the Fung material model is adopted [25]. The strain energy function is defined. The material parameters $c, a_1, \; a_2, \; a_4$ are determined using the data fitting procedure from [19]. Material parameters obtained from the fitting procedure are

$$c = 0.7565[\text{MPa}], \quad a_1 = 0.166, \quad a_2 = 0.084, \quad a_4 = 0.045. \tag{3.24}$$

For the stent material, the alloy of Nitinol is adopted for the definition of the material. The material parameters characterizing this alloy are [19]

$$\begin{array}{llll} E = 60\ 000\ [\text{MPa}] & \nu = 0.3 & & \\ \sigma_s^{AS} = 520 & \sigma_f^{AS} = 750 & \sigma_s^{SA} = 550 & \sigma_f^{SA} = 200 \\ \beta^{AS} = 250 & \beta^{SA} = 20 & \varepsilon_L = 7.5\% & C = 0\ [\text{MPa K}^{-1}], \end{array} \tag{3.25}$$

where all σ and β parameters are in MPa. The material parameters of blood are the density $\rho = 1.05 \times 10^{-3}$[g mm^{-3}] and dynamic viscosity $\mu = 3.675 \times 10^{-3}$ [Pa s].

3.3.5 Stress analysis for stent deployment

According to the boundary conditions and loads mentioned above, the numerical analysis of the material behavior of this complex model is performed. To examine different loading conditions, we apply the hemodynamic flow as well as stent deployment procedure at the arterial wall.

The stent is loaded by an internal uniform radial pressure which varies linearly from 0 to 1 MPa. Due to the artery incompressibility requirement and to avoid locking problems, eight-node brick elements are used in all the analyses [19]. In particular, in the simulations we use up to 232 214 elements and 257 532 nodes, resulting in 666 354 variables. The interaction between the expanding stent and the artery is described as contact between deformable surfaces. As contact conditions, we set finite sliding, no friction, with the constraint enforced by a Lagrange multiplier method. The stenotic segment of the artery which was examined before and after stent deployment is presented in figure 3.9.

Blood flow analysis was performed using the FE method described in the methods section. The shear stress distribution before and after stent deployment is shown in figure 3.10. It can be seen that the stent reduced wall shear stress significantly after deployment, which is caused by opening the artery and reducing the narrowing.

The effective von Mises stress distribution in the stent is presented in figure 3.11. It can be observed that highest stresses are located near the connectors between the stent struts. These parts are subjected to plastic deformation with maximal stress around 180 MPa.

The effective stress distribution in the arterial wall at the two different cross-section locations at the end of stent deployment with maximum deployment pressure is shown in figure 3.12. It can be observed that higher stress exists when wall thickness is reduced during the deployment procedure.

Effective stress distribution for the inflation pressure 1 kPa for stent deployment in the carotid artery is presented in figure 3.13.

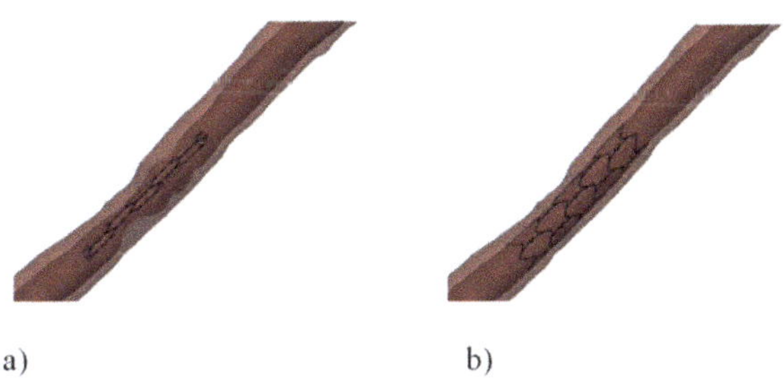

Figure 3.9. Stent positioning before (a) and after (b) stent deployment.

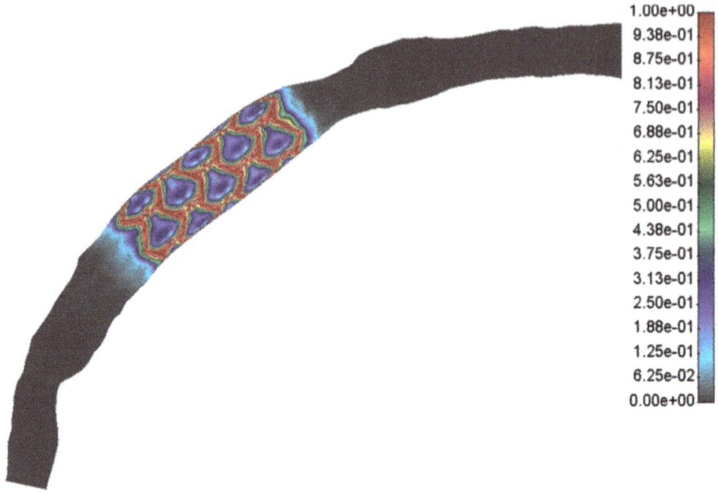

Figure 3.10. Effective stress distribution inside the arterial wall after stent deployment. The units are in MPa.

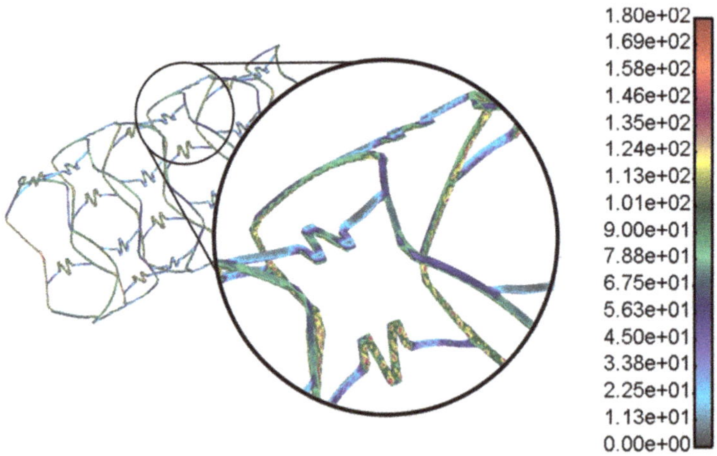

Figure 3.11. Effective von Mises stress distribution for inflation pressure of 1 MPa. The units are in MPa.

3.3.6 Plaque concentration for stented arteries

Plaque progression for a specific patient in the left coronary artery was detected using CTA image analysis at baseline and after 12 months. Volume progression from 50% to 70% was observed with segmentation and registration of CT images. We first examined the baseline and follow-up shear stress distribution (figure 3.14). The boundary conditions for the blood inflow were the same for both the baseline and follow-up studies because we consider there was not significant change. Downstream, the bifurcation level in the second marginal branch showed predominantly low WSS values occurring at baseline (figure 3.15, left panel). A similar situation with the same patient was observed in the right coronary artery in the distal

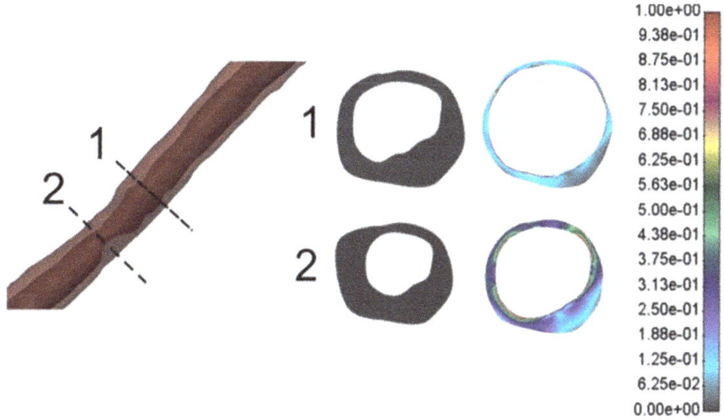

Figure 3.12. Effective stress distribution in the two different cross-section locations inside the arterial wall at the end of stent deployment.

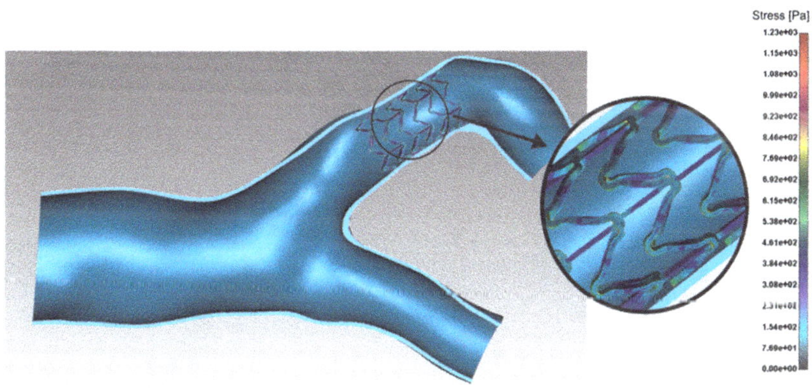

Figure 3.13. Stent deployment in the carotid artery. Stress distribution for the inflation pressure 1 kPa.

portion of the artery (figure 3.15), that showed a progression of the baseline stenosis. The location of the lowest WSS in the distal portion of the vessel corresponded to the site of plaque growth after 12 months. The biomolecular parameters cholesterol, LDL, HDL and triglycerides for the patient at baseline are listed in table 3.1. These parameters are used for the computer simulation. It can be seen that intra-plaque WSS values were lower at baseline compared to the follow-up situation. The red in figures 3.14 and 3.15 denotes the maximal plaque concentration, which directly gives the plaque volume for the left and right specific patient coronary arteries.

3.4 Discussion and conclusions

We analyze stent modeling with plaque formation and progression for specific patients in the coronary and carotid arteries. A coupled 3D artery reconstruction from IVUS and angiography imaging modalities is described, with the ability to

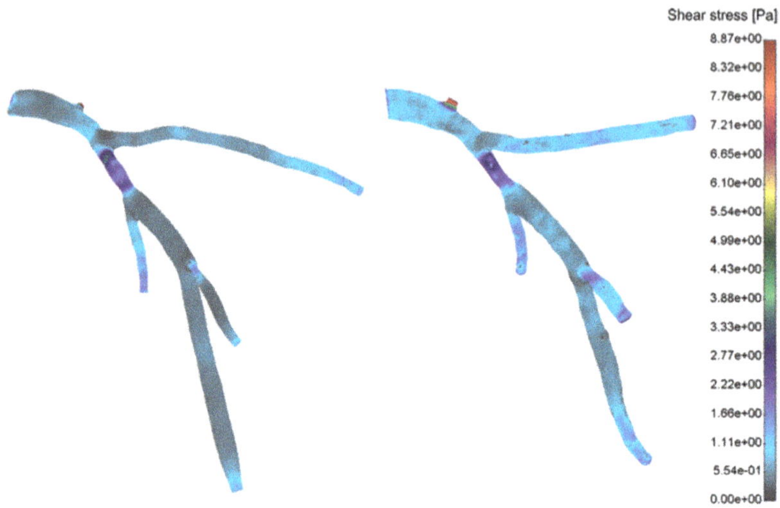

Figure 3.14. Baseline (left) and follow-up (right) shear stress distribution for the left coronary artery.

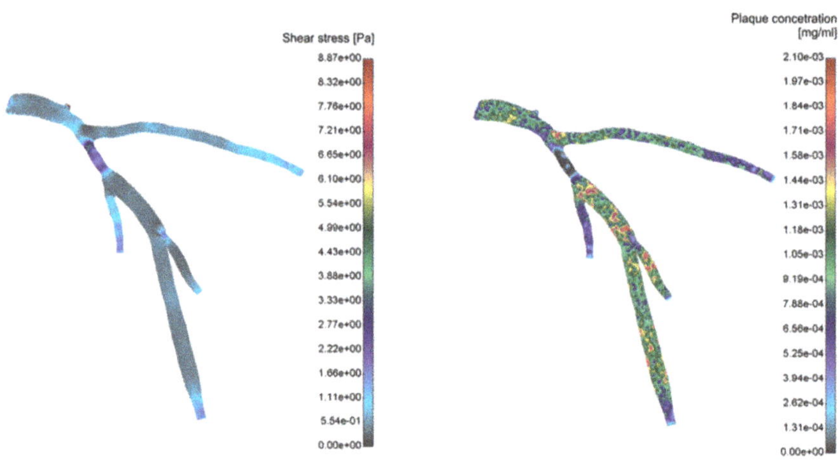

Figure 3.15. Left coronary artery for a specific patient. Left: shear stress distribution. Right: plaque concentration distribution.

Table 3.1. Biomolecular parameters for a specific patient at baseline.

Time	Total cholesterol	LDL	HDL	Triglycerides
Baseline	198	100	36	309

detect luminal narrowing, on the one hand, and generate FE models and process them, on the other. A number of different patients with significant ISR for the same time period of six months follow-up were analyzed. The geometry of the patients for baseline and follow-up has been used for the imaging techniques described in detail. The flow equations are coupled with the transport equation, applying realistic boundary conditions for each patient.

Blood flow simulation is described with the Navier–Stokes and continuity equations. The governing FE equations used in modeling wall tissue deformation with emphasis on the implementation of nonlinear constitutive models are described. The coupling of fluid dynamics and solute dynamics at the endothelium is achieved by the Kedem–Katchalsky equations.

The discrete approach used the DPD method with conservative, dissipative and random forces and an additional attractive force to the arterial wall. Some of the initial results are presented for two patients for the left and right coronary artery. The biomolecular parameters ICAM1, LDL, HDL and triglycerides are used for both patients to calculate plaque concentration. The baseline geometry is used to calculate the shear stress distribution. Follow-up CT studies after 24 months are compared to the simulation results. A good agreement is achieved. This methodology could be validated with retrospective studies from the literature if at least two points in time are available (baseline and follow-up).

The presented methodologies represent patient-specific modeling tools which can be used for clinical treatment decisions. The obtained results are very valuable because they make it possible to visualize and present the spatial distribution of biomechanical quantities, which is practically impossible to obtain without modeling. An additional aim of this chapter was to validate our computer simulation model for plaque progression in patients with stented coronary arteries.

The stress distribution of the artery wall and stent during expansion of occluded zones is analyzed. The shear stress distribution before and after stent deployment is also compared. A better understanding of stent deployment procedures and arterial wall responses, as well as optimal stent design, can be obtained using computer simulation.

Acknowledgment

This study was funded by grants from the Serbia III41007, ON174028 and EC HORIZON2020 689 068 SMARTool project.

References

[1] De Backer G G 2009 The global burden of coronary heart disease *Medicographia* **31** 343–8

[2] Herrington W, Lacey B, Sherliker P, Armitage J and Lewington S 2016 Epidemiology of atherosclerosis and the potential to reduce the global burden of atherothrombotic disease *Circ. Res.* **118** 535–46

[3] Meads C, Cummins C, Jolly K, Stevens A, Burls A and Hyde A 2000 Coronary artery stents in the treatment of ischaemic heart disease: a rapid and systematic review *Health Technol. Assess* **4** 1–153

[4] Serruys P W *et al* 1994 A comparison of balloon-expandable-stent implantation with balloon angioplasty in patients with coronary artery disease *N. Engl. J. Med.* **331** 489–95
[5] Fischman D L *et al* 1994 A randomized comparison of coronary-stent placement and balloon angioplasty in the treatment of coronary artery disease *N. Engl. J. Med.* **331** 496–501
[6] Pache J *et al* 2003 Intracoronary stenting and angiographic results: strut thickness effect on restenosis outcome (ISAR-STEREO-2) trial *J. Am. Coll. Cardiol.* **41** 1283–8
[7] Lee C H *et al* 2007 Sirolimus-eluting, bioabsorbable polymer-coated constant stent (Cura) in acute ST-elevation myocardial infarction: a clinical and angiographic study (CURAMI Registry) *J. Invasive Cardiol.* **19** 182–5
[8] Costa R A *et al* 2006 Angiographic results of the first human experience with the Biolimus A9 drug-eluting stent for *de novo* coronary lesions *Am. J. Cardiol.* **98** 443–6
[9] Yuk S H, Oh K S, Park J, Kim S J, Kim J H and Kwon I K 2012 Paclitaxel-loaded poly (lactide-co-glycolide)/poly(ethylene vinyl acetate) composite for stent coating by ultrasonic atomizing spray *Sci. Technol. Adv. Mater.* **13** 025005
[10] Kim S J *et al* 2011 Development of a biodegradable sirolimus-eluting stent coated by ultrasonic atomizing spray *J. Nanosci. Nanotechnol.* **11** 5689–97
[11] Farooq V, Gogas B D and Serruys P W 2011 Restenosis—delineating the numerous causes of drug-eluting stent restenosis *Circ. Cardiovasc. Interv.* **4** 195–205
[12] Fischman D L *et al* 1994 A randomized comparison of coronary-stent placement and balloon angioplasty in the treatment of coronary artery disease *N. Engl. J. Med.* **331** 496–501
[13] Morice M C *et al* 2002 A randomized comparison of a sirolimus-eluting stent with a standard stent for coronary revascularization *N. Engl. J. Med.* **349** 1315–23
[14] Newman V S, Berry J L, Routh W D, Ferrario C M and Dean R H 1996 Effects of vascular stent surface area and hemodynamics on intimal thickening *J. Vasc. Interv. Radiol.* **7** 387–93
[15] Murata T, Hiro T, Fujii T, Yasumoto K, Murashige A, Kohno M, Yamada J, Miura T and Matsuzaki M 2002 Impact of the cross-sectional geometry of the post-deployment coronary stent on in-stent neointimal hyperplasia: an intravascular ultrasound study *Circ. J.* **66** 489–93
[16] Murphy J and Boyle F 2008 Assessment of the effects of increasing levels of physiological realism in the computational fluid dynamics analyses of implanted coronary stents *3rd Annual Int. IEEE EMBS Conf.*
[17] DePaola N, Gimbrone M A J, Davies P F and Dewey C F 1992 Vascular endothelium responds to fluid shear stress gradients *Arterioscler. Thromb.* **12** 1254–7
[18] Balossino R, Gervaso F, Migliavacca F and Dubini G 2008 Effects of different stent designs on local hemodynamics in stented arteries *J. Biomech.* **41** 1053–61
[19] Simard T, Hibbert B, Ramirez F D, Froeschl M, Chen Y X and O'Brien E R 2014 The evolution of coronary stents: a brief review *Can. J. Cardiol.* **30** 35–45
[20] Lüscher T F *et al* 2007 Drug-eluting stent and coronary thrombosis: biological mechanisms and clinical implications *Circulation* **115** 1051–8
[21] Kimura T *et al* 2010 Comparisons of baseline demographics, clinical presentation, and long-term outcome among patients with early, late, and very late stent thrombosis of sirolimus-eluting stents: observations from the Registry of Stent Thrombosis for Review and Reevaluation (RESTART) *Circulation* **122** 52–61
[22] Mori H, Joner M, Finn A V and Virmani R 2016 Malapposition: is it a major cause of stent thrombosis? *Eur. Heart J.* **37** 1217–9 .
[23] Armstrong E J *et al* 2012 Clinical presentation, management, and outcomes of angiographically documented early, late, and very late stent thrombosis *JACC Cardiovasc. Interv.* **5** 131–40

[24] Tada T *et al* 2013 Risk of stent thrombosis among bare-metal stents, first-generation drug-eluting stents, and second-generation drug-eluting stents: results from a registry of 18,334 patients *JACC Cardiovasc. Interv.* **6** 1267–74

[25] He Y, Duraiswamy N, Frank A O and Moore J E Jr 2005 Blood flow in stented arteries: a parametric comparison in three-dimensions *J. Biomech. Eng.* **22** 637–47

[26] Natarajan S and Mokhtarzadeh-Dehghan M R 2000 A numerical and experimental study of periodic flow in a model of a corrugated vessel with application to stented arteries *Med. Eng. Phys.* **22** 555–66

[27] LaDisa J F, Guler I, Olson L E, Hettrick D A, Kersten J R, Warltier D C and Pagel P S 2003 Three-dimensional computational fluid dynamics modeling of alterations in coronary wall shear stress produced by stent implantation *Ann. Biomed. Eng.* **31** 972–80

[28] Seo T, Schachter L G and Barakat A I 2005 Computational study of fluid mechanical disturbance induced by endovascular stents *Ann. Biomed. Eng.* **33** 444–56

[29] Tortoriello A and Pedrizzetti G 2004 Flow-tissue interaction with compliance mismatch in a model stented artery *J. Biomech.* **37** 1–11

[30] Berry J L, Santamarina A, Moore J E, Roychowdhury S and Routh W D 2000 Experimental and computational flow evaluation of coronary stents *Ann. Biomed. Eng.* **28** 386–98

[31] LaDisa J F, Olson L E, Douglas H E, Warltier D C, Kersten J R and Pagel P S 2006 Alterations in regional vascular geometry produced by theoretical stent implantation influence distributions of wall shear stress: analysis of curved artery using 3D computational fluid dynamics models *Biomed. Eng. Online* **5** 40

[32] LaDisa J F, Olson L E, Guler I, Hettrick D A, Kersten J R, Warltier D C and Pagel P S 2005 Circumferential vascular deformation after stent implantation alters wall shear stress evaluated with time-dependent 3D computational fluid dynamics models *J. Appl. Physiol.* **98** 947–57

[33] Rajamohan D, Banerjee R K, Back L H, Ibrahim A A and Jog M A 2006 Developing pulsatile flow in a deployed coronary stent *J. Biomech. Eng.* **128** 347–59

[34] Nikolsky E *et al* 2003 Stent deployment failure: reasons, implications, and short- and long-term outcomes *Catheter Cardiovasc. Interv.* **59** 324–8

[35] Andreou I *et al* 2016 Atherosclerotic plaque behind the stent changes after bare-metal and drug-eluting stent implantation in humans: Implications for late stent failure? *Atherosclerosis* **252** 9–14

[36] Everett K D *et al* 2016 Structural mechanics predictions relating to clinical coronary stent fracture in a 5 year period in FDA MAUDE database *Ann. Biomed. Eng.* **44** 391–403

[37] Voros S *et al* 2011 Prospective validation of standardized, 3-dimensional, quantitative coronary computed tomographic plaque measurements using radiofrequency backscatter intravascular ultrasound as reference standard in intermediate coronary arterial lesions: results from the ATLANTA (assessment of tissue characteristics, lesion morphology, and hemodynamics by angiography with fractional flow reserve, intravascular ultrasound and virtual histology, and noninvasive computed tomography in atherosclerotic plaques) I study *JACC Cardiovasc. Interv.* **4** 198–208

[38] de Graaf M A *et al* 2013 Automatic quantification and characterization of coronary atherosclerosis with computed tomography coronary angiography: cross-correlation with intravascular ultrasound virtual histology *Int. J. Cardiovasc. Imaging* **29** 1177–90

[39] Athanasiou L *et al* 2016 Three-dimensional reconstruction of coronary arteries and plaque morphology using CT angiography—comparison and registration with IVUS *BMC Med. Imaging* **16** 9

[40] Bourantas C V *et al* 2008 ANGIOCARE: an automated system for fast three-dimensional coronary reconstruction by integrating angiographic and intracoronary ultrasound data *Catheter Cardiovasc. Interv.* **72** 166–75

[41] Plissiti M E, Fotiadis D I, Michalis L K and Bozios G E 2004 An automated method for lumen and media-adventitia border detection in a sequence of IVUS frames *Trans. Inf. Technol. Biomed.* **8** 131–41

[42] de Jaegere P *et al* 1998 Intravascular ultrasound-guided optimized stent deployment. Immediate and 6 months clinical and angiographic results from the Multicenter Ultrasound Stenting in Coronaries Study (MUSIC Study) *Eur. Heart J.* **19** 1214–23

[43] Magnus P C *et al* 2015 Optical coherence tomography versus intravascular ultrasound in the evaluation of observer variability and reliability in the assessment of stent deployment: the OCTIVUS study *Catheter Cardiovasc. Interv.* **86** 229–35

[44] Zhang Y *et al* 2012 Comparison of intravascular ultrasound versus angiography-guided drug-eluting stent implantation: a meta-analysis of one randomised trial and ten observational studies involving 19,619 patients *EuroIntervention* **8** 855–65

[45] Brugaletta S *et al* 2012 Comparison of *in vivo* eccentricity and symmetry indices between metallic stents and bioresorbable vascular scaffolds: insights from the ABSORB and SPIRIT trials *Catheter Cardiovasc. Interv.* **79** 219–28

[46] Wang A *et al* 2013 Automatic stent strut detection in intravascular optical coherence tomographic pullback runs *Int. J. Cardiovasc. Imaging* **29** 29–38

[47] Nakazawa G *et al* 2009 Incidence and predictors of drug-eluting stent fracture in human coronary artery a pathologic analysis *J. Am. Coll. Cardiol.* **54** 1924–31

[48] Scheinert D *et al* 2005 Prevalence and clinical impact of stent fractures after femoropopliteal stenting *J. Am. Coll. Cardiol.* **45** 312–5

[49] Woo J *et al* 2010 Nonlinear registration of serial coronary CT angiography (CCTA) for assessment of changes in atherosclerotic plaque *Med. Phys.* **37** 885–96

[50] Marquering H A *et al* 2008 Coronary CT angiography: IVUS image fusion for quantitative plaque and stenosis analyses *Proc. SPIE* **6918** 69181G

[51] Kojic M, Filipovic N, Stojanovic B and Kojic N 2008 *Computer Modeling in Bioengineering: Theoretical Background, Examples and Software* (Chichester: Wiley)

[52] Filipovic N, Mijailovic S, Tsuda A and Kojic M 2006 An implicit algorithm within the arbitrary Lagrangian–Eulerian formulation for solving incompressible fluid flow with large boundary motions *Comput. Methods Appl. Mech. Eng.* **195** 6347–61

[53] Taylor C A, Hughes T J R and Zarins C K 1998 Finite element modeling of blood flow in arteries *Comput. Methods Appl. Mech. Eng.* **158** 155–96

[54] Nanfeng S, Nigel W, Alun H, Simon T X and Yun X 2006 Fluid-wall modelling of mass transfer in an axisymmetric stenosis: effects of shear-dependent transport properties *Ann. Biomed. Eng.* **34** 1119–28

[55] Filipovic N, Rosic M, Tanaskovic I, Milosevic Z, Nikolic D, Zdravkovic N, Peulic A, Fotiadis D and Parodi O 2012 ARTreat project: three-dimensional numerical simulation of plaque formation and development in the arteries *IEEE Trans. Inf. Technol. Biomed.* **16** 272–8

[56] Filipovic N 2013 *PAK-Athero, Finite Element Program for Plaque Formation and Development* (Serbia: University of Kragujevac)

[57] Boryczko K, Dzwinel W and Yuen D 2003 Dynamical clustering of red blood cells in capillary vessels *J. Mol. Model.* **9** 16–33

IOP Publishing

Vascular and Intravascular Imaging Trends, Analysis, and Challenges, Volume 1
Stent applications
Petia Radeva and Jasjit S Suri

Chapter 4

Current status of computational fluid dynamics for modeling of diseased vessels

Arindam Bit, Himadri Chattopadhyay and Jasjit Suri

Cardiac disorders in association with vascular anomalies are some of the most common diseases, frequently affecting many populations worldwide due to rapid changes in human lifestyles. There is an immense need for early detection of these kinds of disorders using minimally invasive techniques, in order to intervene with early treatment of the disorder, preventing late stage complexity. Computational fluid dynamics (CFD) is one of the few non-invasive techniques for the diagnosis of vascular disorders. At the same time, it provides tools for treatment planning and management, with the most efficient parametric combination for therapeutic solutions. In this chapter, comprehensive descriptions of a few case studies are provided, which reflect the capabilities of this technique to perform modeling of diseased vessels as well as modeling of treatment protocols.

4.1 Introduction

4.1.1 Disease vessel classification

Blood vessels are important components of the circulatory system. A blood vessel experiences sustainable stress conditions in the presence of the continuous flow of blood through its lumen. Cardiovascular diseases (CVDs), such as coronary artery disease and stroke, are among the largest causes of death and disability in the industrialized world. Data from European CVD statistics shows that each year 4 million deaths in Europe occur due to CVD, which is 47% of the total mortality rate [14]. The blood vessels distribute blood to different organs and supply them with nutrition. The arteries, far from being just ordinary conduits, adapt to varying flow and pressure conditions by enlarging or shrinking to meet changing hemodynamic demands. In this chapter, different types of diseases associated with the vascular

doi:10.1088/2053-2563/ab01fach4

network are first described. This is followed by a description of the constitutive equation for transport of blood across the vascular network. Diseased rheological conditions of the transported blood are discussed thereafter. The following part of the chapter deals with the numerical modeling aspects of the transported blood across a diseased vascular network. This is followed by a comprehensive discussion of the various factors and parameters to determine the wall-effect in the presence of shear stress. Finally, the chapter concludes with descriptions of various shear-stress parameters and their influence in the determination of pathological conditions of vascular networks.

4.1.1.1 Stenosed vessel

Diseases in blood vessels are broadly classified as stenoses (figure 4.1) and aneurysms (figure 4.2). Coronary heart disease and stroke are clinical symptoms of atherosclerosis, which is an inflammatory disease in which high plasma concentrations of cholesterol, in particular those of low-density lipoprotein (LDL) cholesterol, are among the principal risk factors.

More precisely, atherosclerosis is a pathological process promoted by inflammation of the inner arterial wall (intima), initiated by an excess of LDL in the blood. The LDL particles, as well as high-density lipoproteins (HDL), become oxidized by ongoing chemical reactions within the body and form ox-LDL, contributing to the atherosclerotic process when the ox-LDL concentration exceeds a threshold. At this stage, endothelial cells activate the immune system (monocytes and T cells) to deal with the problem. Once in the intima, the incoming immune cells instantaneously differentiate into active macrophages, which absorb ox-LDL by phagocytosis. This reaction transforms macrophages into foam cells that should be removed by the immune system, yielding the secretion of a pro-inflammatory signal contributing to the recruitment of new monocytes, and consequently this starts a chronic inflammatory reaction (auto-amplification phenomenon). The inflammation process involves the proliferation and the migration of smooth muscle cells to create a fibrous cap over the lipid deposit, isolating it from the blood flow. The fibrous cap changes the geometry of the vessel and modifies the blood flow. The occurrence of a heart attack or stroke is thus attributed to the degradation and rupture of the cap, the formation of a blood clot in the lumen and the subsequent obstruction of the artery forming stenoses.

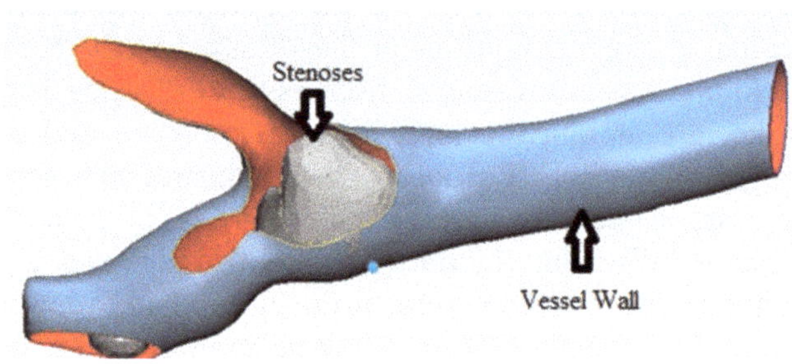

Figure 4.1. Stenosed blood vessel.

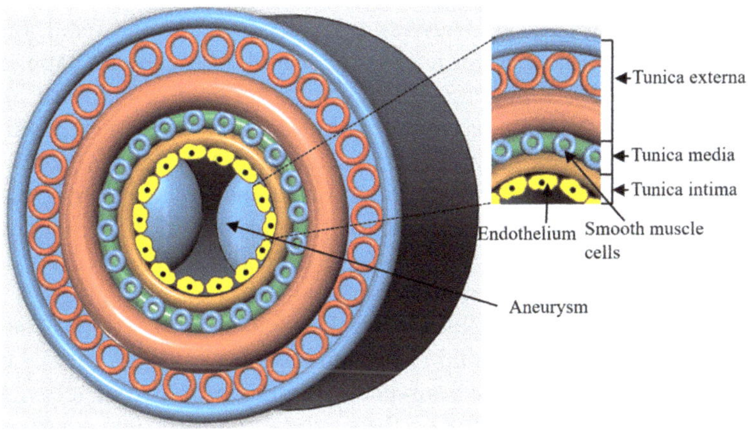

Figure 4.2. Details of an aneurysm.

4.1.1.2 Aneurismal vessel

An aneurysm is a localized dilation, bulging or ballooning of a blood vessel to greater than 1.5 times its original diameter. Aneurysms are typically either fusiform or saccular in shape, occurring most frequently in the abdominal aorta, but can also occur in the thoracic aorta, inter-cranial arteries/capillaries and coronary arteries. They result from weakening of an arterial wall section owing to a variety of genetic, biomechanical, biochemical and hemodynamic factors, such as hereditary conditions, atherosclerosis, inflammation, infection, hypertension, lung disease, smoking and obesity. Thus, the exact causes and sequence of events are not yet fully understood, but are commonly a result of multiple factors. When aneurysm rupture occurs in the cerebral circulation, the clinical manifestation is usually a stroke. However, massive bleeding and circulatory collapse are the results of ruptured abdominal and thoracic aortic aneurysms. In the United States, more than two million people are diagnosed annually with aneurysms and approximately 18 000 Americans are killed by all types of aneurysms every year. A notable victim of aneurysm is none other than Albert Einstein. Although aneurysms can occur in any blood vessel, most, i.e. about 75%, are asymptomatic. When symptoms do occur, they generally result from compression of adjacent structures and can be felt in several ways, such as a pulsating sensation or severe pain, depending on the location of the aneurysm. Figure 4.2 shows the most common form of aneurysm, i.e. saccular.

Thoracic aortic aneurysms (TAAs) occur in the chest. The rupture of a TAA can cause rapid blood loss and death. Clinically, they are not as common as abdominal aortic aneurysms. Hereditary conditions (e.g. Marfan's syndrome) are believed to be the main cause of TAAs. An aortic dissection results from a tear between the tissue layers of the aorta, which is caused by blood flow pumped from the heart, and may acutely dilate causing an aneurysm. The tear usually occurs in the thoracic aorta. Clinically, the aorta is seldom dilated before the dissection occurs. Risk factors include high blood pressure, particularly high diastolic blood pressure, and hereditary disorders such as Marfan's and Ehlers–Danlos syndrome.

Abdominal aortic aneurysms (AAAs) are located below the renal arteries and above the iliac bifurcation. Extension into one or both of the vessels supplying blood to the legs occurs in 40% of patients afflicted with AAAs. Furthermore, as many as 15% of patients with AAAs may also develop aneurysms further down their leg involving the arteries in their groin (femoral arteries) or behind their knees (popliteal arteries). Seventy-five percent of abdominal aortic aneurysms occur in people over 60 years of age. The AAA shapes are irregular, including bulge, prism, zigzag, boat and cylinder. Typically, an AAA is fusiform and asymmetric because the spinal column limits posterior expansion and hence causes anterior bulging.

A brain aneurysm is a weak ballooning in the brain's blood vessels. Clinically, it is also called a cerebral or intracranial aneurysm. Brain aneurysms usually occur at a branch of the brain arteries. If the brain aneurysm reaches a certain size (i.e. >2 cm), the aneurysm may generate pressure on the surrounding tissue and cause progressive problems, and if an aneurysm ruptures and bleeds, stroke or death may follow. Unfortunately, 60% of people with ruptured brain aneurysms die within a year. Compared with aortic aneurysms, heart (or coronary) aneurysms are quite rare. They may occur within the first two weeks after a severe heart attack when much of the heart muscle in the left ventricle (main pumping chamber of the heart) may be dead. The dysfunctional muscle and scar tissue may stretch and dilate to form an aneurysm. Symptoms may include chest pain or pressure, pain in the jaw or arms, trouble breathing, or fainting spells. Rupture of a ventricular aneurysm is usually fatal. Once an aneurysm has reached a critical diameter, with the growth rate and/or other parameter values indicating possible rupture, the treatment options are either open surgery or endovascular repair.

4.2 Constitutive equation of blood flow in a diseased vessel

4.2.1 Mass conservation equation

The equation for mass conservation [3] in a general form is given by equation (4.1) as

$$\frac{\partial \rho}{\partial t} + \frac{\partial(\rho u_1)}{\partial x_1} + \frac{1}{r}\frac{\partial(\rho r u_2)}{\partial x_2} = 0, \tag{4.1}$$

where, x_2, x_1, etc, are defined as follows:

$$\begin{aligned} x_1 &= x \text{ for Cartesian coordinates} \\ &= z \text{ for cylindrical axi-symmetric coordinates} \end{aligned}$$

$$\begin{aligned} x_2 &= y \text{ for Cartesian coordinates} \\ &= r \text{ for cylindrical axi-symmetric coordinates} \end{aligned}$$

moreover,

$$r = 1 \text{ for Cartesian coordinates.}$$

The mass conservation equation for problems involving two-dimensional, Cartesian geometry may be written as

$$\frac{\partial \rho}{\partial t} + \frac{\partial(\rho u)}{\partial x} + \frac{\partial(\rho v)}{\partial y} = 0, \tag{4.2}$$

where x and y are the coordinate directions, and u and v are the velocity components in those coordinate directions, respectively.

For cylindrical, axi-symmetric geometries, the same equation reads [4]

$$\frac{\partial \rho}{\partial t} + \frac{\partial(\rho v_z)}{\partial z} + \frac{1}{r}\frac{\partial(\rho r v_r)}{\partial r} = 0, \tag{4.3}$$

where r is the radial coordinate and z is the axial coordinate. v_r and v_z are the respective velocity components.

4.2.2 Momentum conservation equations

The x momentum equation in Cartesian coordinates may be written as

$$\frac{\partial(\rho u)}{\partial t} + \frac{\partial(\rho uu)}{\partial x} + \frac{\partial(\rho vu)}{\partial y} = -\frac{\partial p}{\partial x} + \frac{\partial(\tau_{xx})}{\partial x} + \frac{\partial(\tau_{yx})}{\partial y}. \tag{4.4}$$

Similarly, the y momentum equation in Cartesian coordinates may be written as

$$\frac{\partial(\rho v)}{\partial t} + \frac{\partial(\rho uv)}{\partial x} + \frac{\partial(\rho vv)}{\partial y} = -\frac{\partial p}{\partial y} + \frac{\partial(\tau_{xy})}{\partial x} + \frac{\partial(\tau_{yy})}{\partial y}. \tag{4.5}$$

In equations (4.4) and (4.5), the viscous stresses appear explicitly and for Newtonian fluids they are given as follows:

$$\tau_{xx} = \mu\left[2\frac{\partial u}{\partial x} - \frac{2}{3}(\nabla \cdot v)\right] \tag{4.6a}$$

$$\tau_{yy} = \mu\left[2\frac{\partial v}{\partial y} - \frac{2}{3}(\nabla \cdot v)\right] \tag{4.6b}$$

$$\tau_{yx} = \tau_{xy} = \mu\left[\frac{\partial u}{\partial y} + \frac{\partial v}{\partial x}\right]. \tag{4.6c}$$

It may be noted here that for incompressible flows, the divergence of velocities, $\nabla \cdot v = 0$, and hence, the expressions for stresses, as given in equation (4.6), assume a much simpler form.

In cylindrical coordinates, for axi-symmetric problems the axial (z) momentum equation is given as

$$\frac{\partial(\rho v_z)}{\partial t} + \frac{\partial(\rho v_z v_z)}{\partial z} + \frac{1}{r}\frac{\partial(\rho r v_r v_z)}{\partial r} = -\frac{\partial p}{\partial z} + \frac{\partial(\tau_{zz})}{\partial z} + \frac{1}{r}\frac{\partial(r\tau_{zr})}{\partial r}. \tag{4.7}$$

Similarly, the radial (r) momentum equation is given as

$$\frac{\partial(\rho v_r)}{\partial t}+\frac{\partial(\rho v_z v_r)}{\partial z}+\frac{1}{r}\frac{\partial(\rho r v_r v_r)}{\partial r}-\frac{\rho v_\theta{}^2}{r}=-\frac{\partial p}{\partial r}+\frac{\partial(\tau_{zr})}{\partial z}+\frac{1}{r}\frac{\partial(r\tau_{rr})}{\partial r}-\frac{\tau_{\theta\theta}}{r}. \quad (4.8)$$

Clearly, for axi-symmetric problems, two additional terms appear in the radial momentum equation. These terms are $\rho v_\theta{}^2/r$ on the left-hand side of equation (4.8), which is essentially an acceleration term (or convection term), and $\tau_{\theta\theta}/r$ on the right-hand side of (4.8), which is a viscous force, arising from the tangential stresses due to the curvature effect.

The non-conservative form of the convective terms is as follows:

$$\underbrace{\rho\left[\frac{\partial\varphi}{\partial t}+v_r\frac{\partial\varphi}{\partial r}+v_z\frac{\partial\varphi}{\partial z}\right]}_{\text{Non-conservative form of the convective terms}}=\frac{\partial(\rho\varphi)}{\partial t}-\varphi\frac{\partial\rho}{\partial r}+\frac{1}{r}\frac{\partial(\rho r v_r\varphi)}{\partial r}$$

$$-\frac{\varphi}{r}\frac{\partial(\rho r v_r)}{\partial r}+\frac{\partial(\rho v_z\varphi)}{\partial z}-\varphi\frac{\partial(\rho v_z)}{\partial z}$$

$$=\underbrace{\frac{\partial(\rho\varphi)}{\partial t}+\frac{1}{r}\frac{\partial(\rho r v_r\varphi)}{\partial r}+\frac{\partial(\rho v_z\varphi)}{\partial z}}_{\text{Conservative form of the convective terms}}-\underbrace{\varphi\left[\frac{\partial\rho}{\partial t}+\frac{1}{r}\frac{\partial(\rho r v_r)}{\partial r}+\frac{\partial(\rho v_z)}{\partial z}\right]}_{\text{These terms are zero by virtue of the continuity equation}}$$

$$=\underbrace{\frac{\partial(\rho\varphi)}{\partial t}+\frac{1}{r}\frac{\partial(\rho r v_r\varphi)}{\partial r}+\frac{\partial(\rho v_z\varphi)}{\partial z}}_{\text{Conservative form of the convective terms}}. \quad (4.9)$$

Therefore, the convective terms may be expressed either in terms of conservative or non-conservative forms and the former is preferred in the present formulation as it is best suited to finite volume formulations. For three-dimensional studies, corresponding three-dimensional forms of the equations are used.

4.3 Viscoelastic models of diseased blood

Most researchers have considered a Newtonian viscosity model for blood flowing through blood vessels. Blood flowing through a diseased blood vessel has certain characteristics which make the viscosity properties of the blood non-Newtonian [2].

4.3.1 Carreau model

The four-parameter non-Newtonian viscosity model proposed by Carreau [1] differs from other models primarily in the curvature of the curve near the transition points between the Newtonian plateaus and the power region as follows:

$$\mu(|\bar{\gamma}|)=\mu_\infty+(\mu_0-\mu_\infty)[1+(\lambda|\bar{\gamma}|)^a]^{(n-1)/a}, \quad (4.10)$$

where $\mu_0 = 0.056$ Pa s is the blood viscosity at a zero shear rate, $\mu_\infty = 0.0032$ Pa s, $\lambda = 3.131$ is the time constant associated with the viscosity that changes with the shear rate, and $n = 0.3568$, $a = 2$.

4.3.2 Power-law model

In [23], a viscosity model for blood is proposed, taking into account hematocrit and total protein minus albumin. It is known as the power-law model, also referred to as the 'best three variable model'. It is represented by

$$\bar{\tau} = k\,|\bar{\gamma}|^{n-1}\bar{\gamma} \tag{4.11}$$

and

$$\mu(|\bar{\gamma}|^{*}) = k\frac{U_{\infty}^{n-1}}{l^{n-1}}\,|\bar{\gamma}|^{*n-1}. \tag{4.12}$$

In [6], Chien *et al* calculated normal blood sample parameters as $k = 14.67 \times 10^{-3}$ Pa s, and $n = 0.7755$. If $n > 1$, the fluid is known as shear-thickening, while fluid is shear-thinning if $n < 1$. The characteristic parameter for a power-law-model-based flow is $\mathrm{Re}_{\mathrm{PL}}$.

As the power-law model does not have the capability of handling Newtonian regions of shear-thinning fluids at very low and high shear rates, Cross [7] proposed a model which can be described as a shear rate dependent viscosity model:

$$\mu(|\bar{\gamma}|) = \mu_{\infty} + \frac{(\mu_0 - \mu_{\infty})}{\left[1 + \left(\frac{\bar{\gamma}}{\bar{\gamma}_c}\right)^{n}\right]}, \tag{4.13}$$

where $\mu_0 = 0.0364$ Pa s is the blood viscosity at a very low shear rate, $\bar{\gamma}_c = 2.63\ \mathrm{s}^{-1}$ is the reference shear rate and $n = 1.45$ is the model constant.

4.3.3 Quemada model

Further considering the viscosity of a concentrated disperse system, Quemada [20] proposed a model based on shear rate and hematocrits. The system of equations of shear stress and effective viscosity in tensorial form and dimensionless form are

$$\bar{\tau} = \mu_F\left(1 - \frac{1}{2}\frac{k_0 + k_{\infty}\sqrt{|\bar{\gamma}|/\gamma_c}}{1 + \sqrt{|\bar{\gamma}|/\gamma_c}}\varphi\right)^{-2}\bar{\gamma} \tag{4.14}$$

and

$$\mu(|\bar{\gamma}|^{*}) = \mu_F\left(1 - \frac{1}{2}\frac{k_0 + k_{\infty}\sqrt{|\bar{\gamma}|^{*}/\gamma_c^{*}}}{1 + \sqrt{|\bar{\gamma}|^{*}/\gamma_c^{*}}}\varphi\right)^{-2}, \tag{4.15}$$

where $\gamma_c^{*} = \frac{\gamma_c}{U_{\infty}/l}$, the viscosity of plasma (the suspending medium), is $\mu_F = 1.2 \times 10^{-3}$ Pa s and hematocrit is $\varphi = 0.45$. The values of other parameters are $\gamma_c = 1.88\ \mathrm{s}^{-1}$, $k_{\infty} = 2.07$ and $k_0 = 4.33$. The characteristic parameters for a Quemada-model-based flow are $\mathrm{Re}_{\mathrm{QU}}$ and γ_c^{*}. The density of blood is considered as 1060 kg m^{-3}, whereas the Newtonian viscosity of blood is considered as 2.02×10^{-6} kg m^{-2} s^{-1}.

4.4 CFD modeling of blood flow in a diseased vessel

4.4.1 Laminar flow model

The laminar flow model of the internal flow regime in closed vessels can be modeled by the semi-implicit pressure linked equation (SIMPLE). It is a procedure for solving the governing equations of fluid transport. The continuity equation can be discretized in this form of the laminar flow model by the following set of equations:

$$[J_e A_e - J_w A_w] + [J_n A_n - J_s A_n] + [J_t A_t - J_b A_b] = 0 \tag{4.16}$$

or

$$\sum_{f}^{N_{\text{faces}}} J_f A_f = 0, \tag{4.17}$$

where fluxes at the control volume faces are

$$J_e = (\rho u)_e,\ J_w = (\rho u)_w,\ J_n = (\rho u)_n,\ J_s = (\rho u)_s,\ J_t = (\rho u)_t,\ J_b = (\rho u)_b. \tag{4.18}$$

To relate the face velocity, u_e, u_w, v_n, v_s, w_t, w_b, to the stored values of velocity at the cell centers, linear interpolation of cell-centered velocities to the faces will result in unphysical checker-boarding of pressure. To avoid checker-boarding, the face values of velocities are not averaged linearly, but using momentum-weighted averaging, as outlined in [21] using weighting factors based on the a_P coefficient. Using this procedure, the face flux for any face of the control volume, J_f, may be written as

$$\begin{aligned} J_f = f_f \Bigg(\rho_f \frac{a_{P,c0} v_{n,c0} + a_{p,c1} v_{n,c1}}{a_{P,c0} + a_{P,c1}} \\ + d_f \Big[\big(p_{c0} + (\nabla p)_{c0} \cdot \vec{r}_0 \big) - \big(p_{c1} + (\nabla p)_{c1} \cdot \vec{r}_1 \big) \Big] \Bigg) \end{aligned} \tag{4.19}$$

$$J_f = \hat{J}_f + d_f (p_{c0} - p_{c1}), \tag{4.20}$$

where

$$\hat{J}_f = f_f \left(\rho_f \frac{a_{P,c0} v_{n,c0} + a_{p,c1} v_{n,c1}}{a_{P,c0} + a_{P,c1}} + d_f [(\nabla p)_{c0}. \vec{r}_0 - (\nabla p)_{c1}. \vec{r}_1] \right). \tag{4.21}$$

With reference to figure 4.3, p_{C0} and p_{C1} are the pressures and $v_{n,C0}$ and $v_{n,C1}$ are the normal velocities, respectively, within the two cells on either side of the face f. The term $\hat{J}_f$ contains the influence of velocities in these two adjacent cells and d_f is a function of the average of the momentum equation. a_P are coefficients for the cells on either side of face f.

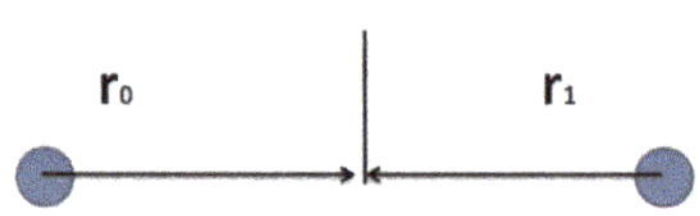

Figure 4.3. Control volume centroids of each control volume on either side of face f.

Accordingly for the control volume, as shown in figure 4.3,

$$J_e = \hat{J}_e + d_e(p_P - p_E) \tag{4.22a}$$

$$J_w = \hat{J}_w + d_w(p_W - p_P) \tag{4.22b}$$

$$J_n = \hat{J}_n + d_n(p_P - p_N) \tag{4.22c}$$

$$J_s = \hat{J}_s + d_s(p_S - p_P) \tag{4.22d}$$

$$J_t = \hat{J}_t + d_t(p_P - p_T) \tag{4.22e}$$

$$J_b = \hat{J}_b + d_b(p_B - p_P). \tag{4.22f}$$

Now for a guessed pressure field p^*, the resulting east face flux from equation (4.22*a*) is

$$J_e^* = \hat{J}_e^* + d_e(p_P^* - p_E^*). \tag{4.23}$$

This does not satisfy the volume continuity equation (4.15), so a correction J_e' is added to the face flux J_e^* so that the corrected face flux J_e becomes

$$J_e = J_e^* + J_e'. \tag{4.24}$$

Similarly, a pressure correction p' is added to the guessed pressure p^* so that the corrected pressure p becomes

$$p = p^* + p'. \tag{4.25}$$

The SIMPLE algorithm states that

$$J_e' = d_e(p_P' - p_E'). \tag{4.26}$$

Substituting J_e' in equation (4.22*a*) we obtain

$$J_e = J_e^* + d_e(p_P' - p_E'). \tag{4.27a}$$

Similarly,

$$J_w = J_w^* + d_w(p_W' - p_P') \tag{4.27b}$$

$$J_n = J_n^* + d_n(p_P' - p_N') \tag{4.27c}$$

$$J_s = J_s^* + d_s(p_S' - p_P') \tag{4.27d}$$

$$J_t = J_t^* + d_t(p_P' - p_T') \tag{4.27e}$$

$$J_b = J_b^* + d_b(p_B' - p_P'). \tag{4.27f}$$

Now putting the value of J_e, J_w, J_n, J_s, J_t, J_b in the continuity equation (4.15),

$$\begin{aligned}&\left[(J_e^*A_e + d_eA_e(p_P' - p_E')) - (J_w^*A_e + d_wA_w(p_W' - p_P'))\right] + \\ &\left[(J_n^*A_n + d_nA_n(p_P' - p_N')) - (J_s'A_s + d_sA_s(p_S' - p_P'))\right] + \\ &\left[(J_t^*A_t + d_tA_t(p_P' - p_T')) - (J_b^*A_b + d_bA_b(p_B' - p_P'))\right] = 0.\end{aligned} \tag{4.28}$$

Rearranging equation (4.13) we can write the equation as follows:

$$a_Pp_P' = a_Ep_E' + a_Wp_W' + a_Np_N' + a_Sp_S' + a_Tp_T' + a_Bp_B' + b, \tag{4.29}$$

where

$$a_P = d_eA_e + d_wA_w + d_nA_n + d_sA_s + d_tA_t + d_bA_b \tag{4.30a}$$

$$a_E = d_eA_e \tag{4.30b}$$

$$a_W = d_wA_w \tag{4.30c}$$

$$a_n = d_nA_n \tag{4.30d}$$

$$a_s = d_sA_s \tag{4.30e}$$

$$a_T = d_tA_t \tag{4.30f}$$

$$a_B = d_bA_b \tag{4.30g}$$

$$b = J_e^*A_e + J_n^*A_n + J_t^*A_t - J_w^*A_w - J_s^*A_s - J_b^*A_b + ({f_P}^0{\rho_P}^0 - f_P\rho_P)\frac{\Delta V}{\Delta t}. \tag{4.30h}$$

Equation (4.29) represents the discretized continuity equation as an equation for pressure correction p'. From equation (4.29) we obtain the pressure correction p' and putting the value of p' in equation (4.26) we obtain the correct pressure field p which satisfies the continuity equation (4.27). Then putting this pressure field in the momentum equation (4.29), we obtain the correct velocity.

The profiles at a particular blockage show similar trends of distribution. The agreement between the power-law model and cross model is remarkable, except for the type II profile at 56% obstruction where the cross model shows a flatter distribution with relatively high magnitude. It can be observed again from the plots that the post-stenotic zone for higher blockage endures a long zone of oscillatory shear stress although the magnitude is relatively less. It is well understood that the flow structure of a stenosed vessel is dominated by vortical structures and the post-stenotic recirculation region [19].

Figure 4.4 shows a contour plot of the time averaged velocity stream function for the type 1 inlet velocity profile at different degrees of stenosis, considering the power-law viscosity model. The comparison is performed at two different Reynolds numbers in figure 4.4, denoted as Re I and Re II. At low Reynolds numbers,

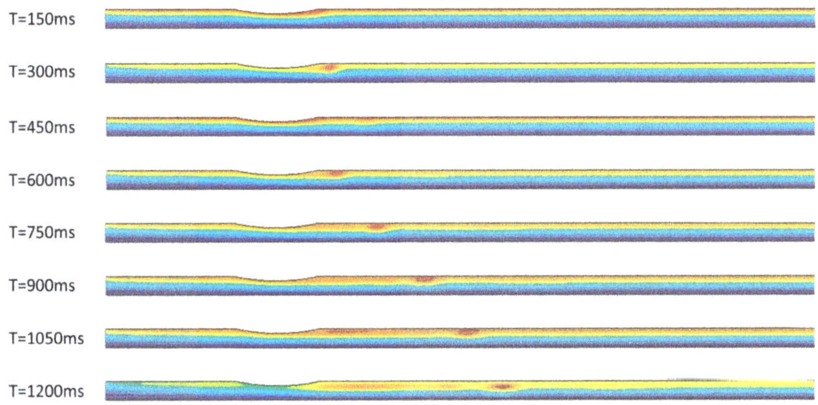

Figure 4.4. Contour view of velocity profiles of blood flowing through mild stenosed vessel at various time steps.

recirculation bubbles propagate away from the region of stenosis with time, producing a lower severity of stenosis (at 25%).

The numerical study of aneurysm was performed using two rheological models, namely the power-law model and Quemada model, to represent the diseased state of blood in a developing flow condition in a straight blood vessel with severe aneurysm of 250% of the mean diameter of the vessel [5]. The results for such a situation of fusiform aneurysms has not been not widely covered. Investigations were performed within the range $690 \leqslant \mathrm{Re} \leqslant 2760$. The responses of two different non-Newtonian viscosity models (namely power-law and Quemada) to different shear rate parameters near the boundaries are compared. Stream lines in the duct of the geometry are shown in figure 4.4, which reflects the development of vortices, considering the power-law model as the viscosity model for blood. As the resolution of the flow increases, the vortex size becomes amplified, signifying the serious affects of the aneurysm on the flow of blood.

A transient nature of flow development occurs in ducts with certain geometry. Such a phenomenon occurs due to the development of a vortex, initiating with offset damping, as depicted in figure 4.5.

4.5 Evaluation of the shear index on the vascular wall

The fluid-mechanical parameters, such as shear stress, vortical structures, pressure profiles and velocity distribution, can be evaluated from the time-dependent primitive variable data. Two important parameters need special mention in this context as they have relevance to the health of arterial tissue, namely the time-averaged wall shear stress (TAWSS) and the oscillator shear index (OSI) as described by [22]. TAWSS can be simply integrated and averaged over a time cycle. Wall shear stress is determined as

$$\mathrm{WSS} = -\mu \frac{\partial u_x}{\partial r}\bigg|_{\mathrm{wall}} \times (1+R'(z)^2). \tag{4.31}$$

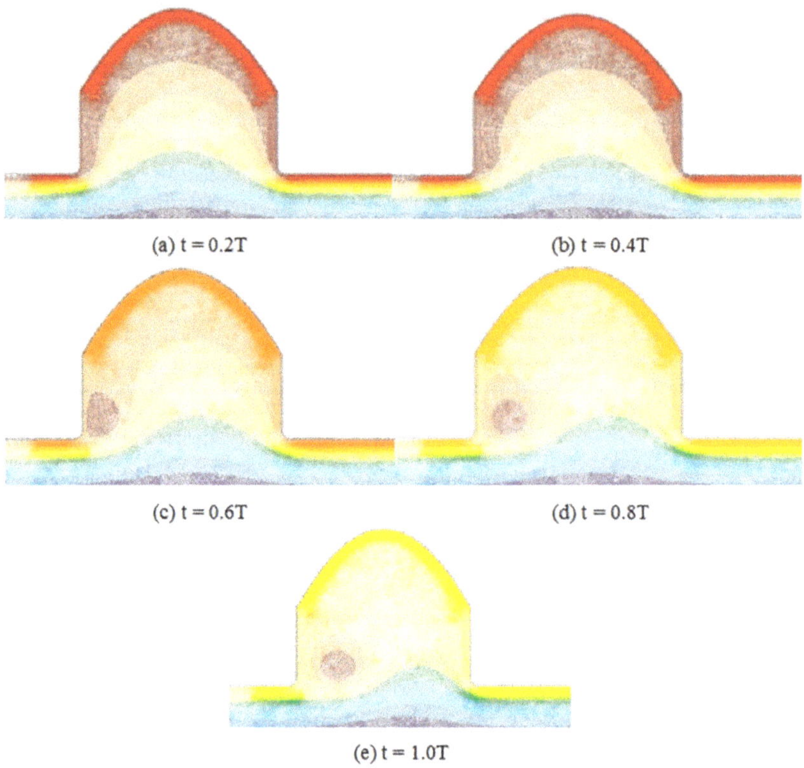

Figure 4.5. Stream line at different time steps at Re I (for the power-law model).

Downstream from the stenosis, $R'(z) = 0$, therefore, WSS $= -\mu \frac{\partial u_x}{\partial r}|_{\text{wall}}$.

The axial component of the velocity u_x is already calculated by equation (4.31).

Let $u_x^* = \frac{u_x}{Q_M / \pi R_0^2}$, $R_*(z) = \frac{R(z)}{R_0}$, $\eta = \frac{r}{R(z)}$ be the non-dimensional variables. The boundary conditions are the following:

The velocity is zero at the wall: $u_x^* = 0$, for $\eta = 1$.

There is symmetry in relation to the z-axis of the tube: $\frac{\partial^3 u_x^*}{\partial \eta^3} = 0$, and $\frac{\partial u_x^*}{\partial \eta} = 0$ for $\eta = 0$.

Let the axial velocity along the z-axis be $u_x^* = w_x^*$ for $\eta = 0$.

Finally, the flow rate is conserved: $Q_* = Q/Q_M = 2R_*(z)^2 \int_0^1 u_x^* \eta d\eta$.

The coefficients A_i of equation (4.16) can also be written as

$$a_0 = w_x^*,\ a_1 = 0,\ a_2 = -4w_x^* + \frac{6Q_*}{(R_*(z))^2},\ a_3 = 0,\ a_4 = 3w_x^* - \frac{6Q_*}{(R_*(z))^2} \tag{4.32}$$

$$\therefore u_x^* = w_x^* + \left(-4w_x^* + \frac{6Q^*}{(R^*(z))^2}\right)\eta^2 + \left(3w_x^* - \frac{6Q^*}{(R^*(z))^2}\right)\eta^4. \tag{4.33}$$

Here, the polynomial degree is limited to four. Since the flow rate is known as a function of time, the determination of the A_i coefficients is equivalent to the determination of the velocity along the z-axis, i.e. u_x^*. The values of w_x^* are given by the experimental values. Finally, as $R^*(z) = 1$ downstream from the stenosis, wall shear stress can now be obtained:

$$-\frac{\partial u_x^*}{\partial \eta} = 12Q^* - 4w_x^*. \tag{4.34}$$

Wall shear-stress plots for vessels with 25% and 50% blockages are calculated using the above equation, and are presented later in this section.

Wall shear stress based descriptors are also used as markers for calculating various states of the endothelial wall of the vessel. Gradient-based descriptors and harmonic-based descriptors are calculated in this chapter. The WSS spatial gradient (WSSG) is a marker of endothelial cell tension. It is calculated from WSS gradient tensor components parallel and perpendicular to the TAWSS vector (m and n, respectively) [8]:

$$\mathrm{WSSG} = \frac{1}{T}\int_0^T \sqrt{\left(\frac{\partial \tau_{w,m}}{\partial m}\right)^2 + \left(\frac{\partial \tau_{w,n}}{\partial n}\right)^2}\, dt. \tag{4.35}$$

Figure 4.6 shows the comparative behavior of WSSG in a diseased vessel under the influence of variations in flow rates.

The maximum absolute rate of change in WSS magnitude over the cardiac cycle is also known as the temporal gradient of WSS (WSST), and it is calculated as follows:

$$\mathrm{WSST} = \max\left(\left|\frac{\partial|\tau_w|}{\partial t}\right|\right). \tag{4.36}$$

Table 4.1 shows transient evaluations of WSST in diseased and healthy arteries at Reynolds numbers Re I, Re II and Re III.

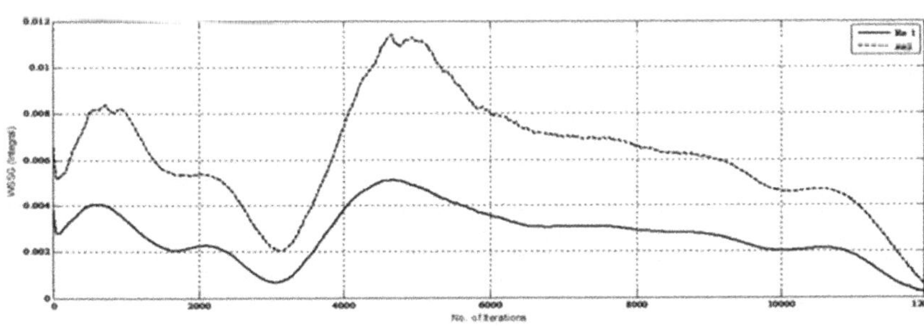

Figure 4.6. Graphical representation of WSSG distribution in diseased blood vessel at different Re.

Table 4.1. Transient form of WSST in both diseased and healthy vessels.

Viscosity model	Flow rate	Healthy vessel WSST	Diseased vessel WSST
Power-law	Re I	0.0147	0.0147
	Re II	0.0127	0.0187
	Re III	0.0094	0.0085
Quemada	Re III	0.0122	0.0101

The behavior of WSST is not similar to that of WSSG for the Quemada model. Here, the Quemada model shows better responses to WSST, but it also depends on flow rate. It is observed that WSST decreases with increased flow rate in a healthy vessel. However, an oscillatory behavior of WSST is found in diseased vessels with increased flow rate.

Figure 4.7 shows a comparative behavior of WSST in a healthy vessel under the influence of variations in flow rates. WSST in the axial direction (x-direction) is found to be more pronounced than WSST in the radial direction (y-direction) at Re I and Re II. However, with a further increase in flow rate to Re II, an oscillatory behavior of WSST is observed in both the x- and y-directions. With a further increase in flow rate to Re III, it is observed that WSST in the radial direction is greater than that in the axial direction.

The harmonic component of WSS waveforms can be a possible metric of disturbed flow. This statement is supported by results revealing that endothelial cells sense and respond to the frequency of the WSS profiles. The time varying WSS magnitude at each node can be Fourier decomposed, and the dominant harmonic (DH) is defined as the harmonic with the highest amplitude [12]. DH is calculated as

$$\text{DH} = \max(F_w(nw_0)), F_w \equiv \text{FFT}(|\tau_w|), \omega_0 = 2\pi/T. \tag{4.37}$$

Table 4.2 shows transient evaluations of DH in diseased and healthy arteries at Reynolds numbers Re I, Re II and Re III. It can be seen that the value of DH increases with increased flow rate in the diseased vessel, whereas it behaves in oscillatory manner in the healthy vessel. However, DH also shows better responses to the flow when considering the rheological properties of the fluid as in the Quemada model.

4.5.1 Oscillatory shear index

The OSI can be defined as

$$\text{OSI} = \frac{1}{2}\left(1 - \frac{\tau_{\text{mean}}}{\tau_{\text{mag}}}\right), \tag{4.38}$$

where τ_{mean} is the time-mean wall shear stress, also known as time-averaged wall shear stress (TAWSS), and τ_{mag} is the time-mean magnitude of the wall shear stress, and they are formulated using

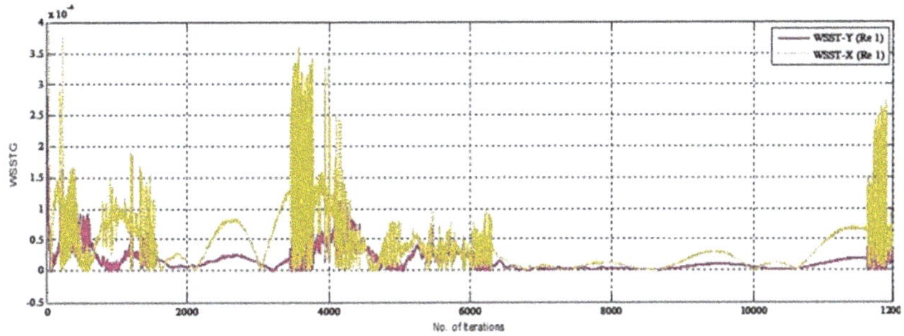

(a) Re I

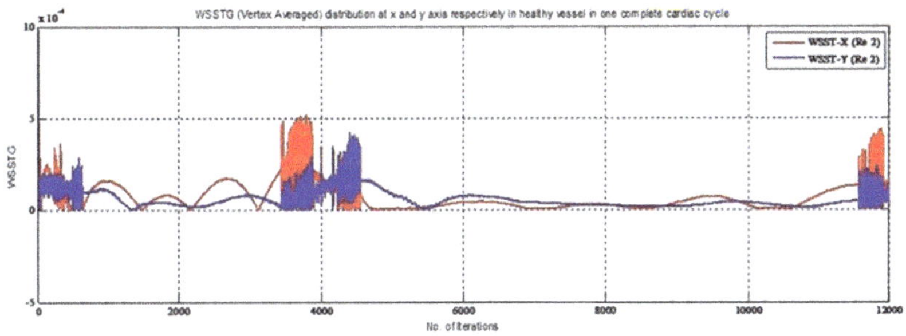

(b) Re II

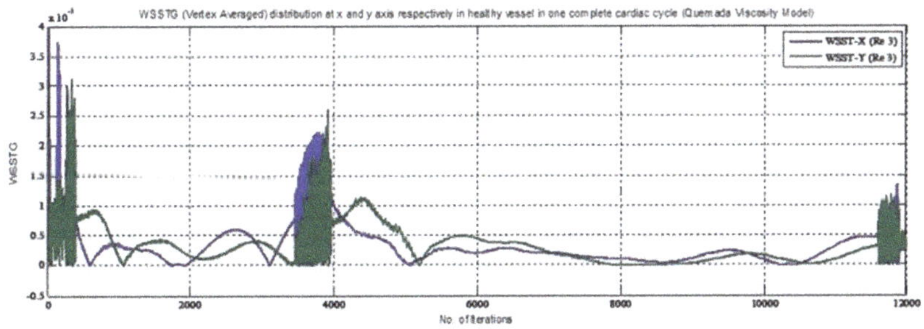

(c) Re III

Figure 4.7. Graphical representation of WSST distribution in a healthy blood vessel at (a) Re I, (b) Re II and (c) Re III.

Table 4.2. DH in both diseased and healthy vessels.

Viscosity model	Flow rate	Healthy vessel DH	Diseased vessel DH
Power-law	Re I	30.6964	30.6964
	Re II	5.5557	70.6169
	Re III	13.2493	82.7616
Quemada	Re III	24.0394	84.4652

$$\tau_{\text{mean}} = \left| \frac{1}{T} \int_0^T \tau_w dt \right| \tag{4.39}$$

$$\tau_{\text{mag}} = \frac{1}{T} \int_0^T |\tau_w| dt. \tag{4.40}$$

A low value of TAWSS (lower than 0.4 Pa) stimulates the pro-atherogenic endothelial phenotype [13], and perturbed endothelial alignments on the walls of vessels are induced at regions where the instantaneous WSS deviates from the main flow direction in a large fraction of the cardiac cycle, and it can be identified as regions of high OSI [11]. The OSI has a range between 0 and 0.5, where 0.5 defines purely oscillatory flow. Areas of high OSI would lead to endothelial dysfunction and atherogenesis and hence the detection of such zones is very important.

Figure 4.8 summarizes the endothelial OSI distribution in vessels containing abnormalities, either in the form of aneurysm or stenosis. Varying flow rates as well

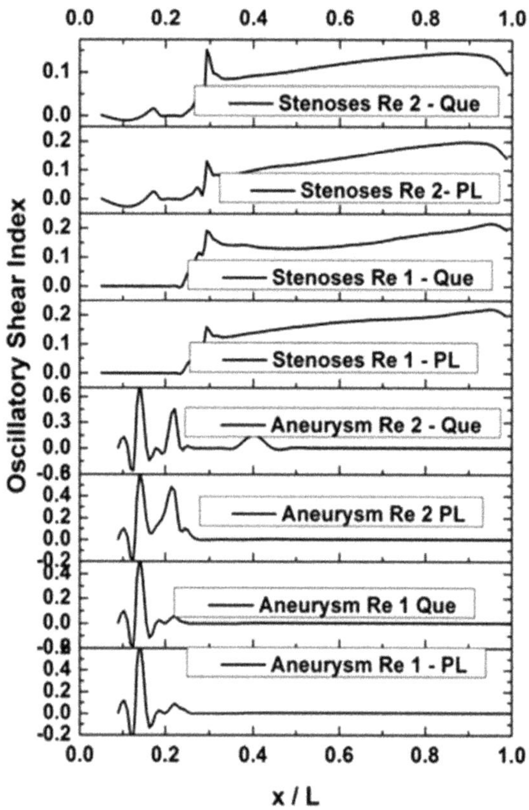

Figure 4.8. OSI distribution plot at different viscosities (PL = power-law, Que = Quemada) and at different flow rates (Re I and Re II).

as different viscosity models (namely the power-law model and Quemada model) are considered for the assessment simultaneously. Insignificant variations of OSI distributions are observed between the power-law and Quemada viscosity models. Modulation of the flow rate induces changes in OSI distribution—dual peaks are observed at higher flow rates in comparison to single peaks at lower flow rates in aneurismal vessels. The peaks of the OSI are found to be higher in magnitude as the flow rate increases in aneurismal vessels, whereas insignificant modulation of the magnitude of the same are observed in stenosed vessels, irrespective of increased flow rates.

4.5.2 Relative residual time

The combination of the OSI and TAWSS is also known as relative residual time (RRT), which is proportional to the residence time of blood particles near the wall:

$$\text{RRT} = \frac{1}{(1 - 2 \times \text{OSI}) \times \text{TAWSS}}. \tag{4.41}$$

Several studies [10, 15, 17, 18] recommended RRT as a single metric of low and oscillating shear.

RRT distributions along the entire length of endothelial linings are shown in figure 4.9. The spatial magnitude of RRT remains several folds higher in vessels with aneurysm than stenosis. The aneurismal vessel exhibits an increase in RRT values with flow rate, whereas RRT decreases with an increase in flow rate in stenosed vessels. Interestingly, an effect of the viscosity model is found in the case of RRT distributions. The peak magnitude of RRT in an aneurismal vessel is found to be higher when considering the Quemada viscosity model (about 300 ms) for a higher flow rate (Re II), whereas the power-law model exhibits a higher value of RRT (about 350 ms) for a lower flow rate (Re I). The stenosed blood vessel has the highest RRT values (about 20 ms and 10 ms for Re I and Re II, respectively) when considering the power-law viscosity model, whereas it attenuates in the Quemada model (about 12 ms and 9 ms for Re I and Re II, respectively). The maximum values of RRT distributions are found at the periphery of the aneurismal vessel, whereas they are found more in the immediate downstream in the stenosed vessel.

4.6 Conclusion

A two-dimensional axi-symmetric geometry of a blood vessel is created containing a stenosis profile, which was pre-defined according to [9]. The severity of the stenoses was varied from 25%–80% and realistic pulsating flow profiles were used to realize influx of blood through the geometry. Non-Newtonian rheological models, namely the Casson model, Carreau model, cross model, power-law model and Quemada model, are generally used along with the Newtonian model to represent the rheological properties of blood in a diseased state. Various shear-stress parameters such as WSS, OSI and RRT are used for qualitative analysis of higher stress distributions and their behavior near the wall of the vessel downstream of the stenosis. The transport phenomena of flow structures in vessels containing severe

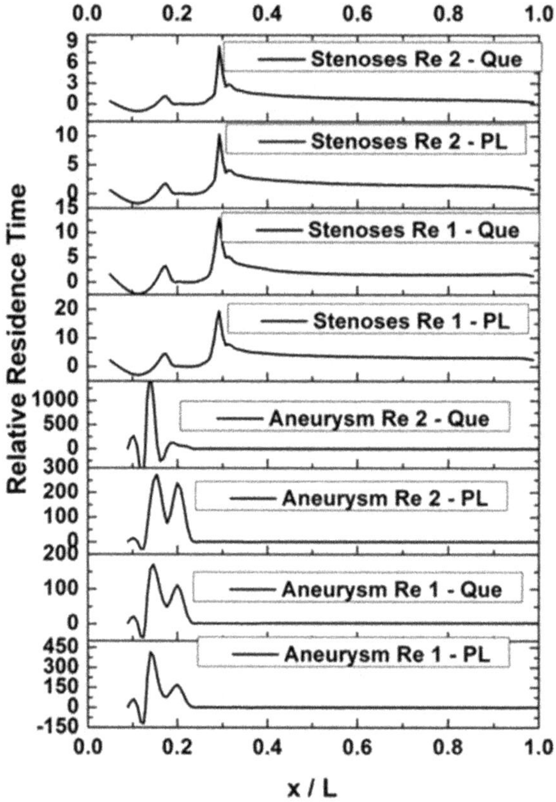

Figure 4.9. RRT distribution plot at different viscosities (PL = power-law, Que = Quemada) and at different flow rates (Re I and Re II).

aneurysms of the saccular type are also presented here. The aneurismal profile was adapted from a pre-defined aneurismal function proposed by [16]. The pulsating flow profiles discussed in this chapter are varied with different Reynolds numbers and the influences of flow rate on the depth of aneurysm are measured in the form of distributions of defined shear-stress markers at the wall i.e. WSS, OSI and RRT. Various parameters, such as mean velocity, r.m.s. velocity, turbulent intensity, velocity flatness, velocity skewness, and maximum velocity and minimum velocity over every cardiac cycle, can also be evaluated as primary parameters for evaluating the probability of secondary stenoses in post-stenotic regions. Some derivative parameters, such as WSS, stenosis length, the pressure drop coefficient and pressure recovery factors, can also be used to validate the results obtained from different numerical investigation of stenosed blood vessels in two-dimensional form.

Biological flow is a complex domain of research involving mechanics, physiology, chemistry, etc. The current chapter addresses certain issues for pathological vessels involving modeling and experiments. The following areas might motivate reader to further study:

- The transition and turbulent regimes of hemodynamics need further attention.
- The investigation of the hemodynamics of blood through smaller capillaries is an unexplored area.
- The interactions of endothelial cells on the intimal lining with the hemodynamics of blood can be investigated by conducting experiments at the cellular level.
- The investigation of changes in cellular properties in extracellular fluids on exposure to high shear rate fluid dynamics can be performed using mathematical modeling and is a potential area of research.
- The cellular diffusion of mass transport across various layers of blood vessel under the influence of high shear rate in a diseased condition of the vessel is another unexplored area.

References

[1] Bird R B, Armstrong R C and Hassager O 1987 *Dynamics of Polymeric Liquids* vol 1 (New York: Wiley)

[2] Bit A and Chattopadhyay H 2018 Acute aneurysm is more critical than acute stenoses in blood vessels: a numerical investigation using stress markers *BioNanoScience* **8** 329–36

[3] Bit A and Chattopadhyay H 2014a Assessment of rheological models for prediction of transport phenomena in stenosed artery *Prog. Comput. Fluid Dyn. Int. J.* **14** 363–74

[4] Bit A and Chattopadhyay H 2014b Numerical investigations of pulsatile flow in stenosed artery *Acta Bioeng. Biomech.* **16** 33–44

[5] Bit A, Ghagare D, Rizvanov A A and Chattopadhyay H 2017 Assessment of influences of stenoses in right carotid artery on left carotid artery using wall stress marker *BioMed. Res. Int.* **2017** 2935195

[6] Chien S, Usami S, Dellenback R and Gregersen M 1967 Blood viscosity: Influence of erythrocyte deformation *Science* **157** 827–9

[7] Cross M M 1965 Rheology of non-Newtonian fluids: a new flow equation for pseudoplastic system *J. Coll. Sci.* **20** 417–29

[8] DePaola N, Gimbrone M A, Davies P F Jr and Dewey C F 1992 Vascular endothelium responds to fluid shear stress gradients *Arterioscler. Thromb.* **12** 1254–7

[9] Drikakis D, Milionis C, Pal S K and Shapiro E 2011 Assessment of the applicability of analytical models for blood flow prediction in reconstructive surgery *Int. J. Numer. Methods Biomed. Eng.* **27** 993–9

[10] He X and Ku D N 1996 Pulsatile flow in the human left coronary artery bifurcation: average conditions *ASME J. Biomech. Eng.* **118** 74–82

[11] Himburg H A, Grzybowski D M, Hazel A, LaMack J A, Li X M and Friedman M H 2004 Spatial comparison between wall shear stress measures and porcine arterial endothelial permeability *Am. J. Physiol. Heart Circ.* **286** 1916–22

[12] Himburg H A and Friedman M H 2006 Correspondence of low mean shear and high harmonic content in the porcine iliac arteries *J. Biomech. Eng.* **128** 852–6

[13] Huang C, Chai Z and Shi B 2013 Non-Newtonian effects on hemodynamic characteristics of blood flow in stented cerebral aneurysm *Commun. Comput. Phys.* **13** 916–28

[14] Jespersen S N and Østergaard L 2012 The roles of cerebral blood flow, capillary transit time heterogeneity and oxygen tension in brain oxygenation and metabolism *J. Cereb. Blood Flow Metab.* **32** 264–77

[15] Lee S W, Antiga L and Steinman D A 2009 Correlations among indicators of disturbed flow at the normal carotid bifurcation *ASME J. Biomech. Eng.* **131** 061013

[16] Molla M M and Paul M C 2012 LES of non-Newtonian physiological blood flow in a model of arterial stenosis *J. Med. Eng. Phys.* **34** 1079–87

[17] Morbiducci U, Gallo D, Ponzini R, Massai D, Antiga L, Redaelli A, Deriu M A and Montevecchi F M 2011 On the importance of blood rheology for bulk flow in hemodynamic models of the carotid bifurcation *J. Biomech.* **44** 2427–38

[18] Morbiducci U, Gallo D, Ponzini R, Massai D, Consolo F, Bignardi C, Deriu M A, Antiga L and Redaelli A 2010 Outflow conditions for image-based haemodynamic models of the carotid bifurcation. Implications for indicators of abnormal flow *J. Biomech. Eng.* **132** 091005

[19] Neofytou P and Drikakis D 2003 Effects of blood models on flow through a stenosis *Int. J. Numer. Methods Fluid* **43** 597–635

[20] Quemada D 1977 Rheology of concentrated disperse systems III. General features of the proposed non-Newtonian model. Comparison with experimental data *Rheol. Acta* **17** 643–53

[21] Rhie C M and Chow W L 1983 Numerical study of the turbulent flow past an airfoil with trailing edge separation *AIAA J.* **21** 1525–32

[22] Tan F P P, Soloperto G, Bashford S, Wood N B, Thom S, Hughes A and Xu X Y 2008 Analysis of flow disturbance in a stenosed carotid artery bifurcation using two-equation transitional and turbulence models *J. Biomech. Eng.* **130** 061008

[23] Walburn F J and Schneck D J 1976 A constitutive equation for whole human blood *Biorheology* **13** 201–19

IOP Publishing

Vascular and Intravascular Imaging Trends, Analysis, and Challenges, Volume 1
Stent applications
Petia Radeva and Jasjit S Suri

Chapter 5

Fast virtual endovascular stenting: technique, validation and applications in computational haemodynamics

Ignacio Larrabide

5.1 Motivation

Although most intracranial aneurysms (IAs) remain asymptomatic, some of them tend to grow and eventually rupture. The rupture of these aneurysms has an incidence of 1%–2% in the adult population [1]. The rupture of an aneurysm leaks blood into the space occupied by cerebro-spinal fluid (CSF). This event is called a sub-arachnoid haemorrhage (SAH), which is associated with significant indices of morbidity and mortality. Between 10% and 20% of SAH patients die before receiving medical attention [2] and approximately one third die in the first 30 days after their intake, resulting in an overall mortality rate of 50% [3]. Of the patients who survive, between a third and half have neurological sequelae.

In addition to symptomatic aneurysms, it is expected that between 0.1%–0.5% of all magnetic resonance imaging (MRI) and computed tomography (CT) studies performed per year will lead to the incidental discovery of asymptomatic IAs in patients arriving at the hospital for other reasons. Therefore, the decision of whether to treat a patient with an IA must take many aspects into consideration. Different risk factors have been associated with an increased likelihood of rupture and often some kind of treatment is required [4, 5]. Neurovascular specialists currently consider many features as important when evaluating unruptured intracranial aneurysms (UIAs). The size of the IA, any history of sub-arachnoid haemorrhage and an AI located in the posterior circulation are the most significant risk factors indicating rupture of UIAs. However, a full understanding of the nature of UIAs is lacking [6].

doi:10.1088/2053-2563/ab01fach5

Taking all the risk factors into consideration, the selection of an appropriate treatment for an IA patient should consider a balance between the risk of aneurysm rupture and the risk of treatment. In the last decade, there have been major advances in the diagnosis and treatment of IAs as a result of major technological developments in diagnostic imaging and intervention as well as a new generation of therapeutic devices [7].

When treating IAs, stents can be used as a scaffold to maintain coils inside the aneurysm cavity when treating broad-neck aneurysms [8]. However, the implantation of neurovascular stents has shown to have an impact on the local curvature of the vessel [9, 10]. Previous studies have proven that, apart from their role as a mechanical support, stents used as scaffolds can also play a role in the diversion of flow away from the aneurysm [11].

In the past few years, computational modelling of intracranial stenting allowed the development of different studies that help in understanding the effects of treatment under different circumstances. The study of local haemodynamics in IAs has proven to be essential in understanding this disease and its various treatment alternatives. Recent advances in computational capabilities have made this possible, leading to a huge development of the field of bio-medical engineering in the study of IAs. Early work by Cebral *et al* [12] was focused on assessing the risk of rupture of IAs, and evaluating the effect of having cyclic topology in the cerebral vasculature [13]. The work of Meng *et al* [14, 15] showed that complex haemodynamics at the apex of an arterial bifurcation induces vascular remodelling resembling aneurysm initiation. In their study, the authors used computational fluid dynamics (CFD) to reproduce haemodynamic conditions at bifurcations which were then compared to biological tissue samples subject to equivalent flow insult. Geers *et al* have focused on studying the sensitivity of computational haemodynamics to different imaging modalities [16], where patient-specific flow simulations were performed from computed tomography angiography (CTA) and three-dimensional rotational angiography (3DRA) for 11 individuals. The effect of steady-state versus transient simulations was also assessed, showing a remarkable reduction in computational time [17].

In addition, flow diversion has gained considerable attention for its high rate of success and simplicity [18–21]. To better understand these mechanisms anatomically and bio-mechanically, different computational techniques have been developed [22, 23], which should be properly evaluated before becoming part of everyday clinical practice. In this text we describe some of the latest advances in IA modelling and its applications in the study of intra-aneurysmal haemodynamics.

5.2 Virtual stenting

A considerable amount of work has been devoted over the past few years to developing computational models of cerebrovascular stents, their physical behaviour and to assess their efficiency for treatment using computational simulation.

The first models for the computational simulation of stents were developed for modelling coronary stents. These approaches were primarily based on the finite element method (FEM) and aimed at modelling the stent's mechanical properties and its interaction with the vessel wall from a strictly mechanical point of view [24, 25]. The fact that coronary stenting is typically done with balloon-inflated stents, posed additional problems for their modelling. In many cases, the treatment of coronaries requires more than one device, which has also been considered more recently [26, 27].

Modelling of cerebral stets has also been considered from a purely mechanical point of view. Initial work by De Beule *et al* was aimed at the optimization of braided cerebral stents, through detailed modelling using the FEM [28]. More recent work by Ma and co-workers presents a methodology for the mechanical FEM simulation of densely braided cerebral stents, which is used for modelling in detail the device mechanics and its individual threads and their behaviour during treatment [29, 30]. These methods are extremely accurate in modelling the mechanical behaviour of the stent and its interaction with the vessel wall. However, their set-up and computational time can be extensive, making their use in daily clinical practice cumbersome.

The early work of Ohta *et al* [31, 32] showed the effects of stents in intra-aneurysmal haemodynamics, proving the feasibility of computational models in assessing the stenting treatment of aneurysms. In the work of Cebral and Lohner [12], further developed by Appanaboyina *et al* [33], a deformable cylinder model is used to adjust an intracranial stent to the patient anatomy. Later, the design of the stent is mapped onto the deformed cylinder to obtain a 3D representation of the deployed stent. Janiga and colleagues [34] proposed a free-form deformation method, which allows the virtual implantation of intracranial stent models into complex patient-specific geometries. This technique was also used in combination with CFD simulations to characterize the inflow and the corresponding residence time in the aneurysm. The work of Peack *et al* has explored the use of deformable models in combination with lineal and torsional spring analogies to deploy different kinds of stents in realistic geometries. Furthermore, they explored the use of thrombosis models to study the occlusion of intracranial aneurysms [35]. These methods make extensive use of simplification assumptions, making them computationally more efficient and simpler. However, they are not capable of representing many of the details of these stents' behaviour and their interaction with the vessel wall.

In this chapter we present results obtained for techniques assuming simplification assumptions, designed for a faster performance. This technique is considered to be simple, keeping in mind its potential use in a clinical context. In the following section the fast virtual stenting (FVS) method is described. This method is based on an extension of simplex deformable models with stent-specific geometrical constraints.

5.3 The fast virtual stenting method

The fast virtual stenting (FVS) method was initially developed to serve as a tool for treatment planning and to provide a fast and simple representation of different stent models inside the patient's own anatomy. FVS is based on simplex deformable meshes and geometrical constraints that account for the shape and design of the stent being modelled, and was initially developed a few years ago [36, 37].

Deformable simplex models have been previously used by Delingette *et al* [38] in object reconstruction and by Montagnat and Delingette for free-form [39] and constrained [40] deformation. The main idea behind this methodology is the use of a second-order partial differential equation for moving a mesh under the effect of internal and external forces. A numerical approximation is obtained by a finite difference discretization, which can be written as

$$\mathbf{p}_i^{t+1} = \mathbf{p}_i^t + (1 - \gamma)\left(\mathbf{p}_i^t - \mathbf{p}_i^{t-1}\right) + \alpha \mathbf{f}_{\text{int}}\left(\mathbf{p}_i^t\right) + \beta \mathbf{f}_{\text{ext}}\left(\mathbf{p}_i^t\right). \tag{5.1}$$

These models are usually discretized using simplex meshes, where at the mesh boundary a free boundary condition is used. In $\mathbb{R}^3$, two-simplex meshes are surface representations that are closely related to triangular meshes. In particular, the underlying graph that defines them is dual (figure 5.1). Complementary definitions and additional information on simplex meshes can be found in the work of Delingette [38].

Additionally, simplex meshes are not appropriate for representing stents as these usually do not comply with the definition of a two-simplex mesh. To overcome this limitation, geometrical information of the stent is also taken into account. This can be obtained from a μ-CT scan of the stent or directly from the stent manufacturer when possible. Geometrical characteristics of the stent in the 'free' state (i.e. expanded outside the vessel) are used to guide the deformation of the mesh. The geometrical characteristics recorded from the free state are set as the reference configuration for the geometrical constraints. Four geometrical constraints are considered:

- *Stent design* (strut pattern): As most stents have a repeating cell design, the stent is modelled as a set of cells (figure 5.1(a)). By the repetition of stent cells, the design of the whole stent is built. This approach allows mapping any stent design on the simplex mesh by a simple repetition process.
- *Strut length*: Total length of a strut between the two ends where it is attached to the stent mesh. This length is measured at the nominal ('free') configuration.

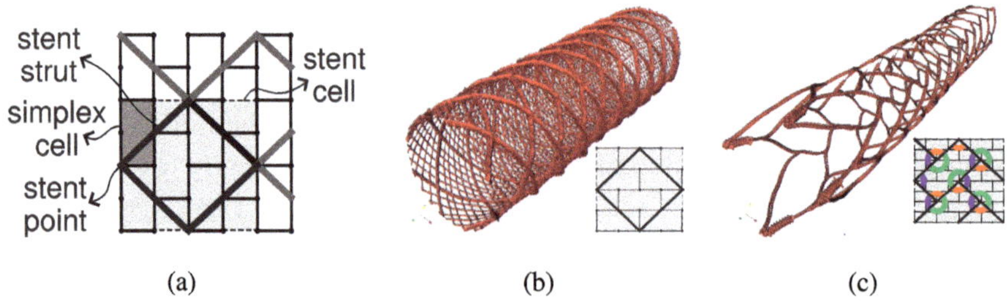

Figure 5.1. (a) Example of a simplex mesh. The stent cells contain the information and description of the stent design. (b) Example of an Enterprise stent (Cordis Neurovascular, Miami Lakes, FL, USA) and its representation. (c) Example of a Silk stent (Balt Extrusion, Paris, France) and its representation.

- *Angle between struts*: Angle between pairs of struts. This angle is measured at the nominal configuration.
- *Deployed stent radius*: Corresponds to the stent radius in the free state configuration and is considered as the equilibrium position for the expanding force.

There are two reasons for using these constraints. First, these parameters are sufficient to describe the global stent geometry if we are not interested in the detailed structural behaviour of the stent, where additional information such as strut cross-sectional shape, as well as distal and proximal stent designs, would be required. Second, this information is relatively easy to obtain for different stents. Such information is stored in a subset of points of the simplex mesh that we call stent points.

The proposed method does not ensure nor force that the final configuration of the stent fully conforms to the nominal stent configuration, implying that these are imposed as 'soft' constraints. In this way, the deformation is stopped when internal and external forces are balanced. The reason for using this simplification is that the stent constraints are measured for the free state when released outside the vessel. When released inside a vessel, the stent does not recover the free state configuration. Then, the use of soft constraints, where a balance between internal and external forces is required, seems more appropriate.

5.4 Validation—how accurate is accurate enough?

The FVS method has been developed as a technique for modelling different types of stents implanted in intracranial aneurysms keeping in mind its use by clinicians. For this reason, its computational efficiency and associated simulation time were specifically taken into account as important factors. This method was also designed to evaluate local haemodynamic alterations after stent implantation, by the use of CFD.

The shape of the stent after implantation is considered for its validation, and the effects of each model on posterior CFD simulations are also evaluated. The FVS method has been validated using FEM models, and later combined with CFD. The validation of FVS is developed in two stages. The FVS method is compared to FEM models with different degrees of complexity, starting with highly detailed descriptions of the mechanics of the stent and vessel wall, which are progressively simplified [41].

5.4.1 FVS versus FEM—mechanics

In this study, the possibility of introducing suitable approximations in the computational models to progressively reduce their complexity and computational time was studied. Two main questions were investigated in this study: (i) how much the stent and vessel wall models have to be simplified to reduce the computational time such that these methodologies can be suitable for the clinical environment and (ii) what information we lose by simplifying these models and what its significance is. It is worth noting that during the interventional procedure a number of variables cannot be precisely controlled, such as the exact position of the stent within the vessel. This issue needs to be taken into account when evaluating the clinical applicability of different computational approaches.

A self-expanding stent, made of a nickel–titanium alloy and resembling the Neuroform stent (Boston Scientific, Natick, MA, USA), was considered. Its geometry was obtained from a μ-CT scan of the real stent (figure 5.2) [42]. The stent is expanded inside an idealized vessel geometry, similar to those harbouring cerebral aneurysms. An idealized situation, where the aneurysm dome is assumed not to significantly affect the released stent configuration, was considered. Thus, only the elliptic aneurysm orifice was reproduced.

Different modelling approaches were considered and compared, characterized by an increasing level of simplification in terms of numerical method (FEM to deformable mesh), geometry (3D to 1D) and material properties (hyper-elastic vessel wall to rigid). Five different FE models were considered. Both 3D and 1D models were adopted for the stent, using eight-node brick elements or two-node linear beam elements for the model discretization, respectively. Figure 5.3(a) shows the simplification in stent geometry with struts and links modelled as 1D beam elements. A total of 64 nodes, having the same geometrical coordinates in the two meshes, are selected as reference points (figure 5.2). The ability of nickel–titanium alloy to recover its original shape (the pseudo-elastic effect) is described by the use of a previously developed user subroutine [43]. Average values for NiTinol are used as material parameters of the material model since the specific properties for the Neuroform stent were not available [25, 44]. For the vessel wall modelling, a single homogeneous layer is considered and discretized by a mesh of three-node shell elements.

Three different constitutive models are chosen to describe the mechanical behaviour of the wall: a hyper-elastic isotropic model whose parameters are derived from experimental data on cerebral vessels [45], a linear elastic isotropic model with a Young's modulus corresponding to the initial behaviour ($\lambda < 1.09$) of the hyper-elastic curve and a rigid body model. Finally, the FVS method is used in the last case. No material property definitions are required by this methodology, and only geometrical information about the stent is needed, as described in the previous section. The six computational approaches are applied to four different neck-stent relative initial positions (positions A–D in figure 5.3(b)), corresponding to various small translations and/or rotations of the stent. The expanded configurations of the

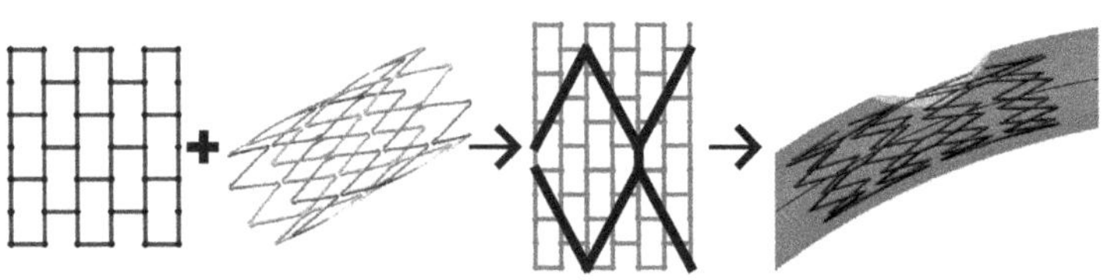

Figure 5.2. The stent geometry is represented by a subset of points on the simplex mesh, which is then expanded inside the vessel.

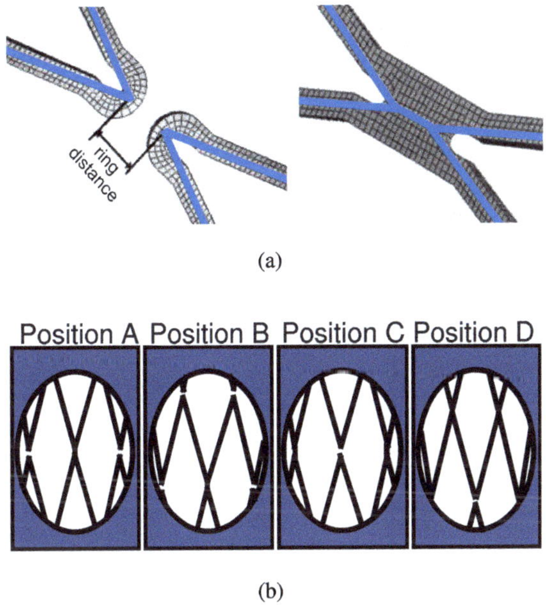

Figure 5.3. (a) Geometry simplification between FEM 3D and FEM 1D models. (b) Details of the four different stent positions evaluated.

3D FEM model with a hyper-elastic wall (FE3H) is selected as the gold-standard, as it represents the most detailed and complex model.

This validation helps in understanding the implications of each simplification while the time complexity of the simulations was decreased. This study showed that:

- Neglecting the mechanical properties of the stent is the main reason for differences in performance both globally and locally (neck area) across different models.
- Neglecting vessel deformability (as in 3D FEM rigid (FE3R) and 1D FEM rigid (FE1R)) also influences the results, implying differences of around 6% across models, mainly in the radial components.
- Considering 3D or 1D struts and links, the models do not induce significant differences in the final configuration of the stent.
- Considering 1D models instead of 3D models allows reduction of the computational cost from 32 727 s (FE3H) to 98 s (FE1R), down to 5 s (FVS).

During the intervention, the orientation of the stent in the vessel is not precisely controlled by the interventional radiologist. Even if the intention of the radiologist is to position the stent in position A, the three other positions investigated (positions B–D, figure 5.3) could be used. We used the four FE3H positions to reproduce the variability in stent location during its implantation. The variability of 35% in the deployed configurations observed in the four FE3H results suggests that all the investigated computational approaches, showing differences lower than 25% in predicting the deployed stent configuration, could provide useful indications from a clinical point of view. Furthermore, simulating the deployment of a Neuroform-like stent may be considered a worst-case scenario for the bench-marked virtual stenting tools, since this stent shows an open-cell design, which highlights the differences in release configurations in the neck region.

The FEM simulations provide very accurate information on the residual stresses and tensions on the stent and the vessel wall. However, the set-up of the simulations is complex and the complexity of the geometry can cause the simulation to end, which is usually related to the convergence and stability of the associated numerical methods.

5.4.2 FVS versus FEM—fluid dynamics

In this section, the FEM and FVS methods for stent deployment described in the previous section are used to obtain the deployed stent representation and CFD simulations are performed for each model. The purpose of this analysis is to understand the influence of the stent modelling approach on simulated intra-aneurysmal haemodynamics.

5.4.2.1 CFD models of stented aneurysmatic vessels

For the generation of CFD models, both the vessel and the stent surface meshes are used. Unstructured tetrahedral elements are generated in ICEM-CFD (ANSYS Inc, Berkeley, CA, USA). The volumetric elements are transferred to the finite volume-based commercial CFD code, CFX (ANSYS Inc., Berkeley, CA, USA). The Navier–Stokes equations are solved with a second-order backward Euler scheme under the assumption of in-compressible, laminar and Newtonian fluid inside a rigid wall boundary. The viscosity and the density of the fluid were matched with experiments at 3.5 cP and 1056 kg m^{-3}, respectively. A pulsatile velocity waveform of a 1 Hz sinus with an average flow rate of 3 cc s^{-1} was imposed at the inlet. The outlets were set to zero pressure (both outlets are at the same distance from the aneurysm). To mimic the effect of contrast injection on the flow rate for each case, the shape of the contrast density curve extracted from the corresponding image sequence was re-scaled to match the volume of 6 cc and superimposed on the flow at the inlet. The same time density curve was imposed at the inlet and the scalar transport equation was time resolved. The initial condition effect on the solution was eliminated by extending the simulation time to three full cardiac cycles. As we are interested in modelling the blood flow in the lumen of a vessel containing a stent, the stent geometry is explicitly meshed and its volume (i.e. the stent struts) is represented as a void within the vessel lumen. A non-slip boundary condition is considered over the surface of the stent and on the surface of the vessel. The stent mesh is cut and the struts lying on the vessel wall are removed. It has been proved that using the patch of the stent over the ostium instead of the whole stent is effective, thus significantly reducing the computational cost of the CFD simulations and preserving the intra-aneurysmal haemodynamics [33].

A qualitative comparison across the five stented cases (intra-position) and between the two stent positions (inter-position, positions A and B in figure 5.3(b)) was performed from the geometrical point of view. First, the hyper-elastic properties of the vessel produced a change of the aneurysm ostium to a more circular shape, and a longitudinal straightening of the vessel in the stented part. Second, FVS showed a different configuration of the stent in both positions compared to the other stented cases, with a greater ring opening and enlarged links. Third, the stent position produced a different stent configuration above the ostium. For example, the asymmetry of the link in position B allowed the struts to protrude into the aneurysm, as is seen for cases FE3H, FE3R and FE1H, but not for cases FE1R and FVS. On the other hand, the symmetric link in posB prevented the struts from protruding and none of the FE cases showed significant differences [41].

Three haemodynamic variables were observed: wall shear stress reduction as a percentage of the pre-treatment condition (WSS%), mean velocity inside the aneurysm after treatment (v%) and mass inflow rate after treatment (mIR%). These results showed a reduction of intra-aneurysm haemodynamic parameters due to the presence of the stents. In position A, the mean values of WSS%, v% and mIR% of the five stented cases were 43%, 40% and 51%, respectively. The intra-position inter-model variability of these parameters ranged between 10% and 15%. In position B, whilst WSS% and v% were comparable with those of position A, mIR% was almost 66%. The inter-model intra-position variability of these parameters ranged from 12% (WSS%) up to 25% (mIR%).

These results indicate that simulating the deployment of a stent in aneurysmatic vessels, depending on the computational approach adopted, allows important effects on intra-aneurysmal haemodynamics to be represented in the succeeding CFD simulations. It was shown that, independent of the stent deployment approach, the insertion of the Neuroform stent model in an idealized aneurysmatic cerebral vessel produced a reduction of average WSS and average velocity inside the aneurysm of almost 50%.

Neuroform is an open-cell stent with no symmetry in the disposition of the links, so the screen effect on blood flow and the possibility of protrusion of struts towards the aneurysm depends on the orientation and position of the stent in the vessel [46]. Hirabayashi *et al* found that the orientation and position of high-porosity stents influence the amount of flow reduction in the aneurysm [47]. In our study, all the cases highlighted inter-position differences in intra-aneurysmal haemodynamics, even though those which combine simplifications (FE1R and FVS) did not show the same trend between position A and position B in all the parameters analysed, as the others did. Furthermore, they resulted in greater inter-position variability.

The present numerical simulation study shows how the choice of computational approach for deploying the stent influences the CFD analysis, particularly in terms of intra-aneurysmal flow. Variability in the intra-aneurysmal haemodynamics existed across the cases, varying according to the parameter analysed and the initial position of the stent considered. The reasons for this variability were discussed and analysed. Average WSS and average velocity were the parameters less affected by the computational approach for deployment and different positioning of the stent. Nevertheless, in all the analyses carried out, an important reduction of intra-aneurysmal flow was clearly induced in all modelled stent–vessel scenarios.

5.4.3 FVS—real versus virtual angiographies

To simulate an angiography, the injection of a contrast agent (dye) was performed by solving the transport (convection–diffusion) equation. The dye was modelled as a massless scalar passively transported by the fluid. In this case, no flow rate change due to the injection of the dye was considered. The temporal terms in the equations were discretized by using an Euler implicit scheme, and the spatial terms were discretized with second-order accuracy.

In figure 5.4, longitudinal and transversal middle cut planes of the vessel show the dye intensity distribution in the parent vessel at three different time steps. The aneurysm filling with the dye (1.125 s) starts impinging the distal part of the ostium and begins a counter clockwise vortex. Then, during the wash out phase (1.7 s), the remaining dye inside the dome is diluted and more layers of the vortex appear towards the aneurysm tip. Two cardiac cycles after the end of the injection (3 s), the vessel dye is completely washed out. However, an average of 0.1% concentration of dye still remains in the dome. The presence of the stent screens the flow entering the aneurysm, decreasing the concentration of dye in the aneurysm. This phenomenon is well represented by all the cases. At 1.7 s, the FE1R and FVS of position A (as in figure 5.3(b)) have some differences to the other cases in terms of the amount and distribution of the dye. Compared to position A, position B shows a generally higher amount of dye flowing inside the aneurysm. In position B, the dye seems to have the same distribution in the FE cases with the same vessel properties. Minor differences were observed for FVS.

5.5 Discussion and future work

FVS has been used for modelling stenting treatment in IAs under different circumstances. In this section we summarize the related work available in the literature. This list is not exhaustive and it is focused on technical studies.

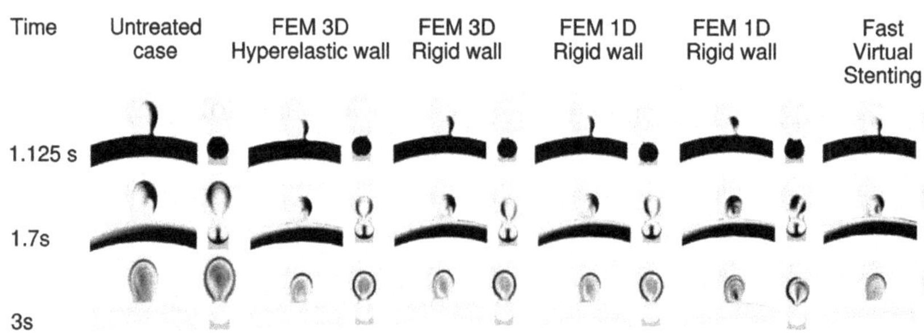

(a)

Figure 5.4. A longitudinal and perpendicular cut across the centre of the aneurysm. The contour plot at each cut plane is coloured by the dye intensity at that point at the instants indicated on the left. Each column corresponds to a different model for virtual stent deployment. It can be observed that similar patterns are presented by the different models.

5.5.1 Comparison of steady-state and transient blood flow simulations of intracranial aneurysms

In the study of Geers *et al* [48], the aim was comparing steady-state simulations to transient simulations for one terminal and one lateral aneurysm. Time-varying CFD simulations capture the variability of blood flow within the cardiac cycle and are commonly used for research purposes, where a detailed analysis of the flow variability is of interest. However, steady-state simulations are less computationally expensive while still providing useful information on the main flow characteristics and WSS distribution under the assumption that the flow phenomena of interest are steady. Such an essential modelling approach might ease the introduction of haemodynamic simulations into clinical practice.

In the cited study, the flow reduction due to placement of endovascular treatment devices for a flow rate waveform (FRW) with an averaged value was evaluated. A SILK stent with 0.06 mm diameter struts (Balt Extrusion, Montmorency, France) was virtually deployed using a deformable model approach constrained by stent and vessel geometry. This type of stent has flow diverting capabilities due to the dense structure of struts.

In figure 5.5, the average WSS on the aneurysm is plotted for different FRWs. The difference between steady-state and transient simulations was in all cases below 5% for the time-averaged WSS. The minimum and maximum WSS differed by less than 20% and were often under- and overestimated, respectively. Generally, the relative difference remained constant with increasing heart rate; it was larger for higher pulsatility indices and smaller for higher average flow rates.

For Reynolds numbers above 300 no steady-state simulations of the lateral aneurysm converged to a steady solution, which is mostly due to the oscillatory nature of flow in such a region. Unless the flow phenomena of interest are steady,

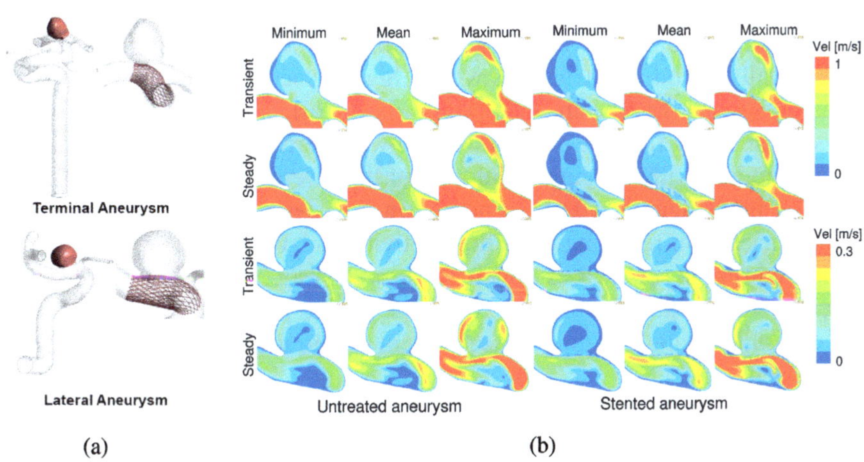

Figure 5.5. (a) Aneurysm models (terminal and lateral) evaluated in the study. The aneurysm and the virtually implanted stent are highlighted in red. (b) Haemodynamic simulation results for the untreated and stent treated case. It can be observed that the differences between the steady and time-averaged simulations are local, not affecting the spatial distribution of maxima and minima.

steady-state simulations show some limitations in such cases. This was thoroughly investigated in follow-up work, but in the absence of endovascular stents [17].

It was found that the haemodynamic information obtained from steady-state simulations is very similar for a number of FRWs, especially in comparison to the current sensitivities in haemodynamic modelling that give rise to large quantitative uncertainties. Although this study showed encouraging results, future work should comprise a larger population to take into account a wider range of possible geometries.

5.5.2 Haemodynamic alterations of intracranial aneurysms induced by virtual stent deployment

It has been recognized that the flow in a stented aneurysm is influenced by multiple factors of the stent geometry, such as strut size and stent porosity. However, the impact of the stent positioning has not been clarified yet. In [49], the effects of various stent axial orientations on aneurysm haemodynamics were studied.

The flow fields obtained from CFD for each aneurysm model were investigated through several haemodynamic parameters. The flow of the parent vessel and the aneurysm were also analysed at the peak systole. In addition to the qualitative comparison of the models, aneurysmal flow was quantitatively examined. To study the influence of stent positioning on the haemodynamic force on the aneurysm wall, the peak systolic WSSs of the aneurysm models were illustrated with the contour plots. The stenting effect of the models with a time-dependent aneurysmal flow velocity, vorticity and WSS variations for an entire cardiac cycle were also compared.

It was observed that because the vessel lumen became narrow after stenting, the computed flow speed in the stented vessel was faster than before placing the stent, with an increase of about 5.4% and 6.3% for the stents tested. Despite the impinging zone WSS being high, the WSS was remarkably low at the dome of the aneurysm, which is usually found in aneurysms with a high aspect ratio.

It was also found that the changes in flow due to orientation are closely related to stent design, showing that the peak systolic flow pattern and WSS distribution of the aneurysm models with varying axial orientation were substantially different for different designs (figure 5.6). Depending on the design, each stent presented a different efficiency in reducing both flow activity and WSS in the aneurysm. It was also observed that in some cases flow into the aneurysm could be increased, because of the effective cross-sectional area reduction at the parent vessel, for some stent designs. This highlights the importance of stent design in achieving the desired effect after treatment.

It was found that the flow speed in the stented artery was faster (1.5%–2.5%) than in the unstented artery. In a similar way, aneurysmal flow activity and haemodynamic forces acting on the wall were reinforced when the scaffolding of the stent was not sufficiently strong.

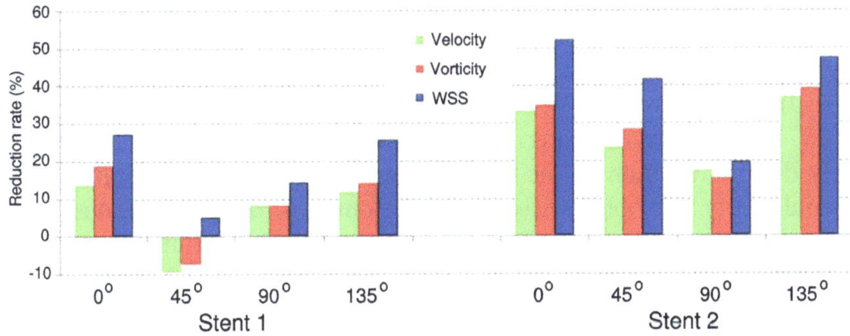

Figure 5.6. Comparison between flow alterations (velocity, vorticity and WSS) for different angulations in steps of 45° for the two stent designs studied. It can be observed that the alterations can be considerable depending on the stent design. Also, increases in flow can be observed in some situations.

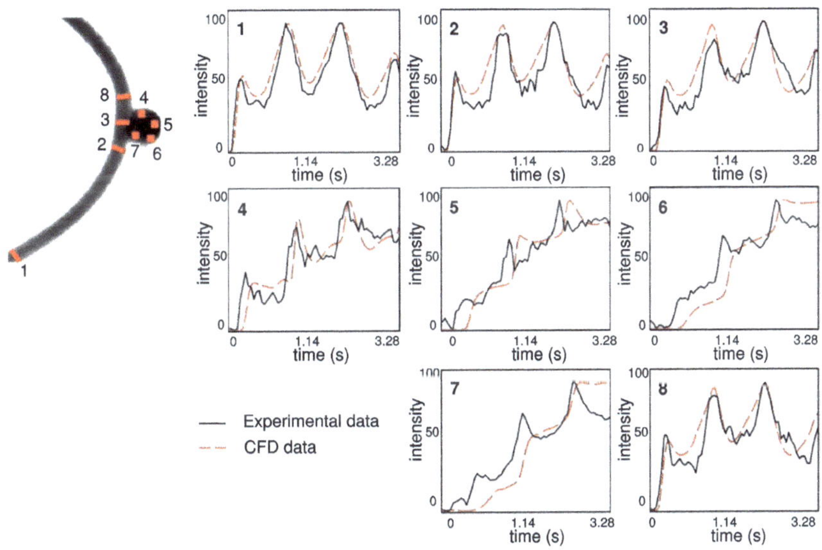

Figure 5.7. In the upper left corner is shown an x-ray image of the phantom used in the experiments when completely filled by contrast. The eight plots on the right of the figure correspond to the TICs extracted from acquired angiograms (black) and virtual angiograms (red) at the eight control points marked on the phantom. The time recordings match for all the plots.

5.5.3 Reproducibility of virtual angiographies by computational haemodynamics simulations in a stented aneurysm model

In the work of Sun *et al* [50], virtual angiographies were used to verify the capability of CFD for predicting the flow inside an aneurysm after flow diverter treatment. For validation, virtual angiograms were quantitatively compared to experimental angiograms using time intensity curves (TICs) in predefined regions of interest in the aneurysm and nearby (figure 5.7). Ground truth flow measurements were obtained from an *in vitro* phantom experiment. Due to the large amount of elements required for an explicit computational mesh, a smaller portion of the virtual stent was used for flow simulation.

The virtual and experimental angiograms show similar flow features, such as the intensity variation between different locations, the impingement site and the rotational flow. However, in the experimental angiogram the contrast is found to be less uniformly distributed than in the virtual angiogram (figure 5.7). Similar trends in terms of pulsatility and bolus arrival time are found for different regions of interest, which correspond to the phantom inlet, aneurysm neck, and upstream and downstream regions to the aneurysm (regions indicated with 1, 2, 3, 4 and 8). The strong match in these regions implies that CFD has the capacity of predicting flow under the assumptions considered. In some cases, in the comparison between the simulated and experimental TICs, mainly at the impingement site, a minor delay is observed. However, the strong pulsatility pattern is still well preserved. In addition, the simulated flow curve is found to be smoother and presents fewer fluctuations than the actual flow curve.

5.5.4 Effect of vascular morphology on haemodynamics after flow diverter placement in intracranial aneurysms

The relation between vascular morphology and the reduction of haemodynamic forces in the aneurysm after flow diverter treatment was studied in [37]. In this work, vascular morphology was studied and quantified following methodologies proposed in previous studies [51].

Vascular morphology was described in terms of the centerline, vessel diameter and curvature using the Vascular Modeling Toolkit (VMTK) package. From the centerline, two variables were considered (figure 5.8(a)):

- D_{pc}: this variable characterizes the distance from the aneurysm ostium (i.e. the origin of the bifurcating branch going into the aneurysm) to the peak curvature before the aneurysm along the vessel centerline.
- a_o: this variable quantifies the angle between the aneurysm vector (i.e. the vector pointing into the aneurysm of the local reference system defined in the aneurysm bifurcation) and the local osculating plane (defined form the local Frenet frame on the parent vessel at the location of the bifurcation).

Also, all vascular geometries were characterized in terms of the length of the model l_S, defined as the length between the proximal end of the ICA visible from the model and the ICA bifurcation.

Figure 5.8 presents the haemodynamic results for two cases that illustrate the differences for different geometrical configurations. For aneurysms far from the curvature peak, the flow into the aneurysm is largely reduced. For the aneurysm near the curvature peak, a strong vortex generated at that location progresses into the aneurysm creating a major flow stream into it. After placement of the flow diverter (FD), the first case presents a stronger cessation of flow motion inside the aneurysm. On the other hand, the inflow in the aneurysm near the curvature peak is not strongly affected by the presence of the FD. For the two exemplary cases

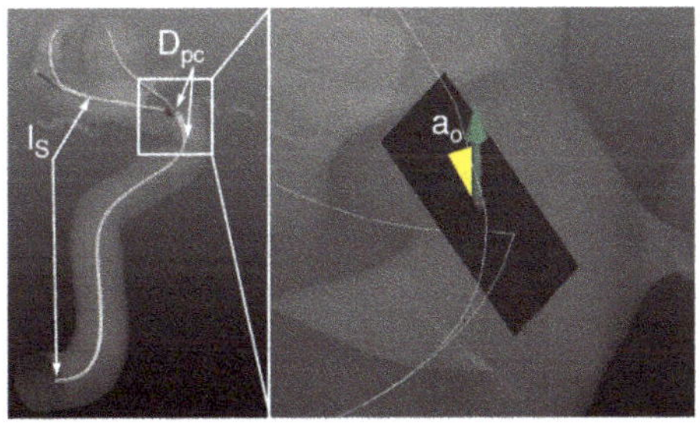

(a)

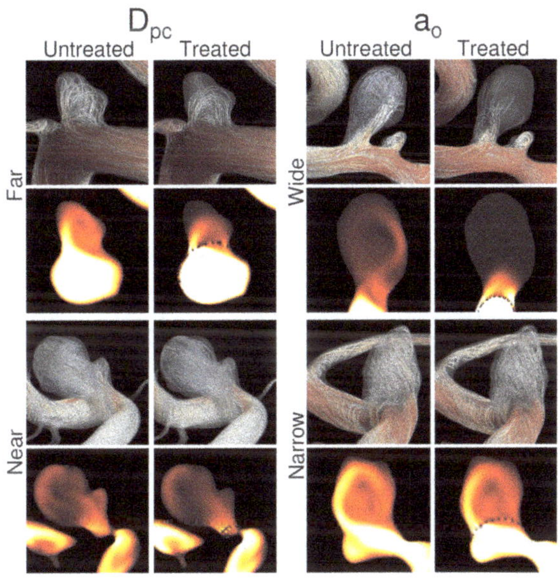

(b)

Figure 5.8. (a) Representation, on an aneurysmatic vessel geometry, of the distance from the aneurysm neck to the curvature peak measured along the centerline (D_{pc}). The red dot represents the location of the aneurysm bifurcation origin. The angle between the osculating plane (dark grey) and the aneurysm vector (green) is also shown. (b) Haemodynamic simulations result for four selected cases. Each group of images presents streamlines (top), velocity magnitude on a cross section plane across the aneurysm (bottom), untreated (left) and treated (right). The left group shows two cases with extreme values of D_{pc} and the right group two extreme cases for a_o. On the left, the top panel shows an aneurysm lying far from the curvature peak (high D_{pc}) and the bottom panel is very near to the peak (low D_{pc}). On the right, the top panel presents a wide angle with respect to the osculating plane (high a_o) and the bottom panel has a narrow angle with respect to it (low a_o).

presented, in one the angle between the aneurysm and the osculating plane is wide (top) and the other has a narrow angle (bottom). We observe for the case on the top (wide angle) that the part of the main flow jet going into the aneurysm is small and the presence of an FD redirects the flow to the parent vessel. When the angle between the aneurysm and the osculating plane is narrow (bottom) the presence of the FD induces smaller changes in the local flow.

It was found that the time-averaged WSS is more reduced in aneurysms far away from the curvature peak. This larger reduction is attributed to the secondary flow being reduced further downstream from the curvature peak. The haemodynamic variable reduction can be correlated to vascular morphology near the aneurysm. This was further studied in a follow-up clinical study [52].

5.5.5 Flow diverter length change and future research

A novel method for the computation of changes in flow diverter length has been proposed recently [53]. This method rapidly computes the length of a braided device when released inside a vessel. This method is designed to aid the interventional neuroradiologist during treatment. The aim is to provide, in real time, a prediction of the change in length of the FD when being placed in the patient's anatomy. The challenge comes with the fact that currently, FDs are braided devices. Because of this, a change in diameter of the device implies a substantial change in its total length. Furthermore, the irregular and tortuous geometry of cerebral vasculature make it very complicated to predict the final length of an FD when placed in the patient anatomy.

The method, initially assessed in [54], is capable of estimating the proximal end point of the device based on quantitative information of the patient anatomy and the distal release position of the stent (figure 5.9(a)). This method has been tested in FDs placed in real patient anatomies. In figure 5.9(b) are shown two views for a Silk stent (Balt Extrusion, Montmorency, France) placed in an internal carotid artery. It can be observed that the total length of the device is accurately estimated, although the

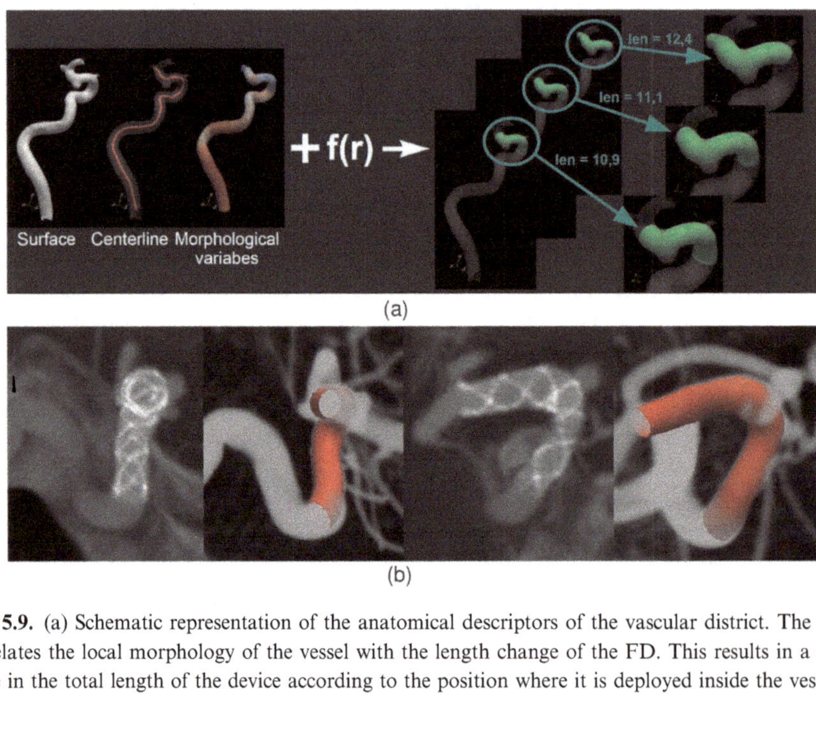

Figure 5.9. (a) Schematic representation of the anatomical descriptors of the vascular district. The function $f(r)$ relates the local morphology of the vessel with the length change of the FD. This results in a different change in the total length of the device according to the position where it is deployed inside the vessel.

vascular anatomy is complex and tortuous. This simulation indicates that a total change of 62% more than the total FD length was observed after placement in the patient anatomy. Its robustness and sensitivity to segmentation of the vessel geometry was also assessed, showing a good performance and tolerance to error in the segmentation threshold [55].

The performance of this method has also been clinically evaluated when used to simulate different brands and types of braided stents, showing an accuracy of over 92% in average, when assessing the final length of the implanted device [56, 57].

Simulation of flow diverter porosity is yet another tool with a promising future in the selection of devices for aneurysm treatment. This technique is still under assessment, and further results will evidence its clinical potential [58]. Furthermore, its combination with CFD has the potential of allowing its use inside the clinic, due to its computationally lower cost [59–61].

The predictive value of computational models is greatly appreciated in the clinic. The ability to plan one or more treatment alternatives and being able to assess their outcome can help in identifying potentially harmful or dangerous situations. Also, the fact that such tools can be used within the intervention room or, equivalently, obtain a response in real time, opens the possibility of them being used in day-to-day clinical practice.

References

[1] Rinkel G J E, Djibuti M, Algra A and van Gijn J 1998 *Stroke* **29** 251

[2] Schievink W I, Schaid D J, Michels V V and Piepgras D G 1995 *J. Neurosurg.* **83** 426

[3] van Gijn J and Rinkel G J E 2001 *Brain* **124** 249

[4] Wermer M J H, van der Schaaf I C, Algra A and Rinkel G J E 2007 *Stroke* **38** 1404

[5] Ishibashi T, Murayama Y, Urashima M, Saguchi T, Ebara M, Arakawa H, Irie K, Takao H and Abe T 2009 *Stroke* **40** 313

[6] Etminan N *et al* 2014 *Stroke* **45** 1523–30

[7] Wiebers D O 2003 *Lancet* **362** 103

[8] Alfke K, Straube T, Dörner L, Mehdorn H M and Jansen O 2004 *Am. J. Neuroradiol.* **25** 584

[9] King R M, Chueh J Y, van der Bom I M J, Silva C F, Carniato S L, Spilberg G, Wakhloo A K and Gounis M J 2012 *Am. J. Neuroradiol.* **33** 1657–62

[10] Biondi A, Janardhan V, Katz J M, Salvaggio K, Riina H A and Gobin Y P 2007 *Neurosurgery* **61** 460

[11] Wanke I and Forsting M 2008 *Neuroradiology* **50** 991

[12] Cebral J R, Castro M A, Burgess J J E, Pergolizzi R S R, Sheridan M M J and Putman C C M 2005 *Am. J. Neuroradiol.* **26** 2550

[13] Castro M A, Putman C M and Cebral J R 2006 *Acad. Radiol.* **13** 811

[14] Meng H, Wang Z, Hoi Y, Gao L, Metaxa E, Swartz D D and Kolega J 2007 *Stroke* **38** 1924

[15] Tremmel M, Xiang J, Hoi Y, Kolega J, Siddiqui A H, Mocco J and Meng H 2010 *Biomech. Model. Mechanobiol.* **9** 421

[16] Geers A J, Larrabide I, Radaelli A G, Bogunovic H, Kim M, Gratama van Andel H A F, Majoie C B, Vanbavel E and Frangi A F 2011 *Am. J. Neuroradiol.* **32** 581

[17] Geers A J, Larrabide I, Morales H G and Frangi A F 2014 *J. Biomech.* **47** 178

[18] Klisch J, Turk A, Turner R, Woo H H and Fiorella D 2011 *Am. J. Neuroradiol.* **32** 627

[19] Kulcsár Z 2010 *Am. J. Neuroradiol.* **23** 20
[20] Nelson P K, Lylyk P, Szikora I, Wetzel S G, Wanke I and Fiorella D 2011 *Am. J. Neuroradiol.* **32** 34
[21] Kallmes D F, Ding Y H, Dai D, Kadirvel R, Lewis D A and Cloft H J 2009 *Am. J. Neuroradiol.* **30** 1153
[22] Jou L D, Quick C M, Young W L, Lawton M T, Higashida R, Martin A and Saloner D 2003 *Am. J. Neuroradiol.* **24** 1804
[23] Steinman D, Milner J, Norley C, Lownie S and Holdsworth D 2003 *Am. J. Neuroradiol.* **24** 559
[24] Petrini L, Migliavacca F, Auricchio F and Dubini G 2004 *J. Biomech.* **37** 495
[25] Migliavacca F and Petrini L 2005 *Med. Eng. Phys.* **27** 13
[26] Chiastra C, Morlacchi S, Gallo D, Morbiducci U, Cárdenes R, Larrabide I and Migliavacca F 2013 *J. R. Soc. Interface* **10** 20130193
[27] Morlacchi S, Colleoni S G, Cárdenes R, Chiastra C, Diez J L, Larrabide I and Migliavacca F 2013 *Med. Eng. Phys.* **35** 1272
[28] De Beule M, Van Cauter S, Mortier P, Van Loo D, Van Impe R, Verdonck P and Verhegghe B 2009 *Med. Eng. Phys.* **31** 448
[29] Ma D, Dargush G F, Natarajan S K, Levy E I, Siddiqui A H and Meng H 2012 *J. Biomech.* **45** 2256–63
[30] Ma D, Dumont T M, Kosukegawa H, Ohta M, Yang X, Siddiqui A H and Meng H 2013 *Ann. Biomed. Eng.* **41** 2143
[31] Ohta M, Wetzel S G, Dantan P, Bachelet C, Lovblad K O, Yilmaz H, Flaud P and Rüfenacht D A 2005 *Cardiovasc. Interv. Radiol.* **28** 768
[32] Hirabayashi M, Ohta M, Rüfenacht D A and Chopard B 2003 *Phys. Rev.* E **68** 021918
[33] Appanaboyina S, Mut F, Löhner R, Putman C and Cebral J R 2009 *Comput. Methods Appl. Mech. Eng.* **198** 3567
[34] Janiga G, Rössl C, Skalej M and Thévenin D 2013 *J. Biomech.* **46** 7
[35] Peach T W, Ngoepe M, Spranger K, Zajarias-Fainsod D and Ventikos Y 2014 *Int. J. Numer. Methods Biomed. Eng.* **30** 1387
[36] Larrabide I, Radaelli A and Frangi A 2008 *Int. Conf. on Medical Image Computing and Computer-Assisted Intervention* **vol 11** pp 790–7
[37] Larrabide I, Kim M, Augsburger L, Villa-Uriol M C, Rüfenacht D and Frangi A F 2012 *Med. Image Anal.* **16** 721
[38] Delingette H 1999 *Int. J. Comput. Vis.* **32** 111
[39] Montagnat J and Delingette H 1998 *Signal Process.* **71** 173
[40] Montagnat J and Delingette H 2005 *Med. Image Anal.* **9** 87
[41] Bernardini A, Larrabide I, Petrini L, Pennati G, Flore E, Kim M and Frangi A F 2011 *Comput. Methods Biomech. Biomed. Eng.* **15** 303
[42] Radaelli A G *et al* 2008 *J. Biomech.* **41** 2069
[43] Auricchio F and Petrini L 2004 *Int. J. Numer. Methods Eng.* **61** 716
[44] Wu W, Wang W Q, Yang D Z, Qi M, Liu X P and Wang W 2007 *J Biomech.* **40** 3034
[45] Monson K L, Barbaro N M and Manley G T 2008 *Ann. Biomed. Eng.* **36** 2028
[46] Hsu S W, Chaloupka J, Feekes J, Cassell M and Cheng Y F 2006 *Am. J. Neuroradiol.* **27** 1135
[47] Hirabayashi M, Ohta M, Rüfenacht D A and Chopard B 2004 *Future Gener. Comput. Syst.* **20** 925

[48] Geers A J, Larrabide I, Morales H G and Frangi A F 2010 *Conf. Proc.: Annu. Int. Conf. IEEE Eng. Med. Biol. Soc.* **2010** 2622
[49] Geers A J, Larrabide I, Morales H G and Frangi A F 2014 *J. Biomech.* **47** 178
[50] Kim M, Larrabide I, Villa-Uriol M C and Frangi A F 2009 *Proc. IEEE Int. Sym. on Biomedical Imaging: From Nano to Macro* (Piscataway, NJ: IEEE) pp 1215–8
[51] Sun Q, Groth A, Larrabide I, Cito S, Aguila M, Frangi A F, Mendes Pereira V, Ouared R, Brina O and Aach T 2011 *Proc. Int. Sym. on Biomedical Imaging* (Piscataway, NJ: IEEE) pp 545–8
[52] Piccinelli M, Veneziani A, Steinman D A, Remuzzi A and Antiga L 2009 *IEEE Trans. Med. Imaging* **28** 1141
[53] Larrabide I, Geers A J, Morales H G, Aguilar M L and Rüfenacht D A 2014 *J. Neurointerv. Surg.* **7** 272–80
[54] Fernandez H, Macho J M, Blasco J, San Roman L, Mailaender W, Serra L and Larrabide I 2015 Computation of the change in length of a braided device when deployed in realistic vessel models *Int. J. Comput. Assist. Radiol. Surg.* **10** 1659–65
[55] Larrabide I 2014 Procedimiento para la determinación de la longitud final de stents antes de su colocación *Patent* https://patentimages.storage.googleapis.com/ab/d4/53/3e834d8c2d2de4/ES2459244B1.pdf
[56] Moyano R K, Fernandez H, Macho J M, Blasco J, San Roman L, Narata A P and Larrabide I 2017 *13th Int. Conf. on Medical Information Processing and Analysis* **vol 10572** (Bellingham, WA: International Society for Optics and Photonics) p 105721H
[57] Narata A P, Blasco J, Roman L S, Macho J M, Fernandez H, Moyano R K, Winzenrieth R and Larrabide I 2018 *Oper. Neurosurg.* **15** 557–66
[58] Joshi K C, Larrabide I, Saied A, Elsaid N, Fernandez H and Lopes D K 2018 *J. Neurosurg.* **1** 1
[59] Fernandez H, Curto A, Ding A, Serra L and Larrabide I 2017 *12th Int. Symp. on Medical Information Processing and Analysis* **vol 10160** (Bellingham, WA: International Society for Optics and Photonics) p 101601C
[60] Dazeo N, Dottori J, Boroni G, Clausse A and Larrabide I 2017 *12th Int. Symp. Medical Information Processing and Analysis* **vol 10160** (Bellingham, WA: International Society for Optics and Photonics) p 101601F
[61] Dazeo N, Dottori J, Boroni G and Larrabide I 2018 *Int. J. Numer. Methods Biomed. Eng.* **2018** e3145

Section III

Vessel and stent segmentation

IOP Publishing

Vascular and Intravascular Imaging Trends, Analysis, and Challenges, Volume 1

Stent applications

Petia Radeva and Jasjit S Suri

Chapter 6

Graph-based cross-sectional intravascular image segmentation

Ehab Essa, Xianghua Xie, Huaizhong Zhang, James Cotton and Dave Smith

We present a fully automatic segmentation approach to detect the media–adventitia border in intravascular ultrasound (IVUS) and the lumen border in optical tomography (OCT) images. A graph-based segmentation method is developed to accurately estimate the borders. Segmentation in IVUS and OCT has been shown to be an intricate process due to the relatively low contrast and various forms of interferences and artifacts caused by, for example, calcification, stents and acoustic shadows. Graph-cut-based methods often require careful manual initialisation and produce inconsistent tracing of the border. We propose unravelling the image and transferring the object segmentation into a height field segmentation in polar coordinates. Thus, the border of interest is obtained by searching a minimum closed set on a node weighted directed graph. We use a double-interface automatic graph cut technique to prevent the extraction of media–adventitia border in IVUS from being distracted by those image features. The cost functions are derived by using a combination of complementary texture features. For OCT, a novel image feature is incorporated into the solution scheme, which is derived from a vector field that takes into account gradient vector interactions across the image domain. In addition, Laplacian diffusion is employed to improve the performance of our method for dealing with excessive noise. Evaluation results demonstrate that our method achieves better performance compared to a number of alternative segmentation techniques.

6.1 Introduction

IVUS and OCT imaging are catheter-based technologies, which show two-dimensional cross-sectional images of the coronary structure. There are two types of borders of interest: the lumen–intima border, which corresponds to the inner

doi:10.1088/2053-2563/ab01fach6

arterial wall, and the media–adventitia border, which represents the outer coronary arterial wall. The appearance of both borders in IVUS or OCT images is affected by various forms of imaging artifacts, such as acoustic shadows caused by the catheter guide-wire, calcium in IVUS, or the stent in OCT.

Among many other techniques, formulating the IVUS and OCT segmentation as a combinatorial optimisation [6, 7, 10, 14, 18, 20, 21, 24, 27] of a cost function based on local image features has been a popular approach. In [18], dynamic programming is used to search a minimum path based on a cost function that incorporates edge information with a simplistic prior relying on assumed echo pattern and border thickness. Manual initialisation is generally necessary. In [21], the border detection is carried out on the envelope data before scan conversion. The authors applied spatio-temporal filters to highlight the lumen, based on the assumption that the blood speckles have higher spatial and temporal variations than the arterial wall, followed by a graph-searching method similar to [18]. However, image features introduced by acoustic shadows or a metallic stent would seriously undermine their assumption. Catheter movement can also cause spatial and temporal fluctuations, which lead to ambiguities. The *s–t* cut method [14] is employed in [24] to segment 3D IVUS data. The vertical intensity pattern along the borders, the Rayleigh distribution and the Chan–Vese minimum variance criterion are used in designing the cost functions. These intensity-based features are susceptible to image variations that commonly exist in IVUS, such as calcification and acoustic shadows.

Several methods rely on user interaction to obtain a good result [1, 2, 10, 20]. However, these methods can be time-consuming and impractical with a large image size and/or a large number of images. For example, in the conventional graph cut [1, 2], user interaction is necessary to infer the unary cost for each pixel. In addition, the definition of smoothness pairwise cost is mainly derived from edge features, which becomes less useful in the obscure regions of the image. In [20], a semi-automatic graph-based method is proposed that repetitively requires the user to interactively correct the segmentation result on the longitudinal view until satisfactory segmentation is achieved.

Li *et al* [14] proposed a terrain-like multiple surface segmentation method by constructing a weighted directed graph that allows imposing some geometrical constraints to define the elasticity of each surface and the inter-relation with other surfaces, and to search for the minimum closed, subgraph set containing the surface on its envelope by utilising the *s–t* cut method to minimise the cost function and without the need for user intervention. This method is well suited to IVUS/OCT segmentation, however, dealing with image artifacts, defining the optimal cost function and adapting the graph construction are the major challenges, as described in [6, 7, 27].

In this chapter, a bottom-up data-driven approach is presented to segment IVUS and OCT images. For IVUS segmentation, a double-interface graph cut segmentation is proposed to delineate the media–adventitia border, in order to achieve reliable results automatically. The impediments, such as stents or fibrotic and calcium plaques, appear inside the media–adventitia border, and the acoustic signal decays rapidly in the adventitia, so there are generally no strong features beyond the media–adventitia border. This observation inspired us to apply an additional interface searching inside the media–adventitia border which links those undesired image features, including partial lumen border, and hence preserves the border of interest. A combination of complementary texture features is used to form the basis of the boundary-based cost functions. For OCT segmentation, a single-interface graph cut segmentation is proposed to delineate the lumen border. Moreover, a novel image feature is incorporated into the cost function, instead of merely using image intensity or the local gradient magnitude. The image feature is derived from the gradient vector interaction across the image domain and possesses the characteristics of regional features.

6.2 Pre-processing

The pre-processing step is to transform images from Cartesian coordinates to polar coordinates and to remove the catheter region from the transformed images. Representing the images in polar coordinates is desirable to facilitate feature extraction with equal emphasis on radial and tangential dimensions. It also facilitates the automated graph cut in searching for minimum closed sets. Moreover, the post-processing can then be carried out more efficiently since it becomes a one-dimensional interpolation instead of two-dimensional.

The catheter generates a blank region which contains no information and is surrounded by a ring-down artifact which may hamper the search process for finding the minimum cost path for the desired border. The ring-down artifact is located in the first rows of the transformed image, and it is approximately a constant. Therefore, a simple thresholding method is used to remove that region, as shown in figure 6.1(c).

6.3 Feature extraction

In IVUS imaging, the media layer largely consists of homogeneous smooth muscle, which exhibits as a dark layer in ultrasound images, and the adventitia layer tends to be brighter, see figure 6.1 as an example. Hence, edge-based features are appropriate to extract the media–adventitia border. In OCT imaging, the lumen appears to be much darker because blood is flushed out before imaging. The intima and other tissues, including plaque, surrounding the lumen have a bright appearance. Hence, the lumen–intima border shows good contrast, i.e. image gradient features may be

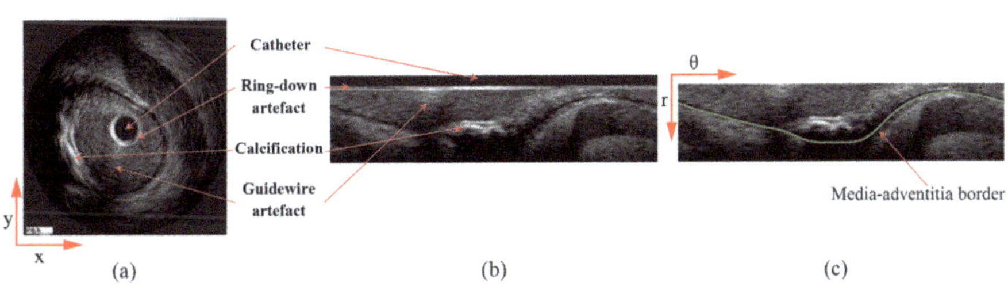

Figure 6.1. (a) An original IVUS image. (b) Polar transformed image. (c) After removing the catheter region (green curve shows the ground-truth of the media–adventitia border).

adopted to highlight the border. However, a guide-wire artifact and other interfering image features commonly exist inside the artery and they cast shadows over the border of interest, disrupting its continuity. Those imaging artifacts generally have large responses to image-gradient-based feature extraction.

6.3.1 Steerable filter

A steerable filter is a linear combination of differently oriented instances of the base filter. A set of n order derivatives of Gaussian (GD) filters $G_n(x, y)$ in different orientations can be used to highlight the edge features along the border. The steerable filters can be defined as a linear combination of a set of Gaussian derivatives [9]:

$$G_n^{\theta}(x, y) = \sum_{j=1}^{M} k_j(\theta) G_n^{\theta_j}(x, y), \tag{6.1}$$

where $G_n^{\theta}(x, y)$ is the rotated version of $G_n(x, y)$ at θ orientation and $k_j(\theta)$, $1 \leqslant j \leqslant M$ are interpolation functions.

Steering derivatives in the direction of the gradient makes them invariant to rotation. These steerable filters are more effective in highlighting oriented structure, e.g. edges, than isotropic band-pass filters, particularly when there is noise interference [9].

6.3.2 The log-Gabor filter

The Gabor filter acts as a band-pass filter that has been used in texture analysis to exploit its similarity with the human visual system [5, 22] and performs multi-channel, frequency and orientation analysis on the visual image. The Gabor filter can achieve optimal joint localisation in the spatial and frequency domains. Gabor filters have two components, a real part and an imaginary part, where the Gabor function is a multiplication of a Gaussian function and a complex sinusoid function in the spatial domain, corresponding to a Gaussian shift from the centre of frequency in the Fourier domain. Here, the log-Gabor filter [8] is used in different scales to enhance the border and to reduce speckles and other image artifacts. The log-Gabor function, $LG(f)$, has a frequency response defined as a symmetric Gaussian on a log frequency axis:

$$LG(f) = \exp\left(-\frac{[\log(f/f_0)]^2}{2[\log(\sigma/f_0)]^2}\right), \tag{6.2}$$

where f_0 is the centre frequency of the filter, and σ is the filter bandwidth. The log-Gabor function has no DC component for any bandwidth filter compared to the Gabor function.

6.3.3 Local phase

Local phase features have been shown to be an effective alternative to intensity derived features to deal with inhomogeneity, low image quality and imaging shadows, which are common in IVUS and OCT images. For example, in [16] local phase features were used to highlight acoustic boundaries in echocardiographic images.

Local phase features are considered as extrema in Fourier phase components, which can be located as peaks in the local energy function obtained by convolving odd and even symmetric log-Gabor filters, $(o_m(x, y), e_m(x, y))$, to remove the DC component and preserve the phase in a localised frequency. Two types of features can be extracted from phase congruency: feature asymmetry and feature symmetry. Feature symmetry favours bar-like image patterns and exists in the frequency components at either the minimum or maximum symmetric points in their cycles, which is useful in extracting the thin media layer in IVUS. Its dark polarity symmetry is used here [11]:

$$\phi_s(x, y) = \max_{\theta} \frac{\sum_m \lfloor [-e_m(x, y) - |o_m(x, y)|] - T_m \rfloor}{\sum_m A_m(x, y) + \varepsilon}, \tag{6.3}$$

where θ and m denote filter orientation and scale, respectively, ε is a small constant, T_m is an orientation-dependent noise threshold, $A_m(x, y) = \sqrt{e_m^2(x, y) + o_m^2(x, y)}$ and $\lfloor . \rfloor$ denotes zeroing negative values.

In contrast, feature asymmetry highlights step-like image patterns and corresponds to the point where all the frequency components are at the most asymmetric points in their cycles. It can be defined as

$$\phi_a(x, y) = \max_{\theta} \frac{\sum_m \lfloor [|o_m(x, y)| - |e_m(x, y)|] - T_m \rfloor}{\sum_m A_m(x, y) + \varepsilon}. \tag{6.4}$$

Phase asymmetry is useful to highlight the lumen border in OCT, where edge features can be seen from the darker lumen layer to the brighter intima layer.

6.3.4 Circulation density features

In the graph cut, the cost function can be generally categorised as edge-based or region-based. Edge-based cost functions assume that the object boundary is largely collocated with image intensity discontinuity, and typically use derivatives of the image intensity function as a local estimation of the likelihood of an object boundary. Region-based cost functions are usually non-edge-based, e.g. a piecewise constant assumption. Quite often, image intensity values are directly used in general image segmentation. Although graph cut algorithms provide global optimality in two-level segmentation, a reliable but also generic image feature that does not assume a strong prior image is desirable for general segmentation that is useful in, for example, object recognition.

We consider intensity discontinuity as perhaps the least constrained and most widely applicable object boundary estimation. Its performance can be easily compromised by image noise, smooth varying intensity at the object boundary, and so on. These shortcomings essentially arise because it is a local measurement and it does not take into account interactions among image gradient vectors. As an example, a region with a relatively large image gradient magnitude but varying gradient directions suggests that it is unlikely to be a location of the object boundary, despite the large magnitude. In contrast, weak gradient vectors that are aligned with each other suggest a greater likelihood of object boundary than what the magnitude itself suggests.

Hence, we present a gradient vector field that is a result of global interactions among original image gradient vectors, in which its circulation density can be used as a reliable image feature for the graph cut. The zero-crossings of this circulation density provide a better indication of the location of the object boundary, and the magnitude of oscillation at zero-crossings indicates the strength of object boundary presence. The signs (positive and negative) of circulation density actually indicate the foreground and background. The derived gradient vector can also be diffused to produce a more coherent circulation density. The image feature is directly derived from edge-based assumptions, but closely resembles region-based methods.

Let $\nabla_i I = f\hat{I}_x$ and $\nabla_j I = f\hat{I}_y$ denote the two components of the image gradient ∇I in the image coordinates (i, j), respectively, i.e. $\nabla I = (\nabla_i I, \nabla_j I)^T$, where f is the edge map (magnitude). A convolution computation is carried out on both components with the kernel $k(\mathbf{x}) = m(\mathbf{x})$. Moreover, the magnitude function m is chosen as an inverse of distance from the origin, i.e. $m(r) = 1/r^{\zeta}$. Thus, the result of this convolution process can be expressed as

$$\begin{cases} G_i(\mathbf{x}) = \nabla_i I * k(\mathbf{x}) = \sum_{\mathbf{s}\neq\mathbf{x}} \dfrac{\nabla_i I(\mathbf{s})}{R_{\mathbf{xs}}} = \sum_{\mathbf{s}\neq\mathbf{x}} f(\mathbf{s}) \dfrac{\hat{I}_x(\mathbf{s})}{R_{\mathbf{xs}}}, \\ G_j(\mathbf{x}) = \nabla_j I * k(\mathbf{x}) = \sum_{\mathbf{s}\neq\mathbf{x}} \dfrac{\nabla_j I(\mathbf{s})}{R_{\mathbf{xs}}} = \sum_{\mathbf{s}\neq\mathbf{x}} f(\mathbf{s}) \dfrac{\hat{I}_y(\mathbf{s})}{R_{\mathbf{xs}}}, \end{cases} \tag{6.5}$$

where $R_{\mathbf{xs}}$ is the distance between $\mathbf{x}$ and $\mathbf{s}$, and $\mathbf{G} = (G_i, G_j)$ denotes the resultant gradient convolution field. Due to the smoothing effect when applying the kernel function, the original image gradient vectors have extended their influence from the immediate vicinity of the edge pixels to a much larger neighbourhood. In fact, the computation in equation (6.5) is across the whole image domain.

The circulation density of this extended gradient vector field is then computed as

$$B = \nabla \cdot \mathbf{G}(\mathbf{x}) = \nabla \cdot (G_i, G_j) = \nabla \times (-G_j, G_i), \tag{6.6}$$

where $\nabla\cdot$ is the divergence operator and $\nabla\times$ is the curl operator. This circulation density has an intrinsic link to the magnetic field used in the MAC model [25, 26] in a variational framework. Specifically, when $\zeta = 1$, B is equivalent to the third and the only effective component of the magnetic field in the MAC model. Hence, the positive and negative values of this circulation density indicate foreground/

background or background/foreground. The zero-crossings of the vector circulation density would indicate the location of object boundaries. This circulation density method is a generalisation of the effective component used in MAC. Moreover, we can refine the computation of this vector circulation density by performing efficient Laplacian diffusion in the extended gradient vector field to overcome, for example, noise interference.

Note that the gradient vector field is actually along the edge direction, so substantial diffusion in the components can result in a significantly improved boundary descriptions. There are various diffusion strategies for this smoothing task. For implementation convenience and less parameter intervention, an isotropic/Laplacian diffusion scheme is used here, which is carried out by solving the following Euler equations:

$$\begin{cases} \dfrac{\partial}{\partial t}\mathcal{G}_i(\mathbf{t}, \mathbf{x}) = p(G_i)\nabla^2\mathcal{G}_i(\mathbf{t}, \mathbf{x}) - q(G_i)(\mathcal{G}_i(\mathbf{t}, \mathbf{x}) - G_i), \\ \dfrac{\partial}{\partial t}\mathcal{G}_j(\mathbf{t}, \mathbf{x}) = p(G_j)\nabla^2\mathcal{G}_j(\mathbf{t}, \mathbf{x}) - q(G_j)(\mathcal{G}_j(\mathbf{t}, \mathbf{x}) - G_j), \end{cases} \tag{6.7}$$

where ∇^2 is the Laplacian operator, $\mathcal{G}_i(0, \mathbf{x}) = G_i(\mathbf{x})$, $\mathcal{G}_j(0, \mathbf{x}) = G_j(\mathbf{x})$, and $p(y)$ and $q(y)$ are weighting functions allowing very little smoothing at strong edges and varying smoothing elsewhere. It is given as

$$p(y) = \exp(-|y|f/K),\ q(y) = 1 - p(y), \tag{6.8}$$

where $f = |\nabla I|$ and K is a constant. The first term on the right side of equation (6.7) is the smoothness term which creates a smoothly varying vector field, while the second term is the data term that encourages the vector field $\mathcal{G}$ to be closed to the gradient of edge map in $\mathbf{G}$.

6.4 Single- and double-interface segmentation

Briefly, a node-weighed directed graph is constructed so that the border extraction is considered as computing a minimum closed set. The search for this minimum closed set is solved by computing a minimum s–t cut in a derived arc-weighted directed graph. For the double-interface segmentation, an additional set of arcs is constructed, taking into account the topological inter-relation between the two interfaces. The associated cost functions for each image modality are defined based on extracted image features. Finally, the desired border, located on the envelope of the minimum closed graph, is smoothed using radial basis function (RBF) interpolation.

6.4.1 Graph construction

A conventional graph cut, such as [1], generally requires user initialisation, and more importantly only deals with one interface, i.e. foreground and background separation. Alternative methods, such as active contour and level set techniques, e.g. [19], can track multiple interfaces. However, they often require user initialisation and do not guarantee a global minimum. Furthermore, since one of the interfaces is affected by image features, such as calcification, which vary from image to image, it does not have consistent shape characteristics. Hence, a deformable model with multiple interfaces, such as [15], may not be suitable.

In [14], the authors proposed a novel graph construction method, which transforms the surface segmentation in 3D into computing a minimum closed set in a directed graph. We adapt this method to a 2D segmentation, which can carry out double-interface segmentation simultaneously in low order polynomial time complexity and does not require user initialisation. This approach also allows us to impose a topological constraint, i.e. the two interfaces in our case cannot intersect or overlap and the media–adventitia border is the outer interface (or lower interface when the IVUS image is transformed to polar coordinates).

For each desired interface, construct a graph $G = \langle V, E\rangle$, where each node $V(x, y), 0 \leqslant x < X$ and $0 \leqslant y < Y$, corresponds to a pixel in 2D image $I(x, y)$ with size $X \times Y$. The graph G consists of two arc types: intra-column arcs and inter-column arcs, see figure 6.2. For intra-column arcs, along each column, every node $V(x, y)$, where $y > 0$, has a directed arc with $+\infty$ weight to the node $V(x, y - 1)$. In the case of inter-column arcs, for each node $V(x, y)$ a directed arc with $+\infty$ weight is established to link with node $V(x + 1, y')$, where $y' = y - \Delta_{p,q}$, and $y \geqslant \Delta_{p,q}$. Similarly, node $V(x + 1, y)$ is connected to $V(x, y')$, where $\Delta_{p,q}$ controls the maximum distance allowed to change between two neighbouring columns p, q in the y-coordinate of the interface $|y - y'| \leqslant \Delta_{p,q}$.

Since the vessel has a cylindrical-like shape, the first and last columns in the polar transformed images are closely connected. Thus, inter-column arcs are added between them in which each node $V(0, y)$ (and also $V(X - 1, y)$) is connected to $V(X - 1, y')$ (and $V(0, y')$, respectively). The nodes in the last row of the graph are connected to each other with $+\infty$ weight to maintain a closed graph.

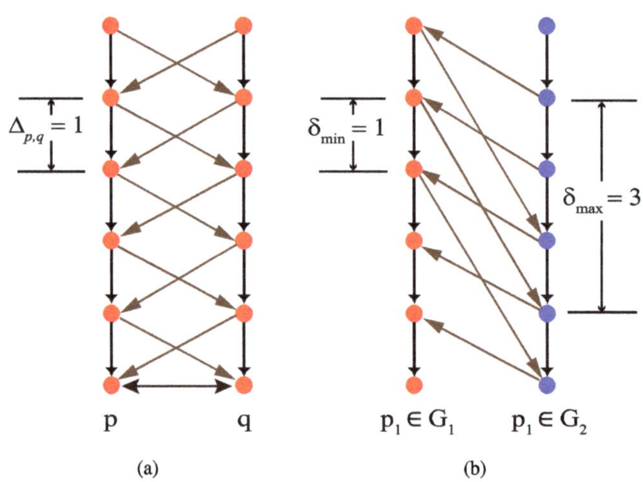

Figure 6.2. Graph construction. (a) Intra-column and inter-column arcs when $\Delta_{p,q} = 1$. (b) Inter-interface constraints when $\delta_{\min} = 1$ and $\delta_{\max} = 3$.

For double-interface segmentation and after constructing the graph for each of the two interfaces to simultaneously segment them, taking into account interrelations between them is necessary and this is achieved by setting up another set of arcs to connect them, as shown in figure 6.2(b). Geometrical and topological constraints can be imposed by setting minimum $\delta_{\min}$ and maximum $\delta_{\max}$ separation distances. The two interfaces thus will not intersect or overlap. This set of arcs, $\mathcal{E}^s$, is defined as

$$\mathcal{E}^s = \begin{cases} \{V_1(x, y),\ V_2(x, y - \delta_{\max}) | y \geqslant \delta_{\max}\} \bigcup \\ \{V_2(x, y),\ V_1(x, y + \delta_{\min}) | y < Y - \delta_{\min}\} \bigcup \\ \{V_1(0, \delta_{\min}),\ V_2(0, 0)\}. \end{cases} \tag{6.9}$$

This graph construction requires the desired interfaces to be open-ended height fields, which in this case means that this will be carried out in polar coordinates.

6.4.2 Cost function

The cost function is defined on the image domain, in which it is inversely proportional to the likelihood of each pixel belonging to the desired border. The cost function can be expressed as $E = \sum_{V \in S} \hat{C}(x, y)$, where $\hat{C}$ denotes the normalised cost function ($\hat{C}(x, y) \in [0.1]$) and S is a path in the directed graph. The formulation of the pre-normalisation cost function, C, is determined as presented below.

6.4.2.1 IVUS

Due to large variations in image features and the correlation between edge information and the media–adventitia border, boundary-based cost functions are used. The cost function indicates the likelihood of each node in the graph belonging to the minimum cost path that represents the desired interface. Two separate cost functions are used to capture the media–adventitia border and an auxiliary interface that is above the media–adventitia, since these two interfaces have different characteristics in image feature and formation.

For the media–adventitia border, three types of features described in section 6.3 are used. It takes the following form:

$$C_1(x, y) = C_d(x, y) + \alpha_1 C_G(x, y) + \alpha_2(1 - \phi_s(x, y)), \tag{6.10}$$

where C_d denotes the term for derivative of Gaussian features, C_G is for log-Gabor, and α_1 and α_2 are constants. The derivatives of Gaussian responses from six different orientations are summed together to form C_d. Similarly, C_G can be obtained by cascading the filtering responses across scales. In addition, more weight can be assigned to coarser scale features so that it presents the connectivity of the media–adventitia border in the presence of an acoustic shadow, e.g. $C_G = G^{(3)} + G^{(4)} + 1.5G^{(5)}$ as used here and $G^{(i)}$ denotes the ith scale. Feature symmetry ϕ_s is useful in enhancing the thin layer of media. It is normalised beforehand, and since the middle of the layer has larger values, $1 - \phi_s$ is used in the cost function so that the interface between the media and adventitia is highlighted. Note that each of the terms in the cost function is normalised.

For the auxiliary interface that is above the media–adventitia, we use a combination of the log-Gabor feature and feature asymmetry:

$$C_2(x, y) = C_G(x, y) + \alpha_3(1 - \phi_a(x, y)), \tag{6.11}$$

where α_3 is a constant. Since the derivative of the Gaussian filter has a relatively stronger response to local intensity variation, it is not included in this cost function. The combination of these two types of features leads the cost function to favour linking globally dominant image features, which very often is distracting for media–adventitia border segmentation.

6.4.2.2 OCT

The zero-crossings of the circulation density feature computed from gradient vector interaction indicate the location of the object boundary. The degree of circulation density oscillation at the zero-crossing suggests the strength of the object boundary. A direct assignment of circulation density to the graph as a nodal cost would be inappropriate, since the minimum or maximum of the circulation density is not an indication of either the location or strength of the object boundary. However, a simple transformation, for instance computing its gradient magnitude, can be applied. Since the decay of circulation density from the object boundary is exponential, a log transformation can be added in order to avoid extreme values being assigned to the graph, i.e. $C = -\log|\nabla B|$.

6.4.3 Compute the minimum closed set

Each graph node is weighted by a value $w(x, y)$ representing its rank to be selected in the minimum closed set graph where the arc costs between graph nodes are infinitive. The weight assignment is carried out according to

$$w(x, y) = \begin{cases} C(x, y) & \text{if } y = 0, \\ C(x, y) - C(x, y - 1) & \text{otherwise.} \end{cases} \tag{6.12}$$

where C denotes any cost function. For a feasible path $\mathcal{S}$ in the graph, the subset of nodes on or below $\mathcal{S}$ form a closed set and it can be shown that the cost of the s–t cut in the graph is equivalent to the cost of nodes in the corresponding subset differing by a constant [14]. Hence, segmenting the border of interest is equivalent to finding the minimum closed set in the directed graph. The s–t cut algorithm proposed by Boykov and Kolmogorov [3] is used to find the minimum closed set, based on the fact that the weight can be used as the base for dividing the nodes into nonnegative and negative sets. The source s is connected to each negative node and every nonnegative node is connected to the sink t, both through a directed arc that carries the absolute value of the cost node itself. The optimal interfaces correspond to the upper envelope of each minimum closed set graph, as shown in figure 6.3. Since the graph has $O(kn)$ nodes and $O(km)$ edges, where k is an integer constant that represents the number of interfaces $1 \leqslant k \leqslant 2$, the minimum closed set can be computed in $T(kn, km)$ time that depends on the choice of the s–t cut algorithm.

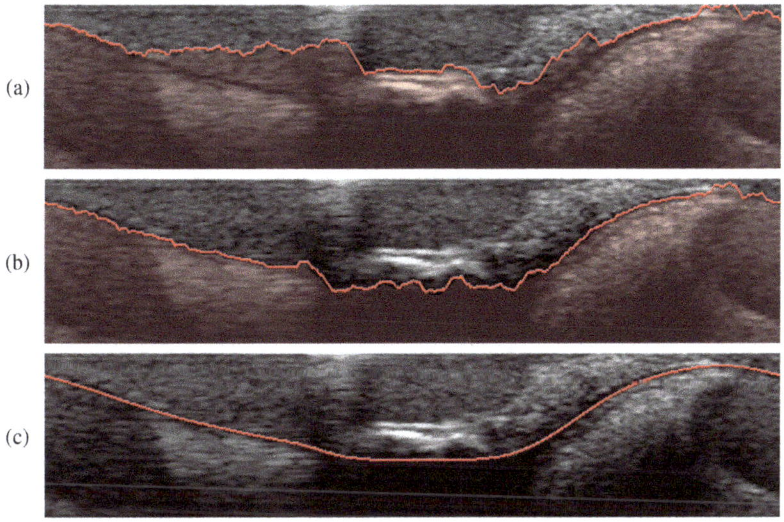

Figure 6.3. The minimum closed set graph highlighted in red: (a) the auxiliary interface, (b) the media–adventitia border and (c) the media–adventitia border after the RBF smoothness.

6.4.4 Post-processing

The smoothing parameter in graph construction prevents sudden drastic changes in the extracted interfaces. However, the segmented interface may still contain local oscillations. Smoothing based post-processing can be adopted to eliminate such oscillations. Here, RBF interpolation using a thin plate based function is used to effectively obtain the final interface. Note that, due to that fact that the images have been transformed into polar coordinates, the RBF processing only needs to be carried out in 1D. Figure 6.3(c) shows the media–adventitia border after applying the RBF smoothness.

6.5 Results: IVUS

IVUS images are acquired using a 40 MHz transducer Boston Scientific ultrasound machine with an Atlantis SR Pro Catheter with a total of ten pullbacks. The ground-truth is formed by manual labelling of the media–adventitia border on every tenth frame, i.e. 3322 frames for quantitative analysis. These images contain various forms of soft and fibrous plaques, calcifications, stents and acoustic shadows. In most of the images, the blood speckle is so prominent that the lumen border is very difficult to see. For all the tested images, ground-truth via manual labelling is available for quantitative analysis. The ground-truth was prepared at the beginning of the project and validated by two clinical consultants. All the parameters are fixed: the minimum and maximum distance between two interfaces, δ_{min} and δ_{max}, are set to be 5 and 140, respectively, and cost function weightings are set as $\alpha_1 = 0.7$, $\alpha_2 = 0.5$ and $\alpha_3 = 0.5$.

In order to comprehensively examine the performance of the proposed method, we use five performance metrics to quantitatively measure the accuracy of the segmentation on all images. These metrics include the absolute mean difference (AMD), Hausdorff distance (HD), area overlap (AO), sensitivity and specificity, which are defined as

$$\begin{aligned} \text{AMD} &= \frac{1}{N}\sum_{i=1}^{N}|y_{\text{AT}}(i) - y_{\text{GT}}(i)|, \\ \text{HD} &= \max_{a\in y_{\text{AT}}}\left\{\max_{b\in y_{\text{GT}}}[\text{dis}(a, b)]\right\}, \\ \text{AO} &= \frac{\text{TP}}{\text{TP} + \text{FN} + \text{FP}}, \\ \text{Sens.} &= \frac{\text{TP}}{\text{TP} + \text{FN}}, \\ \text{Spec.} &= \frac{\text{TN}}{\text{TN} + \text{FP}}, \end{aligned} \tag{6.13}$$

where N is the number of border points, y_{AT} is the automatic border, y_{GT} is the ground-truth border, dis(a, b) is the Euclidean distance between a and b sets of points of the borders y_{AT} and y_{GT}, TP is the true positive area of the vessel, FN denotes false negative, FP denotes false positive and TN is true negative. Note, the area that is within the vessel border is the positive area; outside is negative.

6.5.1 Single-interface segmentation

A single graph is constructed where the value of $\Delta_{p,q}$ is set as a global constant for each pair of neighbouring columns p, q to act as a hard constraint that prevents drastic changes in the border shape. Figure 6.4 shows the effect of the hard geometric constraints $\Delta_{p,q}$ to produce more reasonable results.

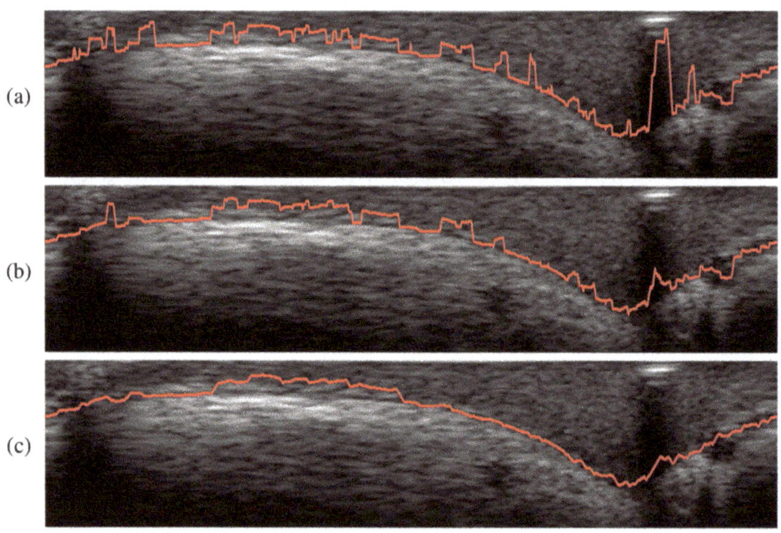

Figure 6.4. The effect of $\Delta_{p,q}$ constraints on single-interface segmentation. These hard constraints are globally set to (a) 10, (b) 5 and (c) 1 pixel distances.

Table 6.1 provides a quantitative comparison between the *s–t* cut, the single-interface segmentation and the proposed double-interface method. It was carried out on a randomly selected subset of 95 images, since manual initialisation for the *s–t* cut method is too labour intensive. We use area overlap (AO) in percentages and absolute mean difference (AMD) in pixels as evaluation measurements. The cost function of the single-interface method is based on the three types of features as defined in equation (6.10). Calcifications, stents or any highly bright patterns in fibrous tissue have strong edge features compared to the surrounding regions, and that is the main reason for the jumbled results of single-interface segmentation in highlighting the media–adventitia border, as shown in figures 6.5(c) and 6.6(b). However, the single-interface segmentation can work properly in ideal images when the artifact that distorted the IVUS image is less, as shown in the first row of figure 6.7. We also run a full test of the single-interface method but using a uniform cost function based on first order (1st) GD. The results are shown in table 6.2 and some qualitative examples can be found in column (c), figure 6.8. However, there is no remarkable improvement in the cases containing artifacts.

6.5.2 Double-interface segmentation

The proposed method was compared against the *s–t* cut [1] and single-interface segmentation with the cost function in equation (6.10). The cost function for the media–adventitia was kept the same. The *s–t* cut method requires manual initialisation, and its result is highly initialisation-dependent. Figures 6.5(a) and (b) shows a typical result achieved using *s–t* cut. Even with reasonable care in initialisation, the result is not satisfactory. The single-interface segmentation gives a partial media–adventitia border, as shown in row (c). However, its performance degrades when there are interfering image structures. The proposed double-interface method achieved better results even without any user interaction, as seen in row (d). More comparative results are given in figure 6.6, which shows the typical performance for each method. The quantitative results are provided in table 6.1.

Table 6.2 shows the result of a full comparison (i.e. 3322 frames) between the single-interface method, the texture-RBF method [17] and the proposed double-interface method. Five evaluation metrics are used, including the absolute mean difference (AMD), Hausdorff distance (HD) in pixel, sensitivity (Sens. %), specificity (Spec. %) and area overlap (AO %) defined in equation (6.13). Papadogiorgaki *et al* [17] proposed an IVUS segmentation method based on discrete wavelet frames to

Table 6.1. Comparison between *s–t* cut, single-interface and double-interface segmentation results.

	s–t cut		Single-interface		Double-interface	
	AO	AMD	AO	AMD	AO	AMD
Mean	78.76	22.61	90.01	12.55	94.16	6.99
Standard deviation	8.90	7.52	11.06	11.45	4.53	4.13

(a)
(b)
(c)
(d)

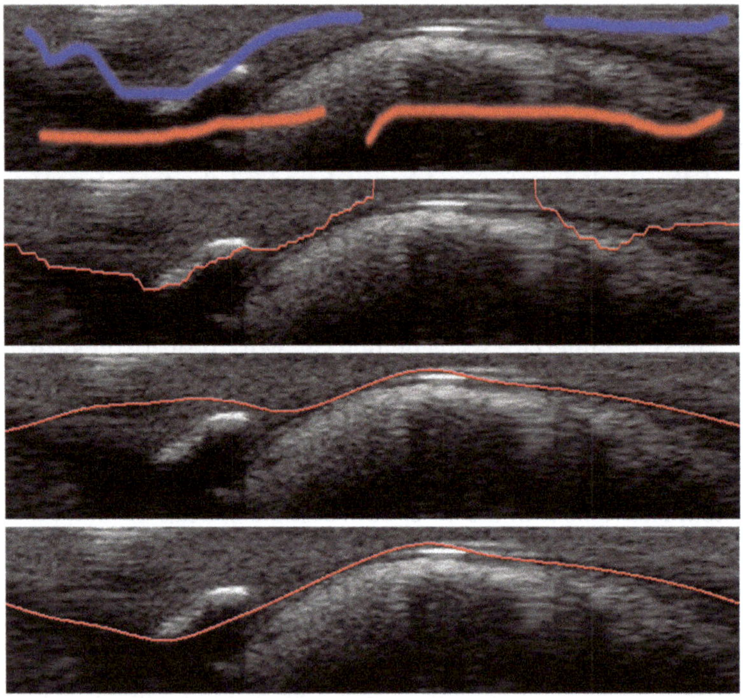

Figure 6.5. (a) Initialisation for the s–t cut and (b) its result. (c) The result for single-interface segmentation. (d) The result for the proposed double-interface method.

construct decomposition trees to identify vessel wall borders. RBF is then used to smooth the initial contour obtained by applying a threshold on those texture features. The texture-RBF method and the single-interface method with 1st GD suffer from the presence of stents or severe calcium plaques and underestimate the media–adventitia border, as shown in columns (b) and (c) of figure 6.8. The proposed method shows better performance, achieving better accuracy and consistency. A qualitative comparison between manual labelling of the media–adventitia border and the proposed method is shown in figure 6.7 and more examples can be found in column (d) of figure 6.8.

6.6 Results: OCT

In our study, to validate the performance of the proposed method in vessel lumen border detection, ten OCT *in vivo* sequences of the human artery were acquired with a frequency domain OCT imaging system (C7-XR, LightLab). Among the images used, there are various forms of fibrous plaques, calcifications, stents and bifurcations which are created from the acquisition process. To establish the ground-truth, the ten pullbacks, i.e. 2283 images in total, are manually labelled to identify the lumen area. In contrast, four recently developed methods are employed to demonstrate the performance of the proposed method. These include the star graph cut [23], VFC [12], the modified Chan–Vese model [4, 28] and DRLSE [13]. Among

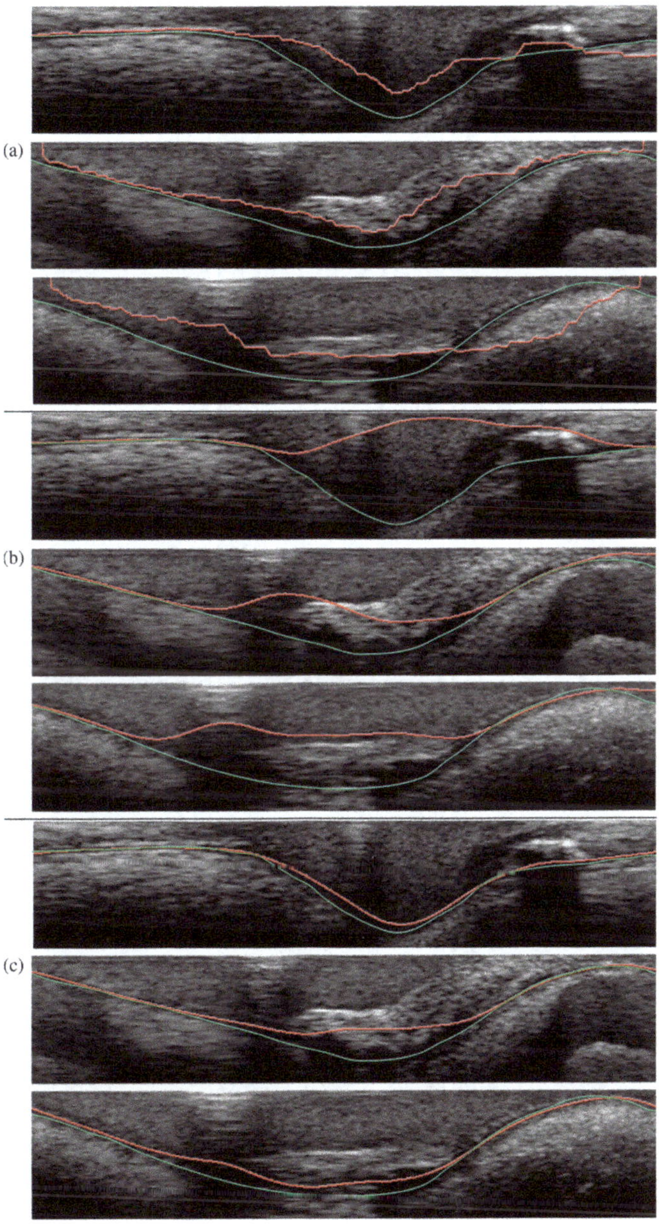

Figure 6.6. Comparison between ground-truth (green) and segmentation results (red): (a) *s–t* graph cut result, (b) single-interface result and (c) double-interface result.

these methods, Zhang *et al* [28] proposed a region-based signed pressure force that combines the Chan–Vese model and geodesic active contour model and utilises a Gaussian filter to avoid re-initialisation of the signed distance function of the generated level set; DRLSE is a typical edge-based method without the need for level set re-initialisation using a distance regularisation term; VFC is a derived active

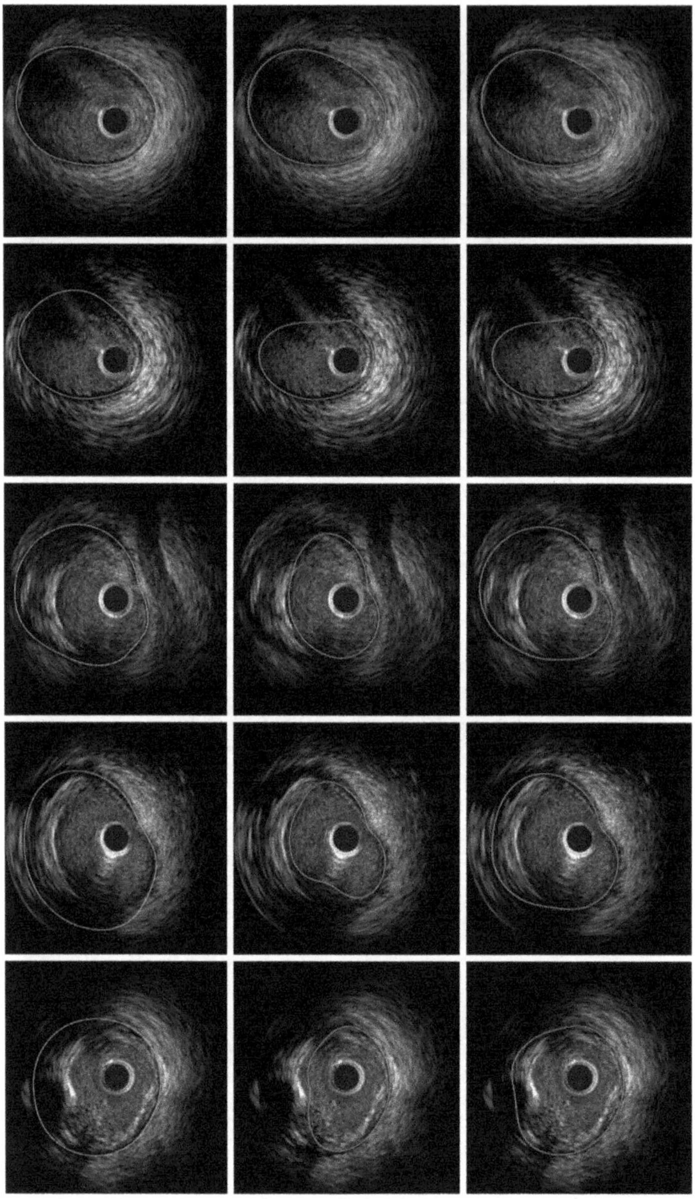
(a) (b) (c)

Figure 6.7. (a) Ground-truth. (b) Single-interface segmentation results. (c) Double-interface segmentation results.

contour model with a proposed vector field convolution as a new external force; and the star graph cut incorporates a star shape prior into the graph cut formulation. In terms of graph-based techniques and shape prior integrations, the proposed method is most similar to the star graph cut in principle. The proposed method is compared to the star graph cut quantitatively and qualitatively with the full acquired data of

Table 6.2. IVUS quantitative comparison. Mean value (standard deviation).

	AMD	HD	AO	Sens.	Spec.
Texture-RBF method [17]	21.68	49.82	83.67	87.92	95.60
	(13.37)	(27.99)	(8.92)	10.14	(4.70)
Single-interface with 1st GD	21.94	53.77	83.57	84.57	98.87
	(19.36)	(39.64)	(13.37)	(13.95)	(1.55)
Proposed method	15.38	39.31	87.91	90.03	97.70
	(9.92)	(23.40)	(6.94)	(6.64)	(5.15)

2283 images. The other methods used in the comparison are all initialisation-dependent and thus we need to choose an appropriate iteration number for the best results, in addition to a careful choice of an initialisation. With these considerations, we randomly select 226 images from the total 2283 images to show their performance in dealing with the OCT segmentation.

In figure 6.9, a set of six OCT images shows the performance of both the star graph cut [23] and the proposed method. The results for the star graph cut and the proposed method are illustrated in columns (c) and (d), respectively, while the original images and their ground-truth are listed in columns (a) and (b). It is obviously apparent that most of the cases in the star graph cut are over-segmented due to the use of 'balloon' force. In contrast, the proposed method generally performs quite well, although the interference of various artefacts exists. However, the proposed method is still affected in some situations due to the adversities in the OCT modality. Several examples with inferior performance are presented in figure 6.10. In row 1, the results show that a serious bifurcation leads to poor performance of the proposed method. In addition, residual blood (shown in row 2) and guide-wire artefacts also cause undermining of border delineation, as shown in rows 3 and 4. The star graph cut performs better than the proposed method in some of these cases.

The quantitative results are presented in table 6.3. The proposed method is superior to the star graph cut in all metrics except for sensitivity. It is understandable that the sensitivity of the star graph cut is a little greater than ours because the star graph cut tends to over-segment.

To compare the proposed method to the deformable methods in capturing the lumen area of OCT images, table 6.4 shows the quantitative results of three edge/region-based methods along with the star graph cut and our method applied to 226 images. As they lack the help of a shape prior, the overall performance of these methods is very poor. In contrast, the proposed method outperforms these techniques significantly. In fact, the Chan–Vese method usually has the advantage over the edge-based method because the region information can be extracted appropriately. However, it is incapable of dealing with an OCT segmentation where the induced artifact is very serious, so its AMD even reaches 39.99 and the AO is merely 38.67%. Among these methods, VFC performs reasonably in terms of the use of the vector field feature, whilst DRLSE cannot detect the lumen properly. In figure

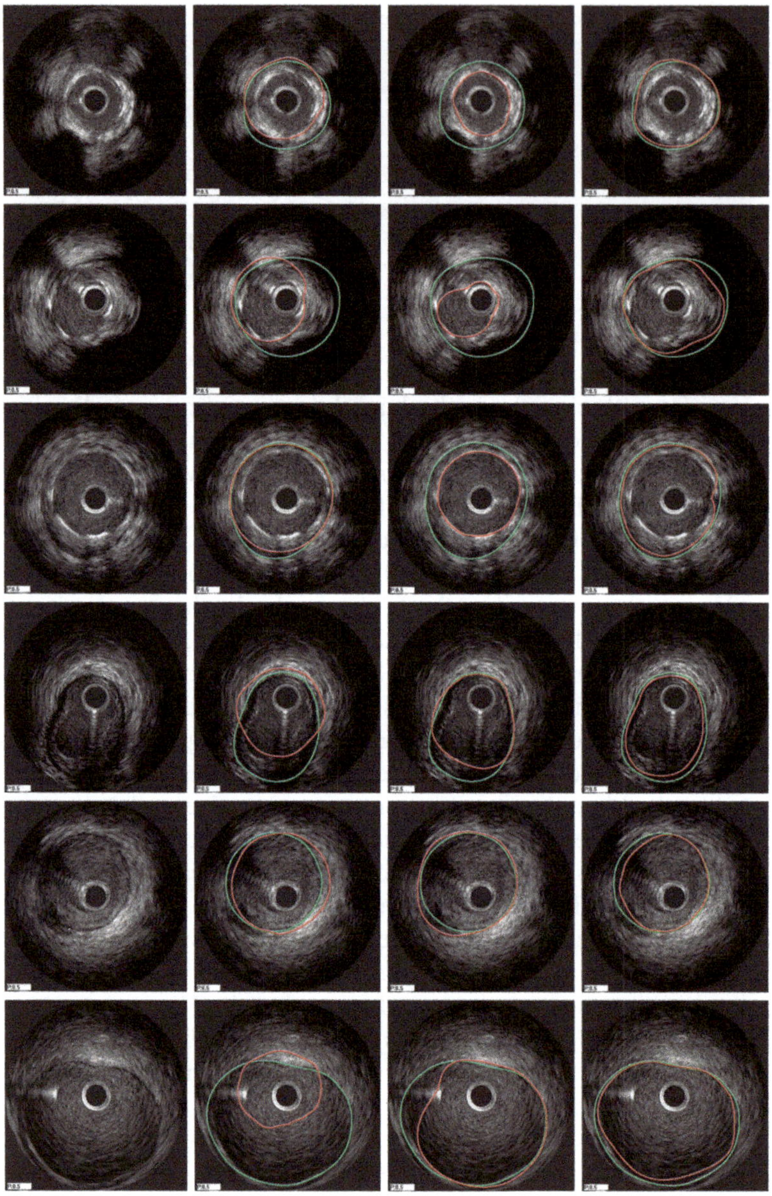

(a) (b) (c) (d)

Figure 6.8. Comparison between ground-truth (green) and segmentation results (red): (a) original image, (b) texture-RBF method, (c) single-interface with 1st GD cost function and (d) proposed double-interface method.

6.11, four examples are presented to illustrate the relevant issues in these methods. In column (c), due to the nature of the Chan–Vese method, the lumen area is always segmented as the background while the bright area is detected. So, the method in [28] is impotent in dealing with the OCT image. In contrast, VFC can perform well in some cases but it meets great difficulties in a situation with serious artefacts, such as

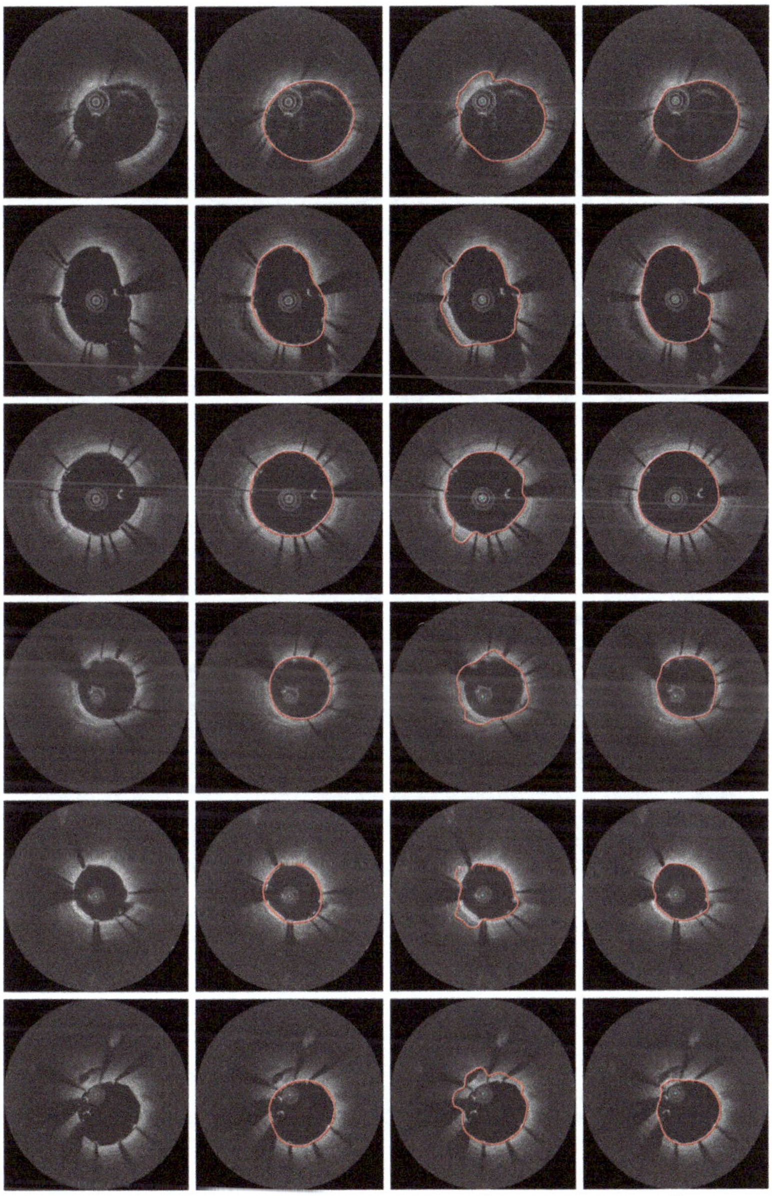

Figure 6.9. Comparison with star graph cut. (a) Original image. (b) Ground-truth. (c) Star graph cut. (d) Proposed method.

the last three cases. A quite similar performance occurs for the method of DRLSE. However, its overall performance is poorer than VFC because it is sensitive to weak edges. It is worth noting that DRLSE and VFC can work well when the artifact interference is acceptable, such as the first case (figure 6.11).

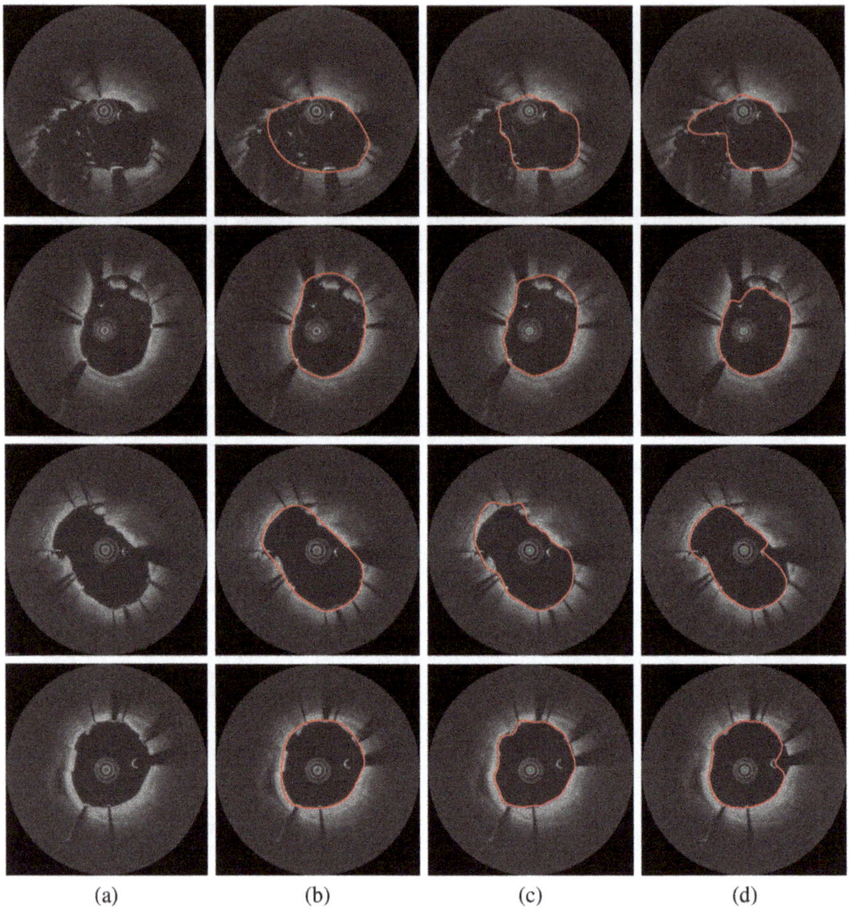

Figure 6.10. Cases with inferior performance of the proposed method. (a) Original image. (b) Ground-truth. (c) Star graph cut. (d) Proposed method.

Table 6.3. Quantitative results with 2283 images for the star graph cut [23] and the proposed method.

	AMD	HD	AO	Sens.	Spec.
Star graph cut [23]	5.85 (4.28)	22.11 (17.91)	91.27 (5.96)	96.52 (4.59)	98.07 (1.65)
Proposed method	4.94 (4.12)	19.09 (20.13)	92.51 (5.43)	96.03 (4.66)	98.85 (1.11)

Table 6.4. Quantitative results with 226 images between the proposed method and the methods in [12, 13, 23] and [28].

	AMD	HD	AO	Sens.	Spec.
Improved Chan–Vese [28]	39.99 (20.54)	95.77 (52.71)	38.67 (30.54)	38.78 (29.36)	99.86 (0.81)
VFC [12]	14.34 (14.69)	50.03 (41.53)	80.05 (16.62)	85.65 (17.72)	97.67 (1.25)
DRLSE [13]	28.44 (9.73)	62.75 (22.56)	68.02 (10.83)	94.72 (9.81)	86.57 (3.65)
Star graph cut [23]	5.45 (3.34)	19.89 (11.45)	91.68 (5.39)	96.77 (3.70)	98.14 (1.03)
Proposed method	4.61 (2.49)	17.08 (12.01)	92.75 (4.45)	96.37 (3.04)	98.83 (1.03)

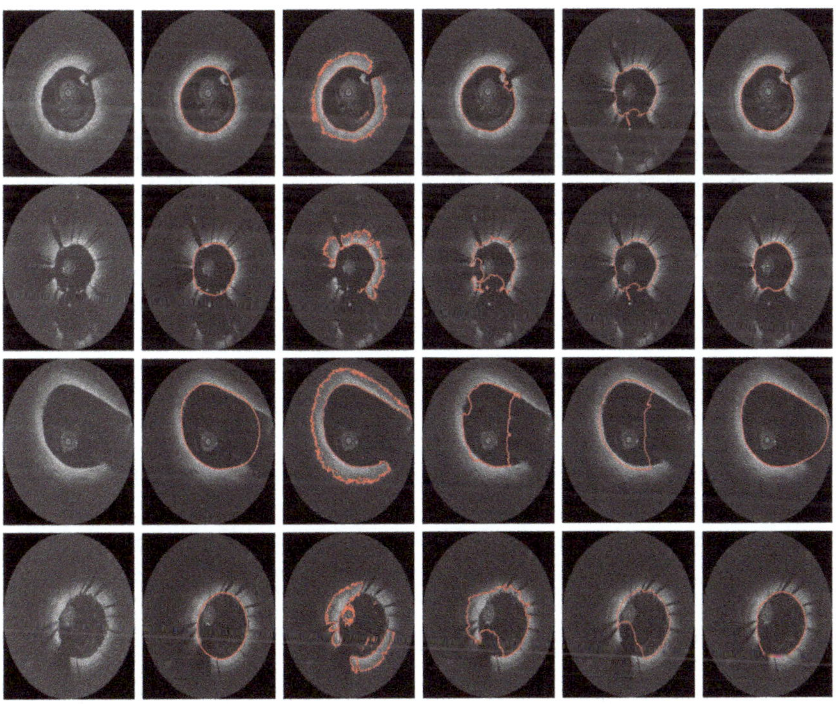

(a) (b) (c) (d) (e) (f)

Figure 6.11. Results of the traditional methods in OCT: (a) original image, (b) ground-truth, (c) improved Chan–Vese method, (d) DRLSE method, (e) VFC method and (f) proposed method.

6.7 Conclusion

Single- and double-interface segmentation methods for OCT and IVUS images were presented. The segmentation problem is defined here as the delineation of the media–adventitia border in IVUS and lumen–intima border in OCT. Images were unravelled to polar coordinates, which facilitate the removing of the catheter ring-down artifact and converting the segmentation problem into finding the minimum closed set graph that implies the border of interest. Steerable Gaussian derivative, Gabor and local phase features are extracted from images that utilise image intensity and texture information to highlight the desired border at different orientations and scales. A new image feature is introduced that is derived from global interactions of gradient vectors across the whole image domain. Laplacian diffusion is employed to refine image features so as to produce more coherent segmentation.

For IVUS segmentation, an automatic double-interface segmentation method is proposed, whose cost functions combine local and global image features and whose geometric constraint is integrated in the graph construction. An auxiliary interface is simultaneously searched to prevent undesirable image features from interfering with the segmentation of the media–adventitia border. Qualitative and quantitative comparison showed superior performance of the proposed method to the traditional graph cut method or single-interface segmentation. For OCT segmentation, a single -interface segmentation is proposed with a cost function defined at the zero-crossing of the circulation density of the gradient convolution field. Experimental results in OCT images demonstrate promising performance in comparison to the star graph cut method. It is also evident that the proposed method takes great advantage of the traditional edge/region-based deformable methods.

References

[1] Boykov Y and Funka-Lea G 2006 Graph cuts and efficient N-D image segmentation *Int. J. Comput. Vis.* **70** 109–31

[2] Boykov Y and Jolly M P 2001 Interactive graph cuts for optimal boundary and region segmentation of objects in N-D images *IEEE Int. Conf. on Computer Vision* (Piscataway, NJ: IEEE) pp 105–12

[3] Boykov Y and Kolmogorov V 2004 An experimental comparison of min-cut/max-flow algorithms for energy minimization in vision *IEEE Trans. Pattern Anal. Mach. Intell.* **26** 1124–37

[4] Chan T and Vese L 2001 Active contours without edges *IEEE Trans. Image Process.* **10** 266–77

[5] Daugman J G 1985 Uncertainty relation for resolution in space, spatial frequency, and orientation optimized by two-dimensional visual cortical filters *J. Opt. Soc. Am.* A **2** 1160–9

[6] Essa E, Xie X, Sazonov I and Nithiarasu P 2011 Automatic IVUS media–adventitia border extraction using double interface graph cut segmentation *IEEE Conf. on Image Processing* (Piscataway, NJ: IEEE) pp 69–72

[7] Essa E, Xie X, Sazonov I, Nithiarasu P and Smith D 2013 Shape prior model for media–adventitia border segmentation in IVUS using graph cut *Medical Computer Vision. Recognition Techniques and Applications in Medical Imaging (Lecture Notes in Computer

Science vol 7766) ed B Menze, G Langs, L Lu, A Montillo, Z Tu and A Criminisi (Berlin: Springer) pp 114–23
[8] Fields D 1987 Relations between the statistics of natural images and the response properties of cortical cells *Opt. Soc. Am.* **4** 2379–94
[9] Freeman W T and Adelson E H 1991 The design and use of steerable filters *IEEE Trans. Pattern Anal. Mach. Intell.* **13** 891–906
[10] Jones J L, Xie X and Essa E 2014 Combining region-based and imprecise boundary-based cues for interactive medical image segmentation *Int. J. Numer. Methods Biomed. Eng.* **30** 1649–66
[11] Kovesi P 1997 Symmetry and asymmetry from local phase *Tenth Australian Joint Conf. on Artificial Intelligence* pp 185–90
[12] Li B and Acton S 2007 Active contour external force using vector field convolution for image segmentation *IEEE Trans. Image Process.* **16** 2096–106
[13] Li C, Xu C, Gui C and Fox M 2010 Distance regularized level set evolution and its application to image segmentation *IEEE Trans. Image Process.* **19** 3243–54
[14] Li K, Wu X, Chen D Z and Sonka M 2006 Optimal surface segmentation in volumetric images—a graph-theoretic approach *IEEE Trans. Pattern Anal. Mach. Intell.* **28** 119–34
[15] MacDonald D, Kabani N, Avis D and Evans A 2000 Automated 3-D extraction of inner and outer surfaces of cerebral cortex from MRI *NeuroImage* **vol 12** 340–56
[16] Mulet-Parada M and Noble A 2000 2D + T acoustic boundary detection in echocardiography *Med. Image Anal.* **4** 21–30
[17] Papadogiorgaki M, Mezaris V, Chatzizisis Y S, Giannoglou G D and Kompatsiaris I 2008 Image analysis techniques for automated IVUS contour detection *Ultrasound Med. Biol.* **9** 1482–98
[18] Sonka M, Zhang X, Siebes M, Bissing M S, DeJong S C, Collins S M and McKay C R 1995 Segmentation of intravascular ultrasound images: a knowledge-based approach *IEEE Trans. Med. Imaging* **14** 719–32
[19] Spreeuwers L and Breeuwer M 2003 Detection of left ventricular epi- and endocardial borders using coupled active contours *Int. Congr. Ser.* **1256** 1147–52
[20] Sun S, Sonka M and Beichel R 2013 Graph-based IVUS segmentation with efficient computer-aided refinement *IEEE Trans. Med. Imaging* **32** 1536–49
[21] Takagi A, Hibi K, Zhang X, Teo T J, Bonneau H N, Yock P G and Fitzgerald P J 2000 Automated contour detection for high frequency intravascular ultrasound imaging: a technique with blood noise reduction for edge enhancement *Ultrasound Med. Biol.* **26** 1033–41
[22] Valois R L D, Albrecht D G and Thorell L G 1982 Spatial frequency selectivity of cells in macaque visual cortex *Vis. Res.* **22** 545–59
[23] Veksler O 2008 Star shape prior for graph-cut image segmentation *Computer Vision—ECCV 2008* (*Lecture Notes in Computer Science* vol 5304) ed D Forsyth, P Torr and A Zisserman (Berlin: Springer) pp 454–67
[24] Wahle A, Lopez J J, Olszewski M E, Vigmostad S C, Chandran K B, Rossen J D and Sonka M 2006 Plaque development, vessel curvature, and wall shear stress in coronary arteries assessed by x-ray angiography and intravascular ultrasound *Med. Image Anal.* **10** 615–31
[25] Xie X and Mirmehdi M 2006 Magnetostatic field for the active contour model: a study in convergence *Proc. of the British Machine Vision Conf.* (Surrey, UK: BMVA Press) pp 14.1–10

[26] Xie X and Mirmehdi M 2008 MAC: magnetostatic active contour model *IEEE Trans. Pattern Anal. Mach. Intell.* **30** 632–46
[27] Zhang H, Essa E and Xie X 2013 Graph based segmentation with minimal user interaction *IEEE Conf. on Image Processing* (Piscataway, NJ: IEEE) pp 4074–8
[28] Zhang K, Zhang L, Song H and Zhou W 2010 Active contours with selective local or global segmentation: a new formulation and level set method *Image Vis. Comput.* **28** 668–76

IOP Publishing

Vascular and Intravascular Imaging Trends, Analysis, and Challenges, Volume 1
Stent applications
Petia Radeva and Jasjit S Suri

Chapter 7

Blind inpainting and outlier detection using logarithmic transformation and total variation

Manya V Afonso and J Miguel Sanches

In this work, we address the problem of image reconstruction with missing pixels or outliers, when the locations of the corrupted pixels are not known and when the noise is multiplicative, which is the algebraic model for ultrasound and synthetic aperture radar imaging. A logarithmic transformation is applied to convert the multiplication between the image, the binary mask and the Rayleigh distributed speckle noise into an additive problem. The image and mask terms are then estimated iteratively with total variation regularization applied on the image, and ℓ_0 regularization on the mask term, which imposes sparseness on the support set of the missing pixels. The resulting alternating minimization scheme simultaneously estimates the image and mask, in the same iterative process. Experimental results show that the proposed method can deal with a larger fraction of missing pixels than two-phase methods, which first estimate the mask and then reconstruct the image. Furthermore, it was experimentally observed that applying the algorithm on radio frequency (RF) images of the carotid artery or intravascular ultrasound images led to an outlier map which clearly delineates the lumen, and can therefore be applicable for segmentation.

7.1 Introduction

Faulty imaging sensors or bit errors during transmission can cause some pixels in an image to be lost or corrupted by impulse noise [14, 38]. In the case of missing pixel values, the corrupted pixels are assumed to have a value equal to zero, and the problem of estimating the complete image is called the inpainting problem [11, 42, 53]. When the image is corrupted by impulse noise, the corrupted pixels have values different from zero, which are drawn from a binary distribution (salt-and-pepper noise), or from a uniform distribution (random valued impulse noise).

doi:10.1088/2053-2563/ab01fach7

Ultrasound images and those from some other coherent imaging modalities are corrupted by a type of noise called speckle noise, which results from interference patterns. Although it is a random process, some works argue that it contains useful information about the microstructure of the tissue and the properties of the incident pressure field [43, 49]. It has been shown that the observed ultrasound RF image can be well approximated as an element-wise multiplication between the image pixels which represent the morphological structure of the organ being imaged, and the speckle field [43]. The statistics of the speckle noise in ultrasound RF images has been assumed to follow the Rayleigh distribution [1, 30, 58]. Other non-Rayleigh distributions such as the gamma distribution [55, 57] and Rayleigh mixture models [52] have also been considered in the literature.

Despeckling methods seek to reduce the speckle noise and make the morphological structures more clearly visible. Denoising methods developed for this modality take into account the multiplicative algebraic relation and the Rayleigh statistics of the noise [4, 13, 50, 64]. Some methods characterize the spiky components of the speckle as outliers which do not fit in the statistical distribution assumed. In [43], an outlier shrinkage step is applied on the log-transformed image to eliminate these outliers. An adaptive window method to compute local statistics and to discard local extrema and replace them by average values based on the local statistics on the B-mode image was proposed in [56]. It was reported in [65] that outliers in ultrasound images resulted from tissue shifting and made image registration difficult.

Image reconstruction and inpainting methods for multiplicative noise generally require the pixel locations of the outliers to be known and therefore cannot be applied to estimate the pixel values at the locations of the outliers. In [5], a new method for blind image inpainting was proposed, which estimates the values of pixels which are missing or corrupted with impulse noise, when their locations are unknown. This method was also extended to non-additive and non-Gaussian noises. In this chapter, we review this method for the case of Rayleigh multiplicative speckle noise, and show that applying it on an ultrasound image can be used as a segmentation method.

The image to be estimated has n pixels and is represented as a vector, say in lexicographic ordering, $\mathbf{x} \in \mathbb{R}^n$. Let $m < n$ be the number of observed pixels or pixels free from impulse noise. The loss of pixels or observing a partial set of m pixels out of n can be represented as an element-wise multiplication of the image with a binary mask in which all but m pixels are zero. In our representation, this observation process is represented as a multiplication of the vector $\mathbf{x}$ with a size $n \times n$ identity matrix $\mathbf{A}$ with the respective diagonal elements corresponding to the $(n - m)$ missing pixels set to zero.

For multiplicative noise, the mapping from $\mathbf{x}$ to the partially observed image $\mathbf{y}$ is given by

$$\mathbf{y} = \mathbf{A}(\mathbf{x} \cdot \eta_S), \tag{7.1}$$

where the speckle noise term η_S is Rayleigh or Gamma distributed, and the multiplication is element-wise.

When the image is corrupted by impulse noise, those pixels of **y** corresponding to the zeros on the diagonal of the observation matrix **A** have a value that corresponds to the noise field η_I,

$$\mathbf{y} = \mathbf{A}(\mathbf{x} \cdot \eta_G) + (\mathbf{I}_n - \mathbf{A})\eta_I. \tag{7.2}$$

Our goal is to estimate the image **x** from the partial observations **y** and also estimate the matrix **A** which indicates which pixels are outliers.

7.1.1 Related work

For standard inpainting, i.e. when the index set of the observed pixels or the observation mask **A** is known, the reconstruction problem can be solved by one of several existing methods for image reconstruction from a sparse set of observations. Many of these methods, such as [2, 9, 10, 22, 32, 37, 41], were developed for the additive and Gaussian noise model and often in the context of compressed sensing [16, 26] reconstruction. However, it must be noted that in compressed sensing the observation operator needs to satisfy conditions to lead to incoherent observations [17]. For the removal of impulse noise, a common approach is to estimate the support set of the noisy pixels using an outlier detection method, to obtain an estimate of **A** and then apply the reconstruction method.

For the additive and Gaussian noise model, there exist several methods for reconstructing an image with missing data and removing impulse noise. Early approaches for estimating the missing values used median filtering, which discards outliers [38]. The adaptive median filter (AMF) [38] and adaptive center weighted median filter [21] were developed to detect the positions of noisy pixels with, respectively, salt-and-pepper and random valued impulse noise. Median filters rely on the accuracy of the neighboring pixels and inherently cannot deal with a large percentage of outliers. In [25] an improved outlier detector based on thresholding, a measure called the rank-ordered logarithmic difference with edge preserving regularization (ROLD-EPR) was proposed, for random valued impulse noise.

Two-phase methods for estimating the image involve a mask estimation step, in which the observation mask **A** is estimated using outlier detection, and a reconstruction step in which a standard convex optimization procedure is used with the estimate of **A** [15, 19]. Another commonly used formulation for denoising with impulse noise is a sum of an ℓ_1-norm data fidelity term and total variation (TV) [20, 48] regularizers, leading to an ℓ_1-TV optimization problem [15]. Sparse regularization using either the ℓ_0 or ℓ_1 norm regularizers on the impulse noise term or support set of the outliers was used in [15, 24, 60] and [62]. An iteratively reweighted least squares (IRLS) based method for mixed impulse and Gaussian noise removal was proposed in [46, 47] with an ℓ_2 data fidelity term corresponding to the observed pixels, an ℓ_1 term corresponding to the noisy pixels and TV regularization on the image.

Several of the above methods are based on alternating minimization, where two or more variables are iteratively estimated through a Gauss–Seidel method [44].

A related approach is the augmented Lagrangian (AL)/alternating direction method of multipliers (ADMM) framework [29], which has been used extensively in recent work on image reconstruction/restoration because of its mathematical elegance and computational speed [37, 63].

For the Poisson noise model, there exist methods for image reconstruction from a partial set of pixels with the observation matrix known, such as [33, 34, 40]. Another method proposed in [8] filled in missing data through the minimization of the image gradient and an approximate solution of the mean curvature flow equation. Patch-based dictionary learning methods for the Poisson model were proposed in [35] for image denoising and in [36] for inpainting.

For the Rayleigh speckle noise model, existing methods such as the classical interpolation methods for ultrasound [54], as well as those based on TV regularization after logarithmic compression [6, 49], all require the sampling matrix to be known. A denoising method for ultrasound with an outlier shrinkage step applied on the log-transformed image was proposed in [43].

7.1.2 Contributions and organization

In [5], we proposed a method to estimate the image $\mathbf{x}$ and the observation mask $\mathbf{A}$, simultaneously, for the additive and Gaussian noise model. We formulated the masking operation as a summation after logarithmic compression, and applied a TV regularizer on the term corresponding to the logarithm of the image, and an ℓ_0-norm regularizer on the term corresponding to the mask. The TV regularizer encourages the estimate of $\mathbf{x}$ to be piece-wise smooth, while the ℓ_0-norm regularizer encourages the mask term to be sparse. The problem was solved iteratively using a Gauss–Seidel alternating minimization scheme. This method was extended to the multiplicative and Rayleigh distributed speckle noise, and Poisson noise models. The data fidelity terms corresponding to these statistical models allow the relation between the image and observation mask to remain additive after logarithmic transformation.

In this chapter, we review the blind inpainting method for multiplicative and Rayleigh distributed noise, and present results for outlier detection in ultrasound images. We show that applying the blind inpainting algorithm on ultrasound images of the carotid artery, without loss of pixels, produced outlier maps which corresponded roughly to the lumen and can be useful for segmenting the images.

We formulate the estimation problem and the blind inpainting algorithm in section 7.2.2. In section 7.3, we present experimental results on inpainting. Subsection 7.3.2 presents results for the application of blind inpainting for segmentation of the lumen.

7.2 Blind inpainting

We begin with the method for blind inpainting for the additive and Gaussian noise model, which is mathematically simpler, and then elaborate the method for multiplicative and Rayleigh distributed noise. In section 7.2.1, the observation model is

$$\mathbf{y} = \mathbf{A}(\mathbf{x} + \boldsymbol{\eta}_G), \tag{7.3}$$

where $\boldsymbol{\eta}_G$ is an additive Gaussian noise term.

7.2.1 Blind inpainting for additive noise

For standard inpainting with TV regularization on the image and with the observation mask **A** known, the problem of estimating **x** as formulated and solved in [2, 22] is

$$\hat{\mathbf{x}} = \arg\min_{\mathbf{x}} \frac{1}{2}\|\mathbf{A}\mathbf{x} - \mathbf{y}\|^2 + \frac{\lambda}{2}TV(\mathbf{x}), \tag{7.4}$$

where $TV(.)$ is the isotropic total variation function and $\lambda > 0$ is the regularization parameter. Note that this problem assumes the additive and Gaussian noise model and has an ℓ_2-norm data fidelity term.

When we need to estimate both the image **x** and the mask **A**, a regularizer $\phi(.)$ is applied on **A**, leading to

$$(\hat{\mathbf{x}}, \hat{\mathbf{A}}) = \arg\min_{\mathbf{x},\mathbf{A}} \frac{1}{2}\|\mathbf{A}\mathbf{x} - \mathbf{y}\|^2 + \frac{\lambda_1}{2}TV(\mathbf{x}) + \frac{\lambda_2}{2}\phi(\mathbf{A}), \tag{7.5}$$

where we now have two regularization parameters, $\lambda_1, \lambda_2 > 0$, for each of the two regularizer terms. The problem (7.5) is difficult to solve because it is not separable for our variables $(\mathbf{x}, \mathbf{A})$.

In [5], a logarithmic transform was used to convert the masking problem into an additive and separable one. Since **A** is a diagonal matrix $\mathbf{A} = \mathrm{diag}(\mathbf{a})$ and the masking operation is element-wise multiplication, the variable of optimization for the observation matrix is the vector of diagonal elements $\mathbf{a} \in \{0, 1\}^n$. When a pixel with index i is observed, the corresponding mask element $a_i = 1$, and when pixel i is lost, $a_i = 0$. Thus, a pixel k in vector **y** is defined as the scalar product,

$$y_i = x_i \times a_i. \tag{7.6}$$

It is not known *a priori* if a given pixel y_k corresponds to an observed one ($a_k = 1$) or not ($a_k = 0$). Rather than have $a_i = 0$ when the pixel is not observed, where a_i is defined to be a small value in the order of 10^{-K} or smaller, K being a positive integer that depends on the dynamic range of the image, typically greater than or equal to 3. Defining $v_i = \log(a_i)$,

$$v_i = \begin{cases} 0, & \text{if } i \text{ is observed} \\ -K, & \text{otherwise} \end{cases}. \tag{7.7}$$

Assuming that **y** and **x** are always positive, applying a logarithmic transformation on equation (7.6) converts it into an additive model,

$$\log y_i = \log(x_i \times a_i), \tag{7.8}$$

$$\log y_i = \log x_i + \log a_i, \tag{7.9}$$

$$g_i = u_i + v_i, \tag{7.10}$$

where $u_i = \log x_i$ and $g_i = \log(y_i + \delta)$. A small positive bias term $\delta > 0$ is added to $\mathbf{y}$ to guarantee positivity. The base of the logarithm used is 10, but we could use the natural logarithm with the only difference being an additive constant term. The problem is now estimating the vectors $\mathbf{u}$ and $\mathbf{v}$, given the log-transformed observation $\mathbf{g}$. We assume that our image $\mathbf{x}$ and therefore its logarithmic transformation $\mathbf{u}$ are piece-wise smooth. We apply a TV regularizer on the log-transformed image $\mathbf{u}$, and the ℓ_0-norm regularizer on the log-transformed mask $\mathbf{v}$. The negative elements of $\mathbf{v}$ therefore correspond to the non-observed pixels and those elements of $\mathbf{v}$ which are equal to 0 correspond to the observed pixels. Since the ℓ_0-norm indicates the number of non-zero elements irrespective of their sign, minimizing $\|\mathbf{v}\|_0$ minimizes the number of non-observed pixels.

The problem therefore becomes

$$(\hat{\mathbf{u}}, \hat{\mathbf{v}}) = \arg\min_{\mathbf{u},\mathbf{v}} \frac{1}{2}\|\mathbf{g} - \mathbf{u} - \mathbf{v}\|_2^2 + \frac{\lambda_1}{2}\mathrm{TV}(\mathbf{u}) + \frac{\lambda_2}{2}\|\mathbf{v}\|_0, \tag{7.11}$$

where $\lambda_1, \lambda_2 > 0$ are the respective regularization parameters.

Since equation (7.11) is a separable problem, we can apply an iterative alternating method as in [12]. We apply an iterative alternating minimization to solve equation (7.11), by isolating the terms in each variable keeping the other fixed, leading to a Gauss–Seidel scheme. Solving for $\mathbf{u}$ at iteration t,

$$\hat{\mathbf{u}}^{(t)} = \arg\min_{\mathbf{u}} \frac{1}{2}\|\mathbf{g} - \mathbf{u} - \mathbf{v}^{(t)}\|_2^2 + \frac{\lambda_1}{2}\mathrm{TV}(\mathbf{u}). \tag{7.12}$$

This is a TV regularized denoising problem, the solution of which can be computed efficiently using an algorithm such as Chambolle's algorithm [18].

Similarly, for $\mathbf{v}$ at iteration t we have

$$\hat{\mathbf{v}}^{(t)} = \arg\min_{\mathbf{u}} \frac{1}{2}\|\mathbf{g} - \mathbf{u}^{(t)} - \mathbf{v}\|_2^2 + \frac{\lambda_2}{2}\|\mathbf{v}\|_0. \tag{7.13}$$

This problem although non-convex, has a solution given by the hard threshold [27]

$$\hat{\mathbf{v}}^{(t)} = H_{\sqrt{2\lambda_2}}(\mathbf{g} - \mathbf{u}^{(t)}), \tag{7.14}$$

where $H_{\lambda_2}(.)$ is the hard threshold operator and is defined element-wise as

$$v_i^{(t)} = \begin{cases} 0, & \text{if } \left(g_i - u_i^{(t)}\right) \leqslant \sqrt{2\lambda_2}, \\ \left(g_i - u_i^{(t)}\right), & \text{otherwise.} \end{cases} \tag{7.15}$$

The steps (7.12) and (7.13) are run alternatingly until the stopping criterion is satisfied. Continuation schemes can be used on the regularization parameters λ_1, λ_2, in which they are multiplied by a factor greater than one, until they reach a certain maximum value, as was done in [59]. The estimates of the image and mask are computed by inverting the logarithmic transformation, $\hat{\mathbf{x}} = 10^{\hat{\mathbf{u}}}$ and $\hat{\mathbf{a}} = 10^{\hat{\mathbf{v}}}$. The conditions for convergence [29, 34] do not require equation (7.12) to be solved exactly, as long as the error sequence decreases and the parameter μ is positive.

7.2.2 Blind inpainting for Rayleigh multiplicative noise

We now extend the method described in the previous sub-section to the multiplicative and Rayleigh distributed noise model. An intuitive way would be to apply the logarithmic transform to convert the observation model (7.1) into an additive one. Then, we could apply the method described in the previous section. However, this approach does not take into account the statistical model of the noise and the appropriate data fidelity term for Rayleigh speckle noise.

We therefore extend the blind inpainting method to Rayleigh distributed multiplicative speckle noise by using the appropriate data fidelity term. For multiplicative noise, multiplying a pixel whose value is 0 will always lead to the corresponding observed pixel being equal to 0 as well. Therefore, we interchange the order of the noisy observation and masking so that our observation $\mathbf{y}$ is the result of observing the masked image $\mathbf{Ax}$ under the noise model. The observation model changes from equation (7.1) to,

$$\mathbf{y} = (\mathbf{Ax}) \cdot \boldsymbol{\eta}_S. \tag{7.16}$$

For the Rayleigh multiplicative noise, the likelihood function is

$$p(\mathbf{y}|\mathbf{Ax}) = \prod_{i=1}^{n} \frac{y_i}{a_i x_i} \exp\left(-\frac{y_i^2}{2(a_i x_i)}\right). \tag{7.17}$$

It is straightforward to show that (see [51] for more details) the associated data fidelity term between $\mathbf{y}$ and $\mathbf{Ax}$ is

$$J_r(\mathbf{y}, \mathbf{Ax}) = \sum_{i=1}^{n}\left(\frac{y_i^2}{2(a_i x_i)} + \log(a_i x_i)\right). \tag{7.18}$$

In equation (7.18), we see that there appears a term with the product $(a_i x_i)$ and a term involving its logarithm. Therefore, as before, we can work with the log-transformed variables $\mathbf{u} = \log \mathbf{x}$ and $\mathbf{v} = \log \mathbf{a}$. Thus equation (7.18) changes to

$$J_r(\mathbf{y}, \mathbf{u}, \mathbf{v}) = \sum_{i=1}^{n}\left(\frac{y_i^2}{2} e^{-(u_i+v_i)} + u_i + v_i\right). \tag{7.19}$$

We now formulate our optimization problem, once again with TV regularization on $\mathbf{u}$ and ℓ_0 regularization on $\mathbf{v}$. The data fidelity term $J(.)$ is changed accordingly. The problem (7.11) for the additive Gaussian noise model changes to the more general problem

$$(\hat{\mathbf{u}}, \hat{\mathbf{v}}) = \arg\min_{\mathbf{u},\mathbf{v}} J(\mathbf{y}, \mathbf{u}, \mathbf{v}) + \frac{\lambda_1}{2} TV(\mathbf{u}) + \frac{\lambda_2}{2} \|\mathbf{v}\|_0. \tag{7.20}$$

Since equation (7.19) involves the sum of a linear term and an exponential term, it is non-separable for **u** and **v**. Therefore, we need to use variable splitting [23] to be able to use the augmented Lagrangian/alternating direction method of multipliers (AL/ADMM) to solve equation (7.20). We therefore introduce two auxiliary variables **z** and **w** to act as the arguments of the TV and ℓ_0 regularizer terms, respectively, leading to the constrained problem

$$\begin{aligned} &\min_{\mathbf{u},\mathbf{v},\mathbf{z},\mathbf{w}} \; J(\mathbf{y}, \mathbf{u}, \mathbf{v}) + \frac{\lambda_1}{2} TV(\mathbf{z}) + \frac{\lambda_2}{2} \|\mathbf{w}\|_0 \\ &\text{subject to} \qquad \mathbf{u} = \mathbf{z}, \; \mathbf{v} = \mathbf{w}. \end{aligned} \tag{7.21}$$

Using the augmented Lagrangian [39, 45], this problem can be shown to be equivalent to the minimization problem

$$\begin{aligned} &\min_{\mathbf{u},\mathbf{v},\mathbf{z},\mathbf{w}} J(\mathbf{y}, \mathbf{u}, \mathbf{v}) + \frac{\lambda_1}{2} TV(\mathbf{z}) + \frac{\lambda_2}{2} \|\mathbf{w}\|_0 \\ &+ \frac{\mu_1}{2} \|\mathbf{u} - \mathbf{z} - \mathbf{d}_z\|_2^2 + \frac{\mu_2}{2} \|\mathbf{v} - \mathbf{w} - \mathbf{d}_w\|_2^2, \end{aligned} \tag{7.22}$$

where $\mu_1, \mu_2 \geqslant 0$ are the penalty parameters, and $\mathbf{d}_z$, $\mathbf{d}_w$ are the so-called Bregman update vectors [37]. This problem is split into four problems at each iteration by gathering all the terms in each variable, and solving for each by keeping the others fixed. Thus, the AL algorithm iterates between minimizing the objective function in equation (7.22) with respect to **f** and **u**, leading to a Gauss–Seidel process (for more details, see [2, 3, 31] and references therein) which at iteration t is summarized as

$$\mathbf{u}^{(t+1)} = \arg\min_{\mathbf{u}} J(\mathbf{y}, \mathbf{u}, \mathbf{v}^{(t)}) + \frac{\mu_1}{2} \left\| \mathbf{u} - \mathbf{z}^{(t)} - \mathbf{d}_z^{(t)} \right\|_2^2 \tag{7.23}$$

$$\mathbf{v}^{(t+1)} = \arg\min_{\mathbf{v}} J(\mathbf{y}, \mathbf{u}^{(t)}, \mathbf{v}) + \frac{\mu_2}{2} \left\| \mathbf{v} - \mathbf{w}^{(t)} - \mathbf{d}_w^{(t)} \right\|_2^2 \tag{7.24}$$

$$\mathbf{z}^{(t+1)} = \arg\min_{\mathbf{z}} \frac{\mu_1}{2} \left\| \mathbf{u}^{(t)} - \mathbf{z} - \mathbf{d}_z^{(t)} \right\|_2^2 + \frac{\lambda_1}{2} TV(\mathbf{z}) \tag{7.25}$$

$$\mathbf{w}^{(t+1)} = \arg\min_{\mathbf{w}} \frac{\mu_2}{2} \left\| \mathbf{v}^{(t)} - \mathbf{w} - \mathbf{d}_w^{(t)} \right\|_2^2 + \frac{\lambda_2}{2} \|\mathbf{w}\|_0 \tag{7.26}$$

$$\begin{aligned} \mathbf{d}_z^{(t+1)} &= \mathbf{d}_z^{(t)} + \mathbf{z}^{(t+1)} - \mathbf{u}^{(t+1)}, \\ \mathbf{d}_w^{(t+1)} &= \mathbf{d}_w^{(t)} + \mathbf{w}^{(t+1)} - \mathbf{v}^{(t+1)}. \end{aligned}$$

As in the case of Gaussian noise, the ℓ_2-TV denoising problem from equation (7.25) is solved using a few iterations of Chambolle's algorithm and the $\ell_2 - \ell_0$ regularized denoising problem from equation (7.26) is solved using the hard threshold. The problems involving $J(.)$, equations (7.23) and (7.24) can be solved approximately using a few iterations of Newton's method [44], after plugging in equation (7.19).

The proposed method for blind inpainting with Rayleigh multiplicative noise is summarized in the following algorithm.

Algorithm. Blind inpainting—non-Gaussian noise
1. Input $\mathbf{y}$.
2. Initialize parameters $\delta > 0$, $K > 0$, λ_1, λ_2, μ_1, μ_2, initial estimates $\mathbf{u}^{(0)}, \mathbf{v}^{(0)}, \mathbf{z}^{(0)}, \mathbf{w}^{(0)}, \mathbf{d}_z^{(0)}, \mathbf{d}_w^{(0)}$.
3. Set $t = 0$.
4. **Repeat.**
5. Compute $\mathbf{u}^{(t+1)}$ using Newton's method to solve (7.23).
6. Compute $\mathbf{v}^{(t+1)}$ using Newton's method to solve (7.24).
7. Compute $\mathbf{z}^{(t+1)}$ using Chambolle's method to solve (7.25).
8. Compute $\mathbf{w}^{(t+1)} \leftarrow H_{\lambda_2/\mu_2}\left(\mathbf{v}^{(t)} - \mathbf{d}_w^{(t)}\right)$.
9. $\mathbf{d}_z^{(t+1)} \leftarrow \mathbf{d}_z^{(t)} + \mathbf{z}^{(t+1)} - \mathbf{u}^{(t+1)}$.
10. $\mathbf{d}_w^{(t+1)} \leftarrow \mathbf{d}_w^{(t)} + \mathbf{w}^{(t+1)} - \mathbf{v}^{(t+1)}$.
11. Update values of λ_1, λ_2.
12. $t \leftarrow t + 1$
13. **Until** the stopping criterion is satisfied.
14. Set estimates $\hat{\mathbf{x}} = e^{\mathbf{u}}$, $\hat{\mathbf{a}} = e^{\mathbf{v}}$.

7.3 Experimental results

In this section we compare our proposed method for blind inpainting, with inpainting using the additive model after logarithmic transformation. In the synthetic experiments with the Lena and Cameraman images, we have the noise free image for reference and use the normalized mean absolute error (NMAE) [28], which is defined as $\|\mathbf{x} - \hat{\mathbf{x}}\|_1 / \|\mathbf{x}\|_1$, the figure of merit. The accuracy of the estimation of the mask is measured in terms of the number of incorrectly estimated mask pixels, which is obtained by the binary exclusive or XOR operation between the estimated mask and the reference. A logical value equal to 1 is obtained at the mask pixels estimated incorrectly, and zero otherwise. Hence, the sum over all the pixels of the logical XOR operation is a measure of the errors in the estimate of the mask. All experiments were performed on MATLAB on an Ubuntu Linux based server with 64 GB of RAM.

Results for the additive and Gaussian noise and Poisson noise models can be found in [5].

7.3.1 Blind inpainting

To test our proposed method, we generate a random binary mask with a fraction of its elements equal to zero and multiply it element-wise to our image corrupted with multiplicative Rayleigh noise. The criteria used to evaluate the accuracy of estimation are the NMAE, the structural similarity index measure (SSIM) [61] and the fraction of incorrectly estimated mask pixels.

We normalize the Lena image by dividing by the maximum pixel value. To compare our method, we use a logarithmic transformation followed by inpainting using a method for inpainting with additive noise. In this case, we use fast two-phase deblurring [15], since AOP [62], although faster, also divides the observed image by 255, and in the case of Rayleigh speckle, the image is already normalized. We summarize our results for the Lena and cameraman images for different fractions of missing pixels, in table 7.1. We can see that taking into account the statistical model offers an improvement in terms of the NMAE. The existing methods for blind inpainting do not always work well for large fractions of missing pixels, above 50%, or take a long time, over 10 min.

For the Lena image, a cropped region from the noisy image with 50% of the pixels missing is shown in figure 7.1(b) and the respective estimates using the proposed

Table 7.1. Inpainting with Rayleigh noise. κ indicates the fraction of missing pixels. (*) The additive model is used after logarithmic transformation [5] (© 2015 IEEE).

		Lena				Cameraman			
κ	Method	Time (s)	NMAE	SSIM	Mask err. (%)	Time (s)	NMAE	SSIM	Mask err. (%)
0.25	Proposed	41	3.12×10^{-06}	0.973	0.664	15.5	1.23×10^{-05}	0.975	11.6
	Additive(*)	11.3	3.81×10^{-06}	0.958	0.000 19	17.3	1.53×10^{-05}	0.961	0.001 14
0.5	Proposed	66.8	3.16×10^{-06}	0.972	0.317	24.4	1.26×10^{-05}	0.974	2.13
	Additive(*)	75.8	3.82×10^{-06}	0.958	4.9	**19.1**	1.53×10^{-05}	0.961	4.29
0.7	Proposed	116	3.17×10^{-06}	0.972	0.0835	156	1.27×10^{-05}	0.973	0.484

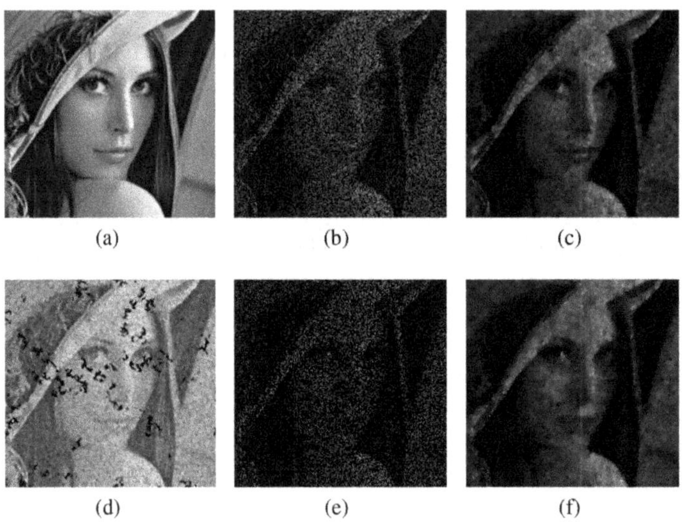

Figure 7.1. Blind inpainting with Rayleigh noise with the Lena image: (a) original image (cropped), (b) observed image with Rayleigh noise and 50% of its pixels missing; (c) estimate from (b) using the proposed method; (d) estimate using inpainting with the additive model after logarithmic transformation; (e) observed image with Rayleigh noise and 70% of its pixels missing; and (f) estimate from (e) using the proposed method [5] (© 2015 IEEE).

method [15] and after logarithmic transformation are shown in figure 7.1(c) and 7.1(d). For a pixel loss of 70%, the observed image and estimate using the proposed method are shown in figure 7.1(e) and 7.1(f). Blind inpainting with Poisson noise for the Cameraman image with 50% and 70% of its pixels missing is illustrated in figure 7.2.

Figure 7.3 demonstrates blind inpainting with the Rayleigh multiplicative noise model for a transversal ultrasound (US) image of the carotid artery. The noisy RF envelope image is shown in figure 7.3(a). The observed image with 75% of the pixels missing is shown in figure 7.3(b). The estimate using the proposed method is shown in figure 7.3(c), with the diagonal profiles shown in figure 7.3(e). We can see from the result of the binary XOR operation between the sampling mask and its estimate shown in figure 7.3(d), that the incorrectly estimated bits are in the region of low pixel values in the RF image. The computation time was 119.3 s for an image of size 201 × 201.

7.3.2 Outlier maps for lumen segmentation

We applied our blind inpainting method on an RF ultrasound image, assuming that it was already masked, to determine which pixels were statistically relevant and which ones had values that did not fit the distribution. The results obtained with the transversal and longitudinal images of the carotid artery are presented in figure 7.4 and 7.5, respectively. The values of the parameters used were the same as those used in the previous section.

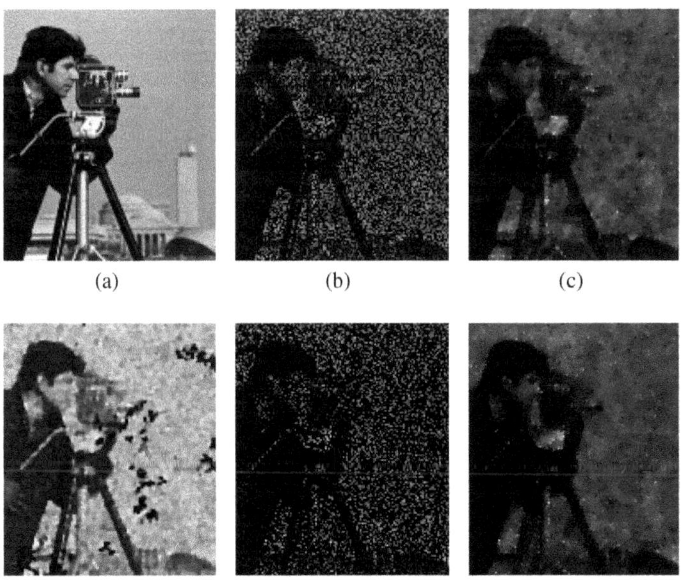

(a) (b) (c)

(d) (e) (f)

Figure 7.2. Blind inpainting with Rayleigh noise with the Cameraman image: (a) original image (cropped); (b) observed image with Rayleigh noise and 50% of its pixels missing; (c) estimate using the proposed method; (d) estimate using inpainting with the additive model after logarithmic transformation; (e) observed image with Rayleigh noise and 70% of its pixels missing; and (f) estimate from (e) using the proposed method [5] (© 2015 IEEE).

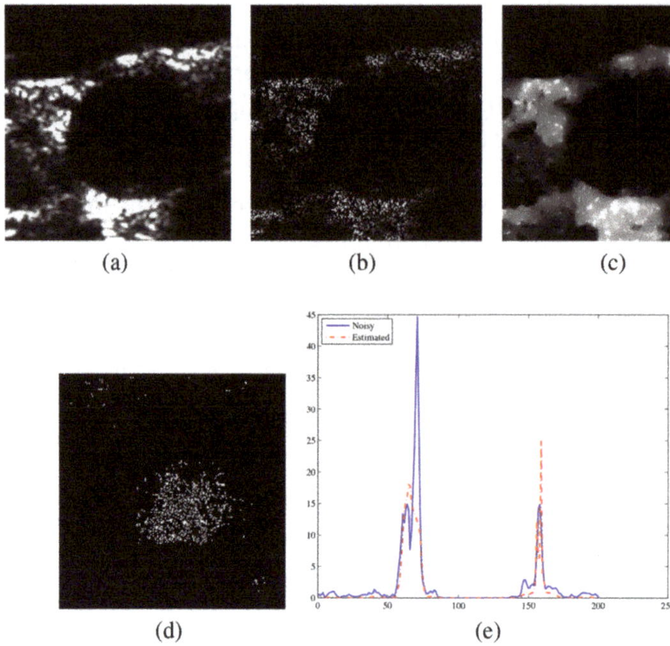

Figure 7.3. Blind inpainting with (Rayleigh) transversal ultrasound image of the carotid artery: (a) noisy radio frequency (RF) image, (b) observed image with 75% of the pixels missing, (c) estimate, (d) result of the binary XOR operation between the mask and its estimate, and (e) diagonal profiles of the noisy and estimated images [5] (© 2015 IEEE).

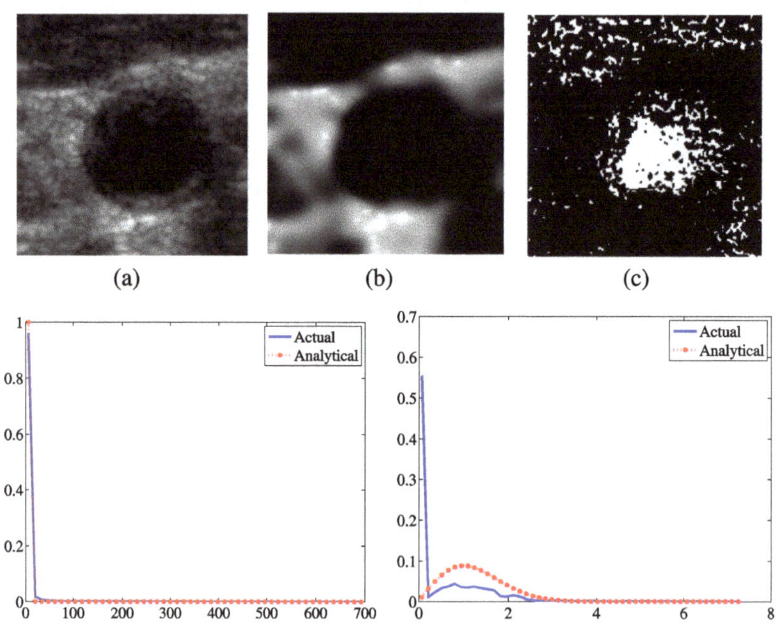

Figure 7.4. Blind inpainting applied on an ultrasound image to detect outliers: (a) transversal RF image of carotid artery, (b) denoised image, (c) positions of detected outliers, (d) histogram of speckle at valid pixels, compared with the Rayleigh distribution, and (e) histogram of speckle at outlier positions, compared with the Rayleigh distribution.

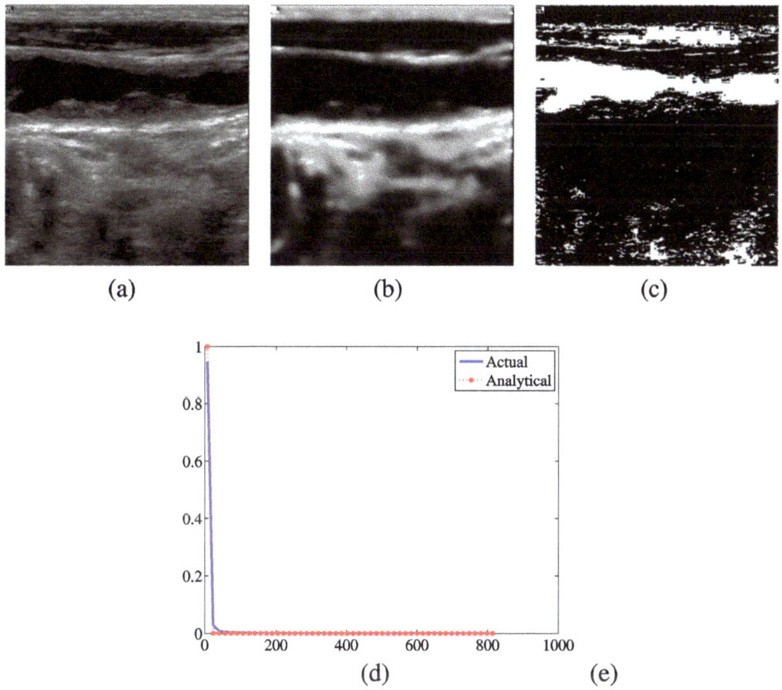

Figure 7.5. Blind inpainting applied on an ultrasound image to detect outliers: (a) longitudinal RF image of carotid artery, (b) denoised image, (c) positions of detected outliers, (d) histogram of speckle at valid pixels, compared with the Rayleigh distribution, and (e) histogram of speckle at outlier positions, compared with the Rayleigh distribution.

Table 7.2. KL divergence of inliers and outliers from ultrasound images.

Image	Fraction outliers	KL div (inliers)	KL div (outliers)
Carotid transversal	0.139	0.074	2.49
Carotid longitudinal	0.21	0.132	3.67
IVUS frame no. 5	0.274	0.0065	4.79
IVUS frame no. 100	0.268	0.0102	5.22

In the estimated outlier maps in figure 7.4(c) and 7.5(c), the white pixels represent the mask pixels estimated incorrectly (the reference mask is assumed to be all ones, i.e. all pixels are observed). Comparing these outlier maps with the respective RF and denoised images, it can be seen that the greatest concentration of outlier values is in the regions that correspond to the lumen. We also present the histograms for the speckle noise field computed by element-wise division of the observed image, by the denoised image $\hat{\boldsymbol{\eta}} = \mathbf{y}/\hat{\mathbf{x}}$. The Kullback–Leibler divergences between the observed histograms and the analytical Rayleigh distributions for the inliers and outliers from the ultrasound images are summarized in table 7.2.

In figure 7.4(d) and 7.5(d), we present the histograms for the noise field over the pixel locations that are considered statistically valid, compared with the analytical probability density function for the Rayleigh distribution with parameter equal to one. For the transversal image, the Kullback–Leibler (KL) divergence between the histogram and the analytical distributions was found to be 0.074, with 13.92% of pixels labeled as outliers. Over the pixels marked as outliers, the KL divergence with respect to the analytical Rayleigh distribution increased to 2.49. For the longitudinal image, 21% of the pixels were marked as outliers, and the KL divergences with respect to the analytical Rayleigh PDF were 0.132 over the set of statistically valid pixels, and 3.67 over the outliers. The difference from the analytical curves can be seen in figure 7.4(e) and 7.5(e).

We also ran the proposed method on two images from the intravascular ultrasound dataset from [7], and the results are presented in figures 7.6 and 7.7. Figures 7.6(a) and 7.7(a) show the RF images, figures 7.6(b) and 7.7(b) show the respective denoised images, and figures 7.6(c) and 7.7(c) show the respective estimated outlier masks. It can be seen from the outlier masks that the outliers are concentrated in the regions corresponding to the lumen in figures 7.6 and 7.7. The histograms of the observed inliers and outliers, along with the analytical Rayleigh distribution are shown in figure 7.6(d) and (e), and in figure 7.7(d) and (e).

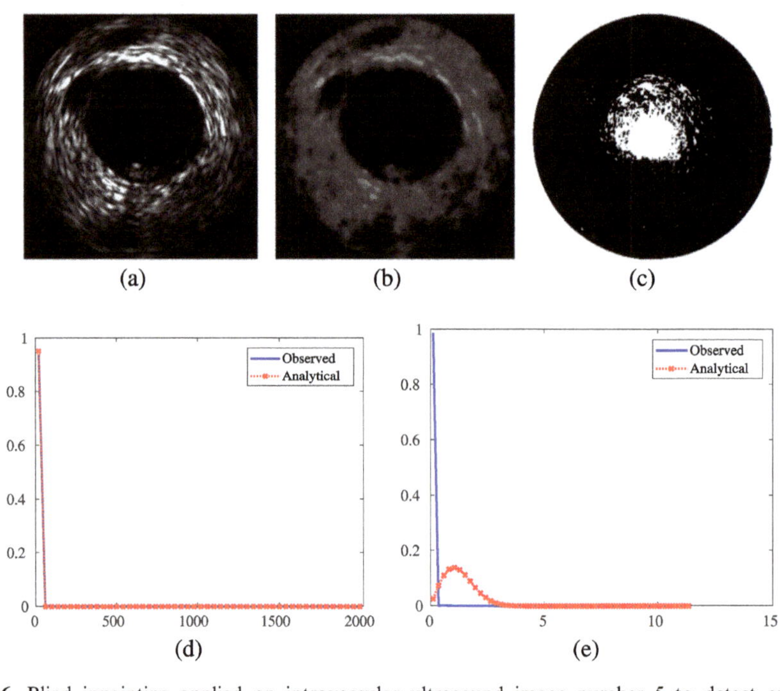

Figure 7.6. Blind inpainting applied on intravascular ultrasound image number 5 to detect outliers: (a) longitudinal RF image of carotid artery, (b) denoised image, (c) positions of detected outliers, (d) histogram of speckle at valid pixels, compared with the Rayleigh distribution, and (e) histogram of speckle at outlier positions, compared with the Rayleigh distribution.

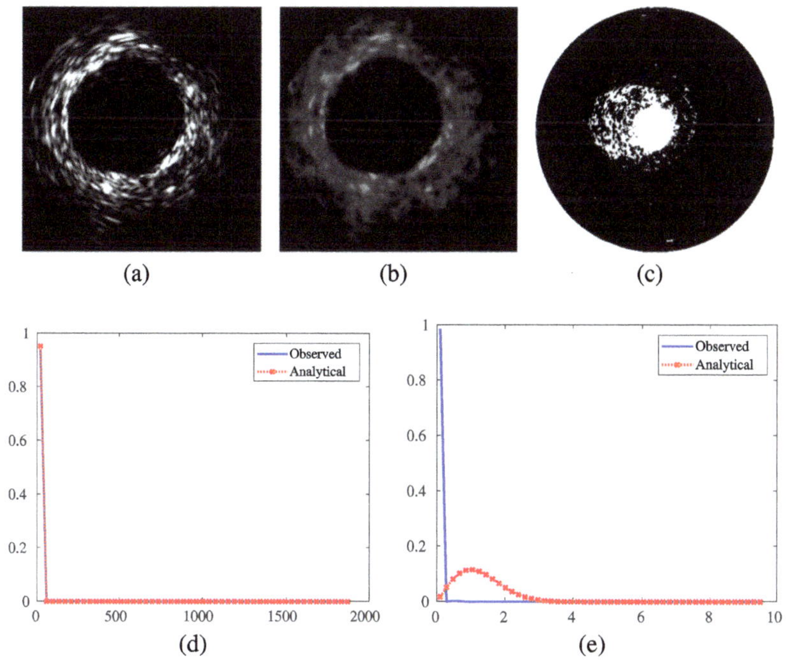

Figure 7.7. Blind inpainting applied on intravascular ultrasound image number 100 to detect outliers: (a) longitudinal RF image of carotid artery, (b) denoised image, (c) positions of detected outliers, (d) histogram of speckle at valid pixels, compared with the Rayleigh distribution, and (e) histogram of speckle at outlier positions, compared with the Rayleigh distribution.

7.4 Conclusions and future work

We have presented an iterative method for image inpainting without knowing the locations of the missing pixels, based on alternating minimization to simultaneously estimate the image and observation mask. The proposed method has been extended to the Rayleigh speckle noise model as well, and was found to be more accurate than transforming the model into an additive one without taking into account the respective statistics. It was experimentally found that applying the inpainting method to ultrasound images of the carotid artery and intravascular ultrasound images without loss of pixels, produced an outlier map which indicated which pixel values are reliable and which pixels are outliers. It was found that the pixels detected as outliers corresponded roughly to the lumen.

Based on the results obtained with real ultrasound images, current and future research includes using the estimation of masks to help in obtaining optimal sampling patterns. A robust mathematical formulation for the segmentation problem is the subject of current and future research.

Acknowledgments

This work was supported by Fundação para a Ciência e Tecnologia (FCT), Portuguese Ministry of Science and Higher Education, through a post-doctoral fellowship (contract no. SFRH/BPD/79011/2011) and FCT project (UID/EEA/50009/2013). The authors thank the authors of [24, 46, 62] for sharing the implementations of their algorithms with us.

References

[1] Abbott J G and Thurstone F 1979 Acoustic speckle: theory and experimental analysis *Ultrason. Imaging* **1** 303–24

[2] Afonso M, Bioucas-Dias J and Figueiredo M 2010 Fast image recovery using variable splitting and constrained optimization *IEEE Trans. Image Process.* **19** 2345–56

[3] Afonso M, Bioucas-Dias J and Figueiredo M 2011 An augmented Lagrangian based method for the constrained formulation of imaging inverse problems *IEEE Trans. Image Process.* **20** 681–95

[4] Afonso M and Sanches J M 2015 Image reconstruction under multiplicative speckle noise using total variation *Neurocomputing* **150** 200–13

[5] Afonso M and Raposo Sanches J 2015 Blind inpainting using ℓ_0 and total variation regularization *IEEE Trans. Image Process.* **24** 2239–53

[6] Afonso M and Sanches J 2013 A total variation based reconstruction algorithm for 3D ultrasound *Pattern Recognition and Image Analysis* (*Lecture Notes in Computer Science* vol 7887) (Berlin: Springer) pp 149–56

[7] Balocco S *et al* 2014 Standardized evaluation methodology and reference database for evaluating IVUS image segmentation *Comput. Med. Imaging Graph* **38** 70–90

[8] Barcelos C A Z and Batista M A 2007 Image restoration using digital inpainting and noise removal *Image Vis. Comput.* **25** 61–9

[9] Beck A and Teboulle M 2009 A fast iterative shrinkage-thresholding algorithm for linear inverse problems *SIAM J. Imaging Sci.* **2** 183–202

[10] Becker S, Bobin J and Candès E 2011 NESTA: a fast and accurate first-order method for sparse recovery *SIAM J. Imaging Anal.* **4** 1–39

[11] Bertalmio M, Sapiro G, Caselles V and Ballester C 2000 Image inpainting *Proc. of the 27th Annual Conf. on Computer Graphics and Interactive Techniques* (New York: ACM Press) pp 417–24

[12] Bioucas-Dias J and Figueiredo M A T 2008 An iterative algorithm for linear inverse problems with compound regularizers *ICIP 2008. 15th IEEE Int. Conf. on Image Processing, 2008* (Piscataway, NJ: IEEE) pp 685–8

[13] Bioucas-Dias J and Figueiredo M 2010 Multiplicative noise removal using variable splitting and constrained optimization *IEEE Trans. Image Process.* **19** 1720–30

[14] Bovik A C 2010 *Handbook of Image and Video Processing* (New York: Academic)

[15] Cai J-F, Chan R H and Nikolova M 2010 Fast two-phase image deblurring under impulse noise *J. Math. Imaging Vis.* **36** 46–53

[16] Candès E, Romberg J and Tao T 2005 Stable signal recovery from incomplete and inaccurate information *Commun. Pure Appl. Math.* **59** 1207–33

[17] Candes E J and Tao T 2005 Decoding by linear programming *IEEE Trans. Inf. Theory* **51** 4203–15

[18] Chambolle A 2004 An algorithm for total variation minimization and applications *J. Math. Imaging Vis.* **20** 89–97

[19] Chan R H, Hu C and Nikolova M 2004 An iterative procedure for removing random-valued impulse noise *IEEE Signal Process. Lett.* **11** 921–4

[20] Chan T, Esedoglu S, Park F and Yip A 2005 Recent developments in total variation image restoration *Handbook of Mathematical Models in Computer Vision* (Berlin: Springer) pp 17–30

[21] Chen T and Wu H R 2001 Adaptive impulse detection using center-weighted median filters *IEEE Signal Process. Lett.* **8** 1–3

[22] Dahl J, Hansen P C, Jensen S H and Jensen T L 2010 Algorithms and software for total variation image reconstruction via first-order methods *Numer. Algorithms* **53** 67–92

[23] Daubechies I, Defrise M and De Mol C 2004 An iterative thresholding algorithm for linear inverse problems with a sparsity constraint *Commun. Pure Appl. Math.* **57** 1413–57

[24] Dong B, Ji H, Li J, Shen Z and Xu Y 2012 Wavelet frame based blind image inpainting *Appl. Comput. Harmon. Anal.* **32** 268–79

[25] Dong Y, Chan R and Xu S 2007 A detection statistic for random-valued impulse noise *IEEE Trans. Image Process.* **16** 1112–20

[26] Donoho D 2006 Compressed sensing *IEEE Trans. Inf. Theory* **52** 1289–306

[27] Donoho D L and Johnstone I M 1995 Adapting to unknown smoothness via wavelet shrinkage *J. Am. Stat. Assoc.* **90** 1200–24

[28] Durand S, Fadili J and Nikolova M 2010 Multiplicative noise removal using L1 fidelity on frame coefficients *J. Math. Imaging Vis.* **36** 201–26

[29] Eckstein J and Bertsekas D 1992 On the Douglas–Rachford splitting method and the proximal point algorithm for maximal monotone operators *Math. Program.* **55** 293–318

[30] Eltoft T 2006 Modeling the amplitude statistics of ultrasonic images *IEEE Trans. Med. Imaging* **25** 229–40

[31] Esser E 2009 Applications of Lagrangian-based alternating direction methods and connections to split Bregman *CAM, UCLA, Tech. Rep.* 09–31

[32] Esser E and Zhang X 2014 Nonlocal patch-based image inpainting through minimization of a sparsity promoting nonconvex functional *UBC, Tech. Rep.* 3: 13

[33] Fessler J A 1995 Hybrid Poisson/polynomial objective functions for tomographic image reconstruction from transmission scans *IEEE Trans. Image Process.* **4** 1439–50

[34] Figueiredo M A and Bioucas-Dias J M 2010 Restoration of Poissonian images using alternating direction optimization *IEEE Trans. Image Process.* **19** 3133–45

[35] Giryes R and Elad M 2013 Sparsity based Poisson denoising with dictionary learning, arXiv:1309.4306

[36] Giryes R and Elad M 2014 Sparsity based Poisson inpainting *Proc. IEEE Int. Conf. Image Processing* (Piscataway, NJ: IEEE) pp 2839–43

[37] Goldstein T and Osher S 2009 The split Bregman method for ℓ_1 regularized problems *SIAM J. Imaging Sci.* **2** 323–43

[38] Gonzalez R C, Woods R E and Eddins S L 2009 *Digital Image Processing Using MATLAB* vol 2 (Knoxville, TN: Gatesmark)

[39] Hestenes M 1969 Multiplier and gradient methods *J. Optim. Theory Appl.* **4** 303–20

[40] Lefkimmiatis S and Unser M 2013 Poisson image reconstruction with Hessian Schatten-Norm regularization *IEEE Trans. Image Process.* **22** 4314–27

[41] Lustig M, Donoho D and Pauly J 2007 Sparse MRI: the application of compressed sensing for rapid MR imaging *Magn. Reson. Med.* **58** 1182–95

[42] Masnou S and Morel J-M 1998 Level lines based disocclusion *ICIP 98. Proc. of 1998 Int. Conf. on Image Processing* (Piscataway, NJ: IEEE) pp 259–63

[43] Michailovich O V and Tannenbaum A 2006 Despeckling of medical ultrasound images *IEEE Trans. Ultrason. Ferroelectr. Freq. Control* **53** 64–78
[44] Nocedal J and Wright S 2006 *Numerical Optimization* 2nd edn (Berlin: Springer)
[45] Powell M 1969 A method for nonlinear constraints in minimization problems *Optimization* (New York: Academic) pp 283–298
[46] Rodriguez P, Rojas R and Wohlberg B 2012 Mixed Gaussian-impulse noise image restoration via total variation *2012 IEEE Int. Conf. on Acoustics, Speech and Signal Processing (ICASSP)* (Piscataway, NJ: IEEE) pp 1077–80
[47] Rodrıguez P and Wohlberg B 2009 Efficient minimization method for a generalized total variation functional *IEEE Trans. Image Process.* **18** 322–32
[48] Rudin L, Osher S and Fatemi E 1992 Nonlinear total variation based noise removal algorithms *Physica* D **60** 259–68
[49] Seabra J C R 2011 Medical ultrasound B-mode modeling, de-speckling and tissue characterization assessing the atherosclerotic disease *PhD dissertation* Instituto Superior Técnico, Lisbon
[50] Seabra J and Sanches J 2008 Modeling log-compressed ultrasound images for radio frequency signal recovery *Conf. Proc. of IEEE Engineering in Medicine and Biology Society* (Piscataway, NJ: IEEE) pp 426–9
[51] Seabra J, Xavier J and Sanches J 2008 Convex ultrasound image reconstruction with log-Euclidean priors *Engineering in Medicine and Biology Society, EMBS'2008* (Piscataway, NJ: IEEE) pp 435–8
[52] Seabra J, Ciompi F, Pujol O, Mauri J, Radeva P and Sanches J 2011 Rayleigh mixture model for plaque characterization in intravascular ultrasound *IEEE Trans. Biomed. Eng.* **58** 1314–24
[53] Shen J and Chan T F 2002 Mathematical models for local nontexture inpaintings *SIAM J. Appl. Math.* **62** 1019–43
[54] Solberg O, Lindseth F, Torp H, Blake R and Nagelhus Hernes T 2007 Freehand 3D ultrasound reconstruction algorithms—a review *Ultrasound Med. Biol.* **33** 991–1009
[55] Tao Z, Tagare H and Beaty J 2006 Evaluation of four probability distribution models for speckle in clinical cardiac ultrasound images *IEEE Trans. Med. Imaging* **25** 1483–91
[56] Tay P, Acton S and Hossack J 2006 Ultrasound despeckling using an adaptive window stochastic approach *2006 IEEE Int. Conf. on Image Processing* (Piscataway, NJ: IEEE) pp 2549–52
[57] Vegas-Sanchez-Ferrero G, Martin-Martinez D, Aja-Fernandez S and Palencia C 2010 On the influence of interpolation on probabilistic models for ultrasonic images *2010 IEEE Int. Symp. on Biomedical Imaging: From Nano to Macro* (Piscataway, NJ: IEEE) pp 292–5
[58] Wagner R, Smith S, Sandrik J and Lopez H 1983 Statistics of speckle in ultrasound B-scans *IEEE Trans. Son. Ultrason.* **30** 156–63
[59] Wang Y, Yang J, Yin W and Zhang Y 2008 A new alternating minimization algorithm for total variation image reconstruction *SIAM J. Imaging Sci.* **1** 248–72
[60] Wang Y, Szlam A and Lerman G 2013 Robust locally linear analysis with applications to image denoising and blind inpainting *SIAM J. Imaging Sci.* **6** 526–62
[61] Wang Z, Bovik A C, Sheikh H R and Simoncelli E P 2004 Image quality assessment: from error visibility to structural similarity *IEEE Trans. Image Process.* **13** 600–12
[62] Yan M 2013 Restoration of images corrupted by impulse noise and mixed Gaussian impulse noise using blind inpainting *SIAM J. Imaging Sci.* **6** 1227–45

[63] Yin W, Osher S, Goldfarb D and Darbon J 2008 Bregman iterative algorithms for ℓ_1 minimization with applications to compressed sensing *SIAM J. Imaging Sci.* **1** 143–68
[64] Yun S and Woo H 2012 A new multiplicative denoising variational model based on *m*th root transformation *IEEE Trans. Image Process.* **21** 2523–33
[65] Zhu L, Ding H, Zhu L and Wang G 2011 A robust registration method for real-time ultrasound image fusion with pre-acquired 3D dataset *2011 Annual Int. Conf. of the IEEE Engineering in Medicine and Biology Society* (Piscataway, NJ: IEEE) 2638–41

IOP Publishing

Vascular and Intravascular Imaging Trends, Analysis, and Challenges, Volume 1
Stent applications
Petia Radeva and Jasjit S Suri

Chapter 8

Differential imaging for the detection of extra-luminal blood perfusion due to the vasa vasorum

E Gerardo Mendizabal-Ruiz and Ioannis A Kakadiaris

The inflammation and disruption of coronary atherosclerotic plaques is the primary cause of acute coronary events such as heart attacks. Several studies have shown that the proliferation of the vasa vasorum (VV) in atherosclerotic plaques is strongly correlated with the degree of plaque inflammation, and it is related to the processes that lead to plaque destabilization and rupture. Intravascular ultrasound (IVUS) is a catheter-based medical imaging system that is capable of providing cross-sectional images of arteries. Contrast agents are injected into the bloodstream during IVUS interventions to trace the blood flow and find any evidence of extra-luminal perfusion, which may be an indication of the VV. The detection of extra-luminal perfusion is performed by comparing the echogenicity of localized regions of a vessel wall and plaque before and after the injection of contrast agents. However, manually performing temporal analysis of variations in the echogenicity is not feasible for more than a handful of IVUS frames due to the amount of labor and concentration involved in assessing changes that may be subtle to the human eye. Computer-aided techniques may be a natural solution to this problem, although they present their own difficulties, which include overcoming the variety of motion artifacts present in IVUS sequences. In this chapter, we present an imaging protocol for contrast imaging in IVUS along with the computational techniques for image stabilization, which allow the detection and localization of changes in echogenicity by differential imaging. We present results on five human cases and four animal cases for which histology was available. These studies illustrate the method's ability to quantify VV density *in vivo*.

doi:10.1088/2053-2563/ab01fach8

8.1 Introduction

Cardiovascular disease (CVD) refers to those disorders that affect the heart and/or vascular system. According to the American Heart Association, CVD accounted for 32.8% (811 940) of all 2 471 984 deaths in the United States in 2008. The most common form of CVD is atherosclerosis, a condition in which the arterial wall hardens and thickens due to the build up and accumulation of plaque [26].

Atherosclerotic processes mainly involve thickening of the intima, and other process such as fibrosis, necrosis, calcification and hemorrhage [10]. The process of atherosclerotic plaque formation is considered to be an inflammatory, response-to-injury phenomenon that is initiated by injury to the endothelium or smooth muscle cells of the artery wall [40]. Although atherosclerosis is a multifocal disease, it is well known that atherosclerotic plaques are not similar to one another in composition, progression rate, stability or thrombogenicity.

In the past, it was believed that the increase of plaque and the consequent narrowing of the coronary arteries was the cause of fatal coronary events. Currently, it is known that the inflammation and disruption of coronary plaques with superimposed thrombosis is the primary cause of acute coronary events. It has been shown that for up to 75% of acute ischemic coronary syndromes, atherosclerotic plaque rupture is the underlying pathological mechanism [2, 7]. Pathology studies indicate that certain plaques are more prone to develop acute coronary events than others. In this context, the field of cardiology has introduced the term 'vulnerable plaque' (VP), which refers to those plaques with a high likelihood of rupture, thrombotic complications and the consequent rapid progression to stenosis [29, 33–35].

Although there is no broad consensus on what characteristics define a VP, autopsy studies have provided useful indicators of the features exhibited by certain plaques immediately before rupture. The histopathologic characteristics of ruptured plaques have been well defined [43]. The most consistent findings include: (i) a large lipid (necrotic) core composed of free cholesterol crystals; (ii) cholesterol esters and oxidized lipids impregnated with tissue factor; (iii) a thin fibrous cap depleted of smooth muscle cells and collagen; (iv) an outward (positive) remodeling; (v) inflammatory cell infiltration of the fibrous cap and adventitia (mostly monocyte/macrophages, some activated T cells and mast cells); (vi) intra-plaque hemorrhage; and (vii) the formation of new microvessels (neoangiogenesis or neovascularization) at the arterial wall adventitia, and within the atherosclerotic plaque (i.e. the vasa vasorum) [44].

8.1.1 The vasa vasorum

In normal conditions, the vasa vasorum (VV) may be present in the adventitial layer of large vessels such as the aorta. However, recent evidence has suggested that the presence and proliferation (increase in density) of VV in the plaque (i.e. vasa plaquorum, VVP) [13] is correlated to the processes which lead to the destabilization of the plaque (figure 8.1) [1, 5, 9, 19, 25].

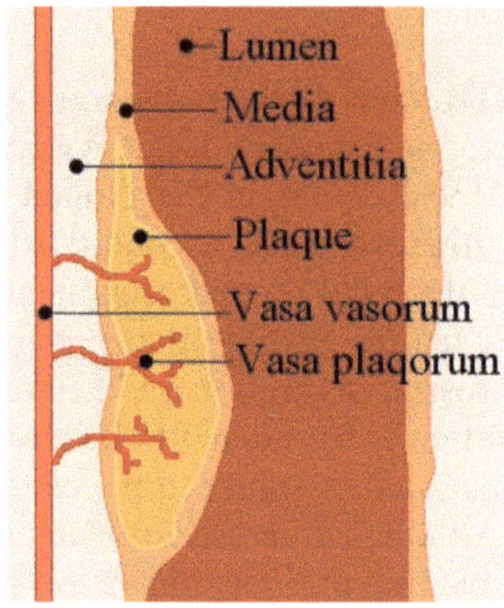

Figure 8.1. Depiction of atherosclerotic plaque and neovascularization in a vessel.

Additional findings indicate that: (i) the microvessel density is greater in ruptured plaques than nonruptured plaques, (ii) the microvessel density is correlated to macrophage infiltration and (iii) microvessel density within the plaque is correlated to plaque rupture [32]. These findings suggest that the proliferation of the VV and VVP can be used as a marker of plaque inflammation and a preceding or concomitant factor associated with plaque rupture and instability [21, 23]. Therefore, the *in vivo* detection of extra-luminal perfusion due to microvasculature can enable the development of an index of plaque vulnerability.

8.1.2 Intravascular ultrasound

IVUS is a catheter-based imaging technique that provides high-resolution, cross-sectional images of the interior of blood vessels in real time *in vivo*. The IVUS imaging technique consists of steering a guidewire with a small diameter (about 0.84 mm) into the blood vessel branch to be imaged. The ultrasound catheter is then slid in over the guidewire and positioned within a target segment of interest. The IVUS system starts acquiring and displaying the images, usually at 30 frames/second.

The IVUS catheter consists of a miniaturized transducer (about 0.06 mm in diameter) which transmits ultrasound pulses and receives an acoustic radio frequency (RF) echo signal at a discrete set of angles (commonly 240–360). These signals are then processed to reconstruct an image that is meaningful to the physicians (i.e. the B-mode image). The B-mode reconstruction process consists of the detection of the positive envelopes of each A-line, time-gain compensation (TGC) of the signal, stacking of the signals along the angular direction, quantization of the signal and 8 bit gray scale mapping. The image generated by this process is known as the polar B-mode image. Finally, the polar B-mode image is geometrically transformed to obtain the familiar disc-shaped image known as the Cartesian B-mode image.

Although IVUS provides reliable cross-sectional images of the coronary arteries, the *in vivo* imaging of the coronary VV and VVP remains a great challenge due to their small size (reported diameters of human artery VV ranged from 11.6 to

36.6 μm, capillary VV from 4.7 to 11.6 μm and venous VV from 11.6 to 200.3 μm [24]), echo transparency and the presence of different IVUS artifacts. Since the detection of the VV and VVP can be posed as the detection of microcirculation beyond the lumen border (i.e. extra-luminal perfusion), IVUS is used in combination with contrast agents (contrast-enhanced IVUS, CE-IVUS) as tracers of blood flow. Then, if extra-luminal perfusion is detected, this may be an indication of the presence of microvasculature. The use of CE-IVUS has proven useful for assessing the amount and distribution of neovessels within atherosclerotic lesions [20].

Modern ultrasound contrast agents consist of solutions of gas-filled spheres that are surrounded by a shell designed to aid their longevity in the bloodstream. The scale of these microbubbles (diameter: 1–10 μm) is similar to the scale of red blood cells (diameter: ~8 μm), and hence they may be used as tracers of blood flow. Depending on the energy and frequency of the ultrasound beam, the contrast agent microbubbles may present either linear or nonlinear oscillations. Linear oscillations occur when equal-amplitude contraction and relaxation of the microbubbles is induced by the ultrasound signal. Nonlinear oscillations occur when the microbubbles expand above their baseline diameter at a greater scale when compared to their ability to compress below it. In the case of linear oscillations (fundamental mode), the microbubbles produce echo signals with the same frequency as the ultrasound transducer (i.e. the fundamental frequency). In the case of nonlinear oscillations, the microbubbles will produce the fundamental frequency and multiples of this frequency, known as harmonics, sub-harmonics and ultra-harmonics.

The feasibility of using harmonic and sub-harmonic IVUS for the detection of microbubbles using a prototype nonlinear IVUS system and commercially available contrast agents has been investigated [16–18]. This method is capable of providing microbubble-specific imaging by detecting nonlinear signals. The prototype nonlinear IVUS system consists of a custom-built, single-element transducer that is mechanically rotated and has sophisticated pulse sequences generated using pulse inversion, methods for tissue and catheter motion compensation, and specially designed signal filters for processing the received signal. A tissue harmonic imaging (THI) system which consists of a dual-frequency transducer element mounted on an IVUS catheter was also proposed [11, 12]. As a result, this prototype IVUS system can operate in both the fundamental frequency and the second-harmonic imaging modes. This system uses a conventional, continuously rotating, single-element IVUS catheter that is operated in the fundamental 20 MHz, fundamental 40 MHz and harmonic 40 MHz modes (transmit 20 MHz, receive 40 MHz). The use of a focused broadband miniature polyvinylidene fluoride–trifluoroethylene (PVDF–TrFE) ultrasonic transducer for IVUS second-harmonic imaging was also investigated [4]. This study demonstrated that focused transducers are capable of producing second harmonics faster and stronger at specific depths. Unfortunately, these methods for contrast imaging remain experimental and require non-commercially available IVUS hardware (e.g. harmonic imaging systems and catheters), non-standard contrast agents, or both.

In this chapter, we present a computer-aided technique that allows the detection of extra-luminal perfusion using CE-IVUS imaging to be accomplished with standard, commercially available IVUS systems and off-the-shelf microbubble contrast agents (namely, those normally used for echocardiographic purposes). Toward this end, we introduce a number of techniques for IVUS image stabilization which enable the use of difference imaging to detect those changes which occur in the IVUS imagery due to the perfusion of an intravascularly injected contrast agent into the plaque and vessel wall.

8.2 Methods

8.2.1 Data acquisition protocol

The proposed image acquisition protocol for the detection of the VV using contrast-enhanced IVUS consists of placing the IVUS catheter within a plaque of interest and fixing its position during the whole recording sequence. Baseline IVUS images are acquired over an initial period of time. Then, a bolus injection of contrast agent is made near the catheter, and finally more images are acquired over a period of time after the injection. In most cases the concentration of bubbles in the blood is sufficient for the the lumen to become temporarily echo-opaque until bolus passage. Consequently, the IVUS sequence consists of three periods: a pre-injection period (30–60 s), a brief during-injection period (< 5 s) and a post-injection period (30–60 s).

If there exists microcirculation beyond the lumen, we expect that the microbubbles will increase the echogenicity of those perfused regions. One way to detect this increase of echogenicity consists of comparing the IVUS images corresponding to the periods before and after the contrast agent injection. Then, if there exists a positive change in the intensity on the post-injection IVUS images compared to the pre-injection images over a certain region, this could be an indicator of perfusion.

8.2.2 Computer-aided detection of perfusion

If there is no motion present in the sequence, the detection of the increase of echogenicity in the region beyond the lumen due to perfusion could be accomplished simply by subtracting a frame corresponding to the period before the injection of contrast agent (i.e. pre-contrast frame) from a frame corresponding to the period after the injection of the contrast (i.e. post-contrast frame). However, despite the efforts to maintain the ultrasound sensor as stable as possible while imaging within the coronary arteries, inter-frame motion variability can be observed, mostly due to cardiac cycle motion, making it impossible to perform the detection of enhancement using this technique directly. Consequently, to detect enhancement in the IVUS image due to perfusion of contrast agent, sequence stabilization must be performed. Thus, the proposed method consists of three parts:

Algorithm 1. Detection of extra-luminal perfusion by differential imaging.

Part 1. Sequence stabilization.

Step 1.1. Stabilization with respect to catheter and wall motion.

Step 1.2. Alignment of pre- and post-contrast images.

Part 2. Detection of enhancement by differential imaging.
Part 3. Quantification of enhancement.

The details of each step are presented next.

8.2.2.1 Sequence stabilization

The goal of sequence stabilization is to approximate pixelwise correspondence between a region of interest in each frame of the IVUS sequence. This is a challenging task considering the constant natural expansion and contraction of the artery wall (i.e. wall motion), and the possible changes in the position of the catheter within the artery (i.e. catheter motion) due to the cardiac and respiratory cycles, which result in undesired motion artifacts (figure 8.2).

A common practice to stabilize IVUS data is by synchronizing the IVUS sequence with the electrocardiogram signal (i.e. ECG-based gating). This procedure consists of decimating the IVUS data by selecting those frames corresponding to a given peak on the ECG which may correspond to the same instant of the cardiac cycle. However, the use of this method results in the rejection of many frames with possible valuable information with no guarantee that the structures of the vessel depicted in the gated frames have an exact correspondence to the same anatomical position. Another option for the stabilization of the sequences is to employ image-based gating methods (e.g. [14, 15, 36–38]). These methods perform frame selection based on the analysis of the similitude between the gray-level intensity distributions of the structures of the vessel depicted in the IVUS B-mode reconstruction among the frames of the sequence. In general, these methods are successful in grouping frames from different instants of the cardiac cycle, since they are able to discriminate between frames with large differences in the structures of the vessel. However, to find a good anatomical correspondence between the pre- and post-contrast frames, these methods may not be sufficient since significant changes in the gray-level intensities of the images are expected in the case of enhancement due to extra-luminal perfusion, and because the enhancement of the lumen area due to the contrast agent may remain present during a period of time after the injection of microbubbles

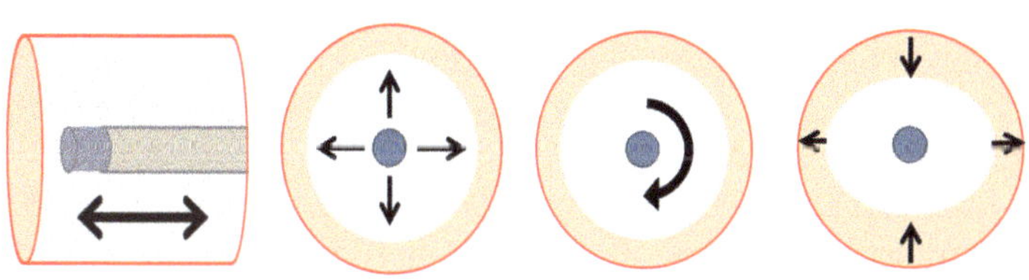

(a) (b) (c) (d)

Figure 8.2. Sources of motion artifacts: (a) axial catheter motion, where the catheter moves along the vessel axis, perpendicularly to the imaging plane; (b) translation parallel to the imaging plane; (c) rotation around the vessel axis; and (d) elastic wall motion. Note that elastic transformations are not uniform but may be more extreme in some locations than other.

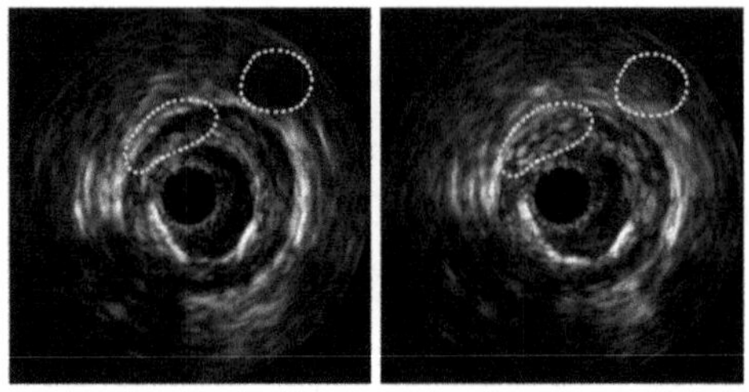

(a) (b)

Figure 8.3. Example of a case with evident enhancement. (a) Frame corresponding to the pre-contrast period and (b) frame corresponding to the post-contrast period. The annotations indicate the places where the enhancement occurred.

(figure 8.3). Therefore, it is necessary to perform additional stabilization of the sequence to find those frames that correspond to the same anatomical position.

An example of this limitation is depicted in figure 8.3. This example corresponds to a 20 MHz sequence of a human coronary artery case for which the enhancement in the indicated regions of plaque and adventitia is evident. The multi-dimensional scaling (MDS)-based gating method presented in [38] was employed to find the correspondence of pre- and post-contrast frames. In this method, image-based gating is accomplished by the transformation of the image sequence to a Euclidean frame similarity space in which each frame is represented by a particular, although not necessarily unique, point. Clustering this space provides ensembles of stabilized frames and plotting it provides a visual overview of the events occurring in the sequence. Figure 8.4 depicts the plot of the clustering result using K-means on the MDS-transformed frame data. In this graph, the red elements correspond to the pre-contrast frames while blue elements correspond to the post-contrast frames. Note that this method does not provide compact clusters that contain pre- and post-injection frames for all values of k different to one.

Therefore, it is necessary to perform a different type of analysis of the sequence to find those frames that are likely to correspond to the same anatomical position. In this work, we propose to perform sequence stabilization by an analysis of the morphological characteristics of the lumen region. The rationale is that frames corresponding to the same anatomical position will depict similar lumen characteristics. Our method consists of two steps: (i) stabilization with respect to catheter and wall motions and (ii) alignment of pre- and post-contrast images. Next, the details of each step are explained in detail.

Step 1.1. *Stabilization with respect to wall and catheter motions.* The first step of our stabilization method requires the identification of the lumen/wall interface (i.e. lumen segmentation) on each of the pre- and post-contrast frames in order to compute the statistics regarding the area and the similarity of shape. Segmentation of the lumen is a common task in the analysis of IVUS data since it allows the assessment of the morphological characteristics of the vessel and plaque (e.g. lumen diameter, minimum lumen cross-section area and total atheroma volume). This

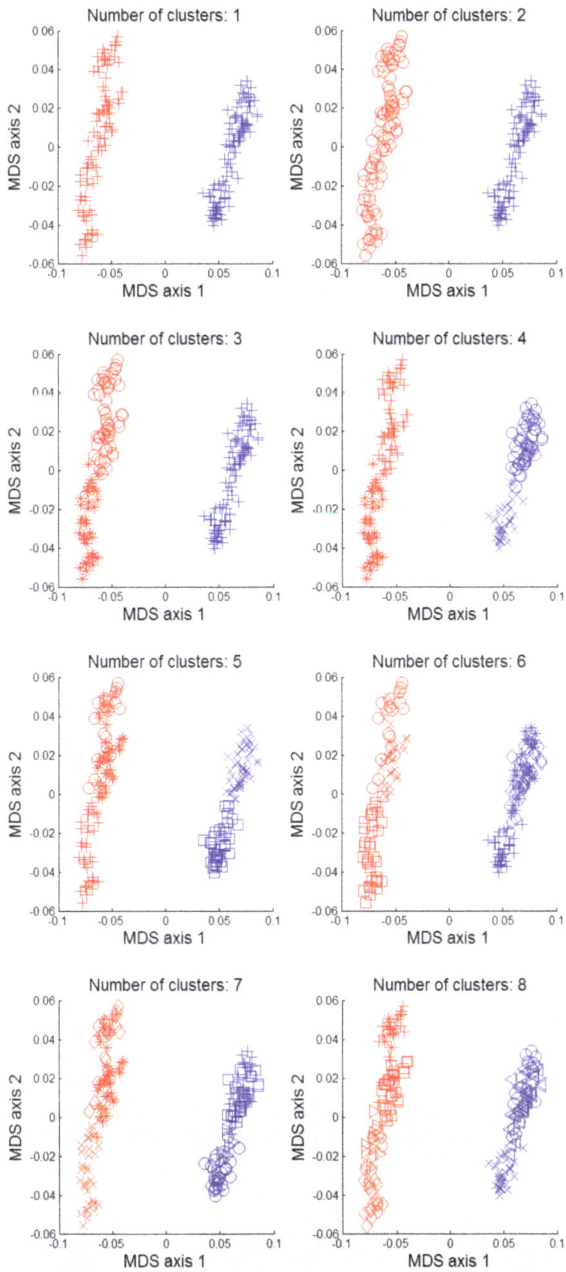

Figure 8.4. Example of clustering results using the MDS method proposed in [38]. Red elements correspond to frames from the period before the injection while blue elements correspond to frames from the period after injection.

information is crucial for making decisions such as whether a stent is needed to restore blood flow in an artery and to determine the characteristics of the stent. Other applications include the study of mechanical properties of the vessel wall, characteristics of the plaque and 3D reconstruction of the vessel. Segmentation of IVUS images can be performed manually by an expert observer. However, considering the large number of images in an IVUS sequence, manual segmentation is a tedious task that may be excessively time-consuming. Thus, several methods have been proposed to perform automatic segmentation of the IVUS data [3, 6, 22, 27, 28, 30, 39, 42, 45]. The result of the segmentation process is a binary image (i.e. segmentation image) for each frame on which the pixels of the regions corresponding to the lumen are set to a value of one while the rest of the pixels have a value of zero (figure 8.5(b)).

Two frames corresponding to the same anatomical location at the same wall contraction–expansion cycle instant may look different if a change of the position in the catheter occurs (figure 8.6). However, the lumen area depicted in both frames should be similar. Therefore, the first step of our method consists in finding those frames from the pre- and post-contrast periods with a high similarity of the depicted lumen areas. Thus, we compute the area corresponding to the lumen for each frame using the lumen segmentation. Then, the area values are clustered using the k-means method employing different values of k. The clustering results for each value of k are presented to the user who chooses the cluster to be analyzed using, as the criterion, the presence of a compact cluster with a similar number of pre- and post-contrast frames with a high similarity of areas (figures 8.7 and 8.8).

Step 1.2. *Alignment of pre- and post-contrast images.* Apart from the cardiac and respiratory cycles, another possible source of catheter motion is due to the injection of the contrast agent that is performed manually using the IVUS catheter. Therefore, it is necessary to perform a stabilization of the pre- and post-contrast frames separately. Thus we divide the similar-area frames into two classes: pre- and post-contrast frames (F^b and F^C, respectively).

For each frame F_i^z in a class z we compute the Dice similarity coefficient $d_{i,j}^z$ between its corresponding segmentation S_i^z and the segmentation of all the other frames in the group $S_j^z \forall \{j \neq i\} \in z$:

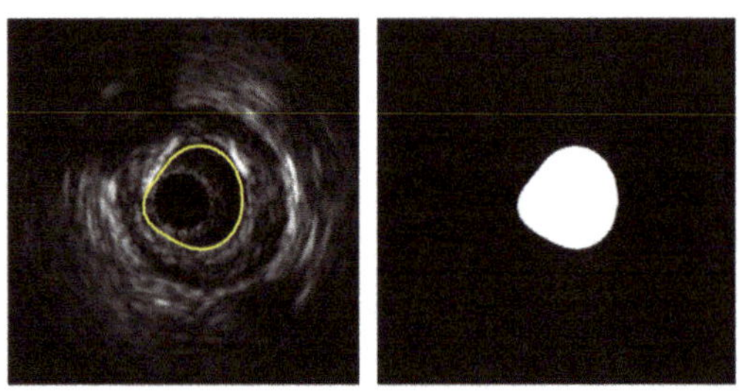

(a) (b)

Figure 8.5. Depiction of the segmentation of the lumen contour in (a) a Cartesian B-mode image and (b) its corresponding binary segmentation image.

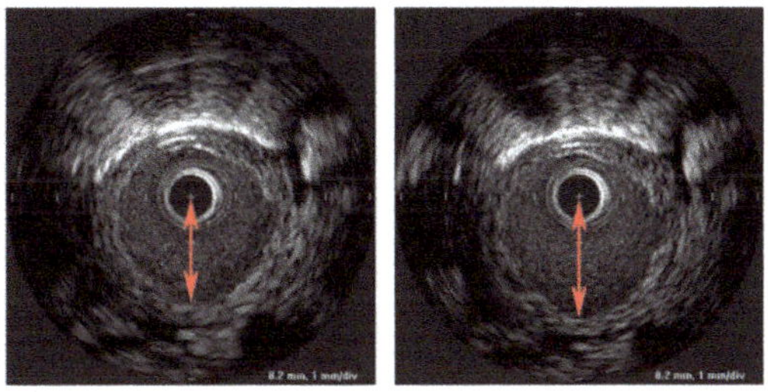

(a) (b)

Figure 8.6. Example of catheter motion in two frames with similar lumen areas. The arrow indicates the differences of the distances between the center of the catheter and a corresponding point in the lumen border.

$$d^z_{i,j} = \frac{2|S_i \cap S_j|}{|S_i| + |S_j|}.$$

Two frames are considered to have a high lumen-shape similarity if the resulting Dice coefficient $d^z_{i,j}$ is above a given similarity threshold $\tau_d \in [0\ 1]$. We select the largest set of frames with high lumen-shape similarity for each class. The result of this analysis is two groups of pre- and post-contrast frames with similar lumen morphological characteristics among each group. A final fine alignment to remove the catheter motion is necessary to perform the differential imaging. A pre-injection baseline image is generated by computing the mean value for each pixel in the N^b pre-contrast analysis Cartesian B-mode frames F^b:

$$B(i, j) = \frac{1}{N^b}\sum_{k=1}^{N^b} F^b_k(i, j). \tag{8.1}$$

Similarly, a mean post-injection image C is generated by computing the mean intensity of each pixel in the N^C post-contrast analysis frames F^c:

$$C(i, j) = \frac{1}{N^C}\sum_{k=1}^{N^C} F^c_k(i, j). \tag{8.2}$$

Finally, we perform a fine alignment by applying a non-rigid registration of both images using $C(i, j)$ as the fixed image. The registration is performed using the B-spline registration method presented in [41] using the square of the pixel-intensity differences as the registration metric. It is important to note that the lumen region has been removed from all the frames in the set in order to prevent possible misalignments in the registration procedure due to the variability of the gray-level intensities from the lumen region.

8.2.2.2 Detection of enhancement by differential imaging

The local difference of echogenicity for each pixel D is obtained by subtracting the gray-level intensity value of each pixel in the post-injection image C from the corresponding pixel value on the pre-injection baseline image B:

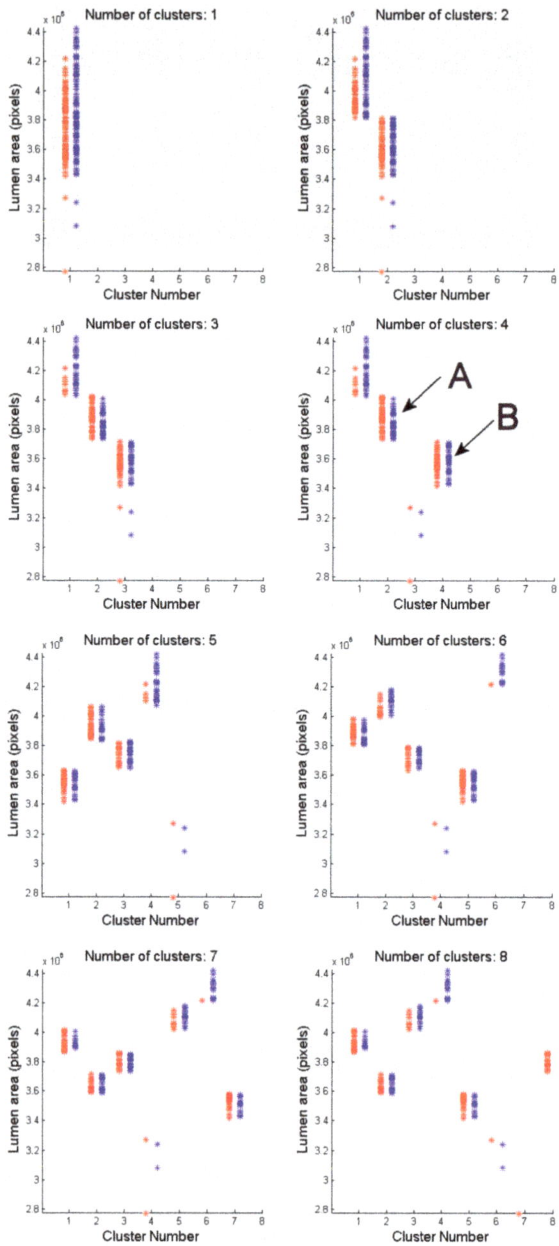

Figure 8.7. Example of luminal area clustering result: selection of the number of clusters k to use. The arrows indicate the two candidates for analysis in this example.

$$D(i, j) = C(i, j) - B(i, j). \tag{8.3}$$

The significance of the difference between the intensity values from the pre- and post-injection pixels is evaluated using a one-tail t-Student's significance test at a

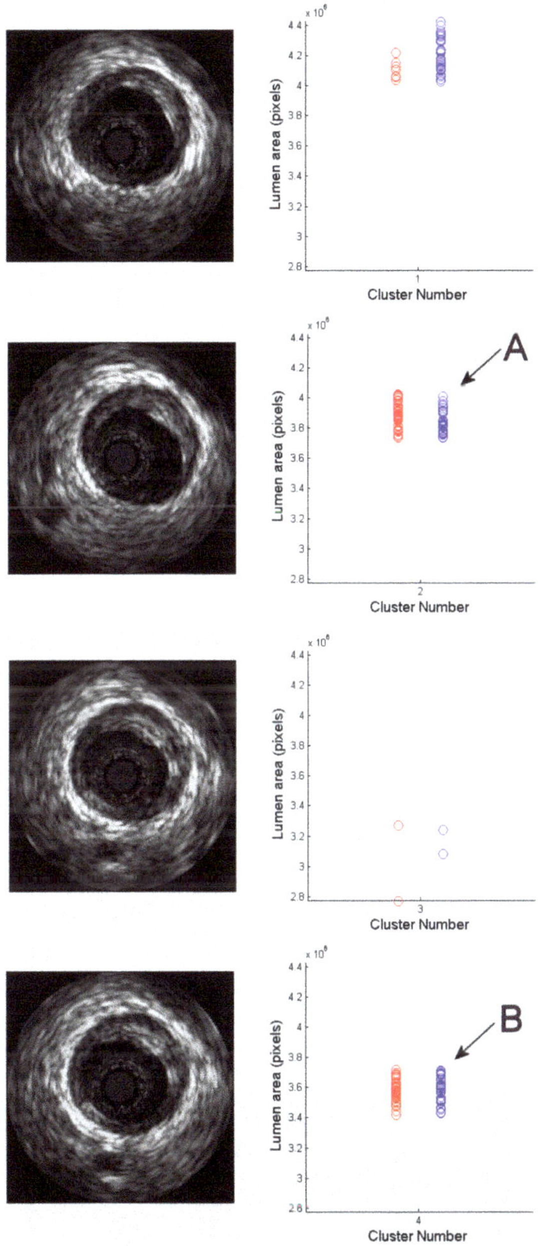

Figure 8.8. Example of the luminal area clustering result: selection of the cluster to analyze. The arrows indicate the two candidates for analysis in this example.

significance level of $\alpha = 0.005$. For this test, the null hypothesis is that the observed value of the pixel in the post-injection image $C(i, j)$ is not statistically different from its corresponding value in the pre-injection image $B(i, j)$. We consider that a change of intensity in a pixel is significant if the null hypothesis for the pixel statistics is rejected. Then, only pixels for which the null hypothesis is rejected are considered for analysis. Finally, an enhancement image E is obtained by applying a threshold τ_e to the pixels of D:

$$E(i, j) = \begin{cases} D(i, j), & \text{if } D(i, j) \geqslant \tau_e \\ 0, & \text{otherwise.} \end{cases} \tag{8.4}$$

8.2.2.3 Quantification of enhancement

The quantification of enhancement analysis is performed on a region of interest (ROI) defined by the user in a frame of the sequence to analyze (figure 8.9). Visualizations are created by mapping the differential image ROI D into the domain of the original IVUS images F and overlaying them in a standard manner (e.g. using color-mapping) so that enhancement may be viewed in its anatomical context.

Enhancement is quantified by computing the total enhancement area in pixels (Γ) of those regions in the defined ROI:

$$\Gamma = \sum_{i,j} D(i, j). \tag{8.5}$$

Additionally, the maximum and mean enhancement values corresponding to the ROI are reported.

8.3 Results

In this section we present results for five cases acquired from human coronary arteries using a solid-state array 20 MHz Volcano Therapeutics, Inc., Invision IVUS system, and four cases acquired from rabbit aortas using a rotating 40 MHz catheter with a Galaxy 2 Boston Scientific IVUS system. Recordings were performed as follows. For the coronary artery of interest, an IVUS pullback was initially obtained and the maximally stenotic point in the vessel located. The IVUS catheter was then repositioned at this point and held steady over a matter of minutes. Baseline images were acquired during a period of approx. 30 s, then a bolus injection of contrast was administered through the guiding catheter (i.e. proximally to the imaging sensor)

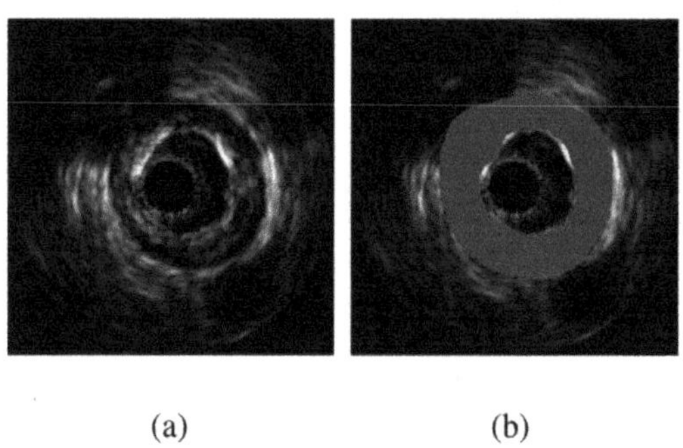

Figure 8.9. Example of (a) a frame corresponding to a sequence to be analyzed and (b) the ROI selected for enhancement analysis (i.e. plaque and media).

and, finally, more images were acquired over 2 min. For all cases the contrast agent used was Optison^{TM}, a commercially available contrast agent whose constituent microspheres are composed of octafluropropane gas surrounded by an albumin shell. The mean bubble diameter is 3.7 μm with 95% of the bubbles being smaller than 10 μm [31]; in comparison, the approximate diameter of a red blood cell is 8 μm [8]. It is important to note that during the injection of the contrast agent, the lumen region will depict a great echogenicity due to the passing of the microbubbles (figure 8.10). However, it is common that the other structures of the vessel are no longer visible during the injection since the majority of the ultrasound energy is reflected by the microbubbles. Therefore, the proposed analysis is performed on the frames corresponding to a selected period of time of 10 s before the first frame on which the microbubbles can be detected in the lumen, and 10 s after the lumen is visible again. The values for the Dice similarity threshold and the enhancement threshold were empirically set to $\tau_d = 0.95$ and $\tau_e = 30$, respectively. Table 8.1 lists the resulting total enhancement areas for each case.

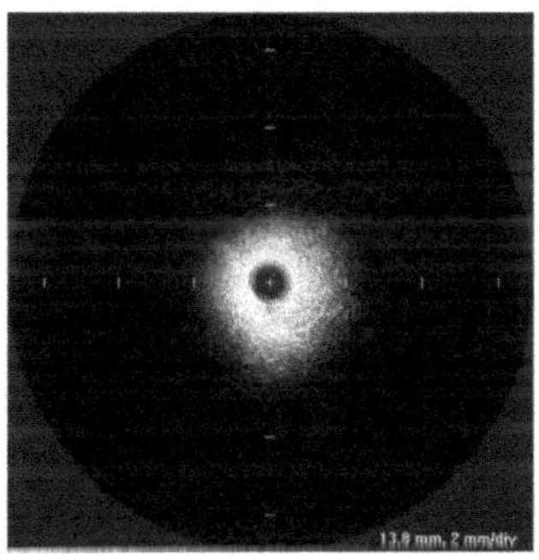

Figure 8.10. Example of a frame corresponding to the period during the injection of contrast agent.

Table 8.1. Quantitative enhancement-detection results. μ stands for maximal enhancement while Γ stands for total enhancement area.

Case Id	Subject	IVUS frequency	μ	Γ
1	Human	20 MHz	179.2	2551
2	Human	20 MHz	90.2	989
3	Human	20 MHz	70.6	69
4	Human	20 MHz	43.2	30
5	Human	20 MHz	50.3	41
6	Rabbit	40 MHz	66.9	1007
7	Rabbit	40 MHz	123.5	488
8	Rabbit	40 MHz	188.2	1987
9	Rabbit	40 MHz	182.0	144

8.3.1 Human cases

All human patients had indications for coronary percutaneous intervention and intravascular ultrasound imaging. Written informed consent was obtained from all patients and the study protocol was approved by the ethical committees of our institutions.

Figure 8.11 depicts the results from case 1. Note that there exist multiple large regions in the plaque and media/adventitia region, which depicts a large enhancement after the injection of contrast agent, suggesting the presence of extra-luminal perfusion due to VV and VVP. In addition, there is some evidence of direct plaque/microbubble interaction at the 12 o'clock region of the luminal border, where the bubbles persist in a dense concentration. This could be evidence of a leaky plaque (i.e. one with a disrupted cap).

Figure 8.12 depicts the results from case 2. In this case, the results suggest the presence of extra-luminal perfusion in the media/adventitia region which may be an indication of VV. Additionally, evidence of enhancement can be observed in a

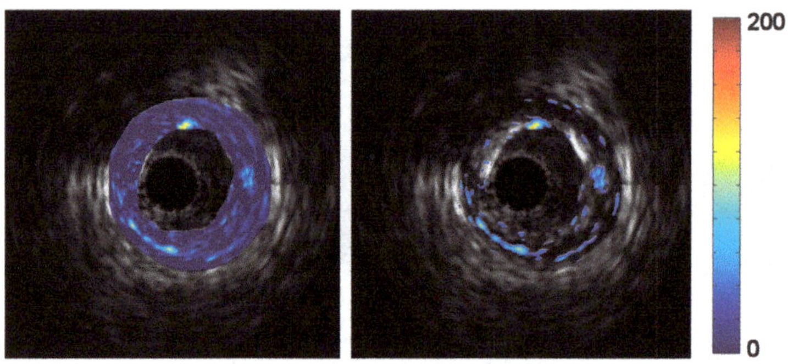

(a) (b)

Figure 8.11. Enhancement detection for case 1. (a) ROI enhancement before thresholding and (b) overlay of detected thresholded enhancement in the mean post-injection image.

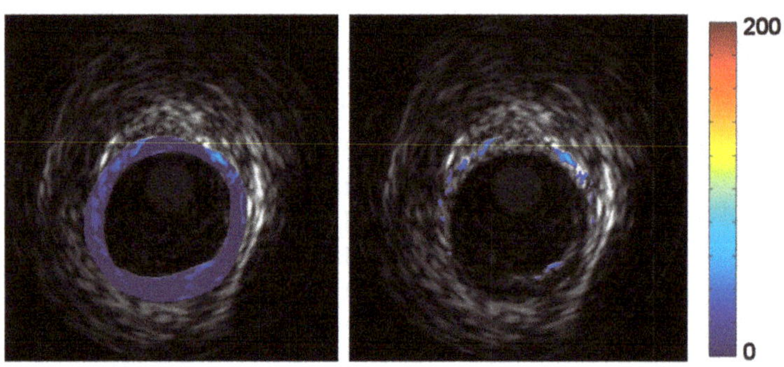

(a) (b)

Figure 8.12. Enhancement detection for case 2. (a) ROI enhancement before thresholding and (b) overlay of detected thresholded enhancement in the mean post-injection image.

region of plaque near the lumen border (between 5 and 6 o'clock). While this may indicate VVP, it also could be the result of endothelial adhesion of the contrast agent.

Figures 8.13, 8.14 and 8.15 depict the results for cases 3, 4 and 5, respectively. While there is some evidence of enhancement in certain regions we cannot ascertain the presence of perfusion due to the small size and low enhancement value. Figures 8.14 and 8.15 depict the results for cases 4 and 5, respectively. In these cases, the evidence of enhancement is not strong enough to assume the presence of perfusion.

8.3.2 Animal cases

New Zealand white male rabbits were fed an atherogenic diet for a period of three months to develop atherosclerotic plaques. The plaques under investigation were marked with surgical clips inserted externally by the surgeon on the aortic wall under

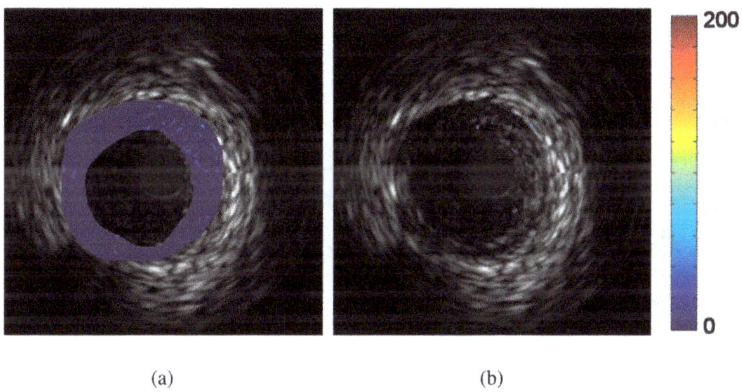

Figure 8.13. Enhancement detection for case 3. (a) ROI enhancement before thresholding and (b) overlay of detected thresholded enhancement in the mean post-injection image.

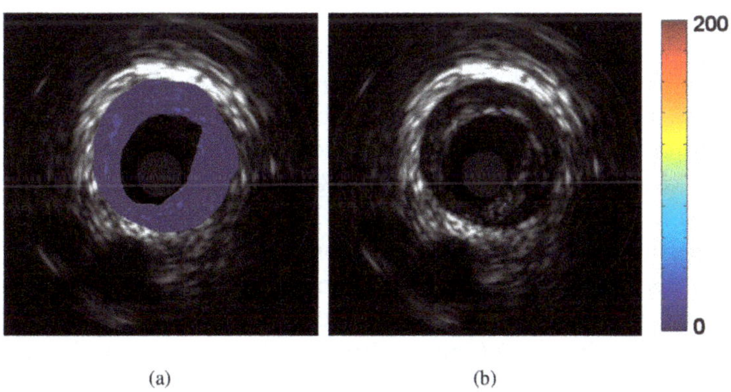

Figure 8.14. Enhancement detection for case 4. (a) ROI enhancement before thresholding and (b) overlay of detected thresholded enhancement in the mean post-injection image.

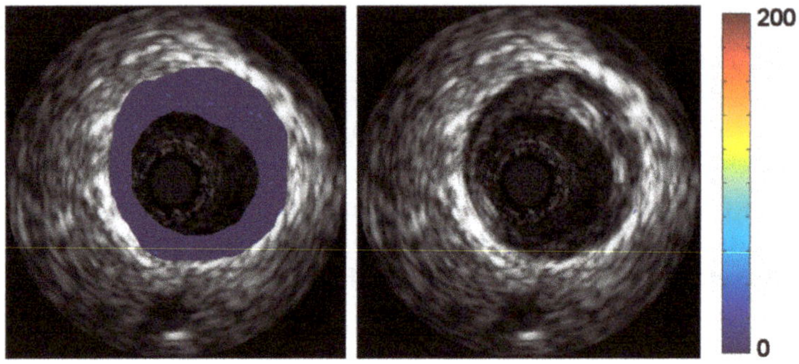

(a) (b)

Figure 8.15. Enhancement detection for case 5. (a) ROI enhancement before thresholding and (b) overlay of detected thresholded enhancement in the mean post-injection image.

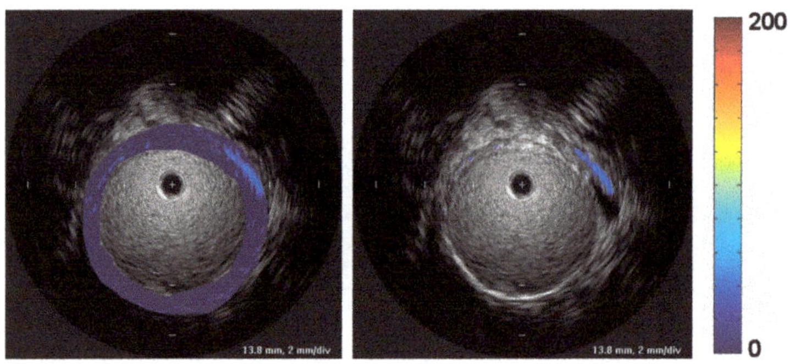

(a) (b)

Figure 8.16. Enhancement detection for case 6. (a) ROI enhancement before thresholding and (b) overlay of detected thresholded enhancement in the mean post-injection image.

fluoroscopic and IVUS guidance. CD31 was used in the histology as stain for endothelial cells.

Figure 8.16 depicts the results for case 6. Note that there exists strong evidence of enhancement in the media/adventitia region between 1 and 2 o'clock, and moderate evidence of enhancement behind the plaque between 9 and 11 o'clock. Figure 8.17 depicts the histological slide corresponding to this case. As can be noted, ROI A depicts a large vasculature in the adventitia region. Similarly, there exists evidence of large perfusion in the adventitia on the ROI B, which appear to correlate with the results of the proposed enhancement-detection method.

Figure 8.18 depicts the result for case 7. For this case, there exists some evidence of enhancement in multiple sections of the media/adventitia region. By visual comparison with the histology (figure 8.19), correlation between the enhancement-detection results and the histological evidence of extra-luminal perfusion can be noted.

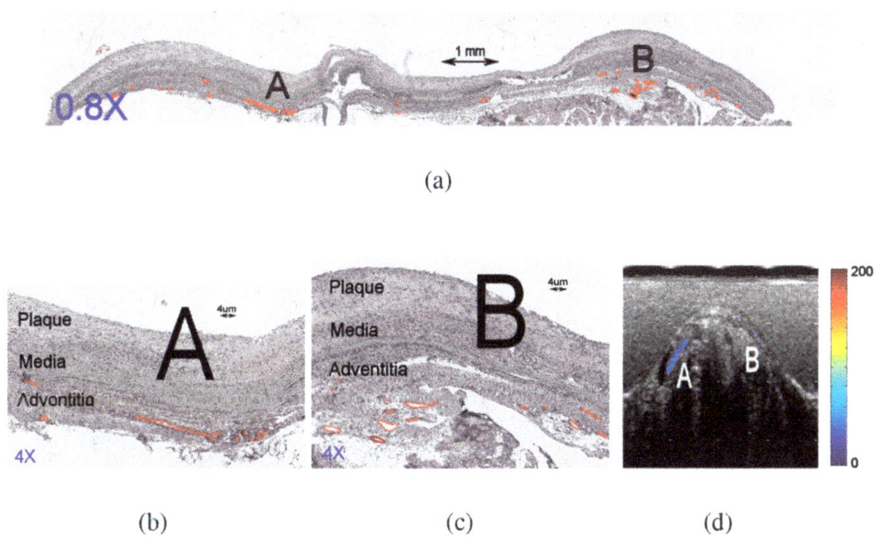

Figure 8.17. Qualitative comparison of histology with the enhancement-detection of case 6. (a) Complete vessel histology slide, (b) zoom on ROI A, (b) zoom on ROI B and (c) enhancement-detection result in the polar B-mode image.

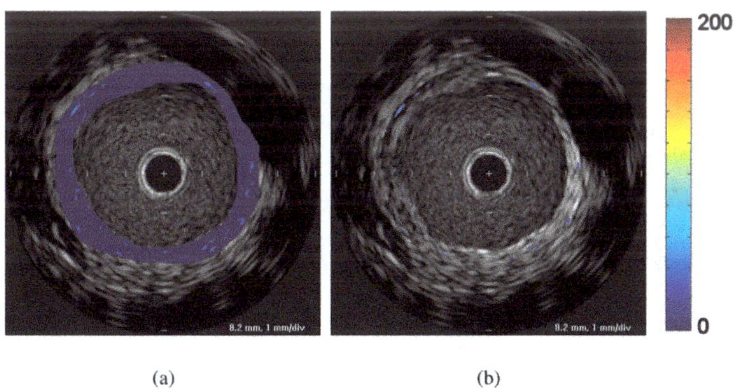

Figure 8.18. Enhancement detection for case 7. (a) ROI enhancement before thresholding and (b) overlay of detected thresholded enhancement in the mean post-injection image.

Figure 8.20 depicts the result for case 8. This case depicts a high density of evidence of enhancement in the media/adventitia regions which correlates with the high density of VV in the adventitia regions in the histology (figure 8.21). It is important to note that there exists some evidence of enhancement in some regions near the lumen which may be due to endothelial adhesion of the contrast agent.

Figure 8.22 depicts the results for case 9. In this case, the proposed enhancement-detection method did not find strong evidence of enhancement in any region. These results also appear to correlate with the histological slide which depicts a poor presence of VV (figure 8.23).

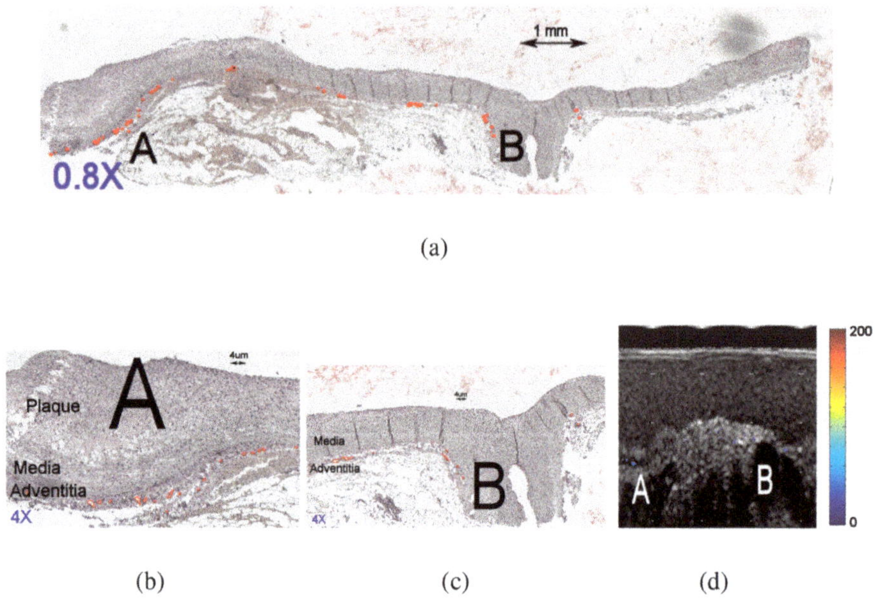

Figure 8.19. Qualitative comparison of histology with the enhancement detection of case 7. (a) Complete vessel histology slide, (b) zoom on ROI A, (b) zoom on ROI B and (c) enhancement-detection result in the polar B-mode image.

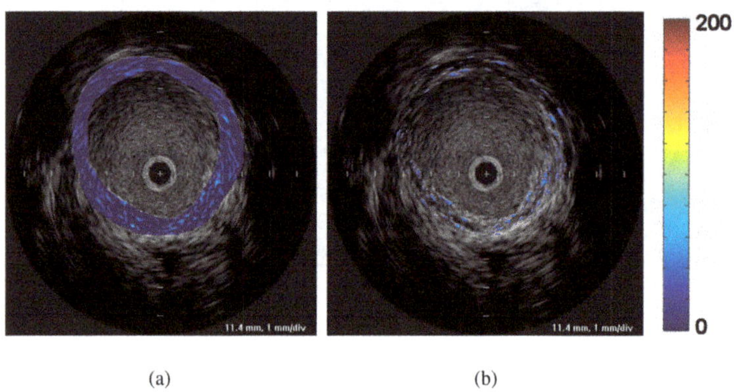

Figure 8.20. Enhancement detection for case 8. (a) ROI enhancement before thresholding and (b) overlay of detected thresholded enhancement in the mean post-injection image.

8.4 Discussion

The significant changes in the IVUS signal after microbubble passage leave no doubt as to its ability to show contrast enhancement. Compared with the other techniques proposed for detecting VV on IVUS, the advantage of our method lies in the fact that no special hardware or contrast agents are necessary (as in harmonic IVUS). Instead, our method is able to detect perfusion within the ROI by using the data

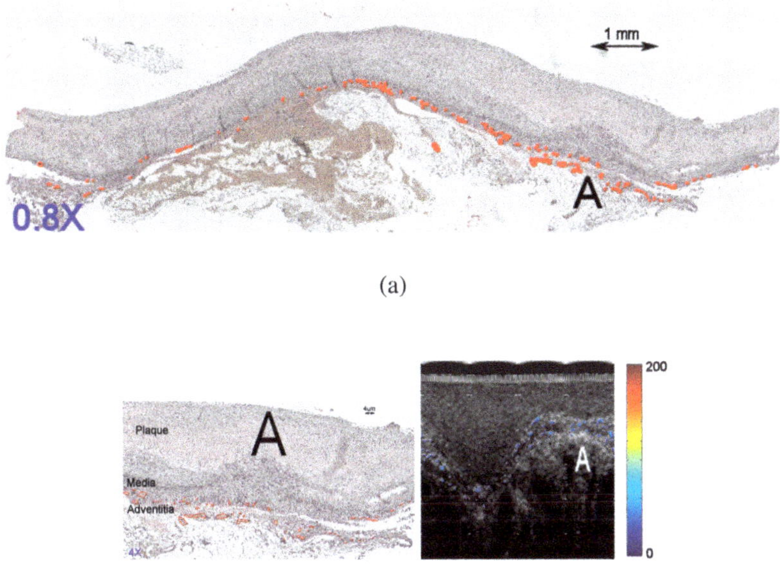

(a)

(b) (c)

Figure 8.21. Qualitative comparison of histology with the enhancement detection of case 8. (a) Complete vessel histology slide, (b) zoom on ROI A and (c) enhancement-detection result in the polar B-mode image.

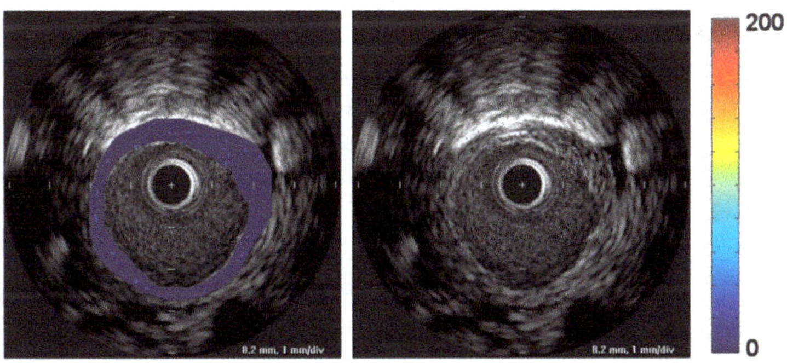

(a) (b)

Figure 8.22. Enhancement detection for case 9. (a) ROI enhancement before thresholding and (b) overlay of detected thresholded enhancement in the mean post-injection image.

extracted from existing commercially available IVUS systems and contrast agents. It is important to note, however, that due to the size of the microvasculature and its elastic characteristics with respect to blood pressure, our method is most likely to detect microvasculature with relatively large lumen areas or bundles of small-sized microvessels. The primary limitation of our method is the requirement that we image every area of interest twice: once before and once after the injection of contrast.

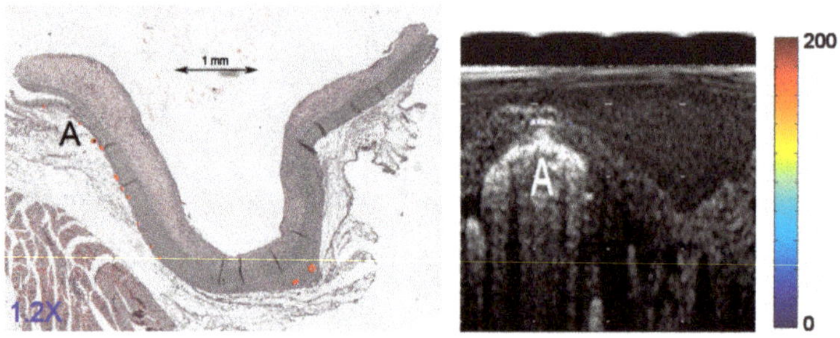

(a) (b)

Figure 8.23. Qualitative comparison of histology with the enhancement detection of case 9. (a) Complete vessel histology slide and (b) enhancement-detection result in the polar B-mode image.

However, this limitation is necessitated by our desire to restrict ourselves to currently available IVUS hardware and standard contrast agents. A second limitation is that our method relies on accurate lumen segmentation on the frames to be analyzed. However, this can be performed either manually or by one of the many different methods proposed in the literature.

8.5 Conclusion

We have presented a method that enables *in vivo* imaging of extra-luminal perfusion under IVUS using commercially available contrast agents. Current evidence and knowledge suggest that this perfusion is related to the presence of VV microvessels which, in turn, are a potential marker for plaque inflammation and consequent vulnerability. As such, contrast-enhanced IVUS presents a promising imaging approach to the assessment of plaque vulnerability.

References

[1] Balakrishnan K R and Kuruvilla S 2006 Role of inflammation in atherosclerosis: immunohistochemical and electron microscopic images of a coronary endarterectomy specimen *Circulation* **113** e41–3

[2] Burke A P, Farb A, Malcom G T, Liang Y H, Smialek J and Virmani R 1997 Coronary risk factors and plaque morphology in men with coronary disease who died suddenly *N. Engl. J. Med.* **336** 1276–82

[3] Cardinal M, Soulez G, Tardif J C, Meunier J and Cloutier G 2010 Fast-marching segmentation of three-dimensional intravascular ultrasound images: a pre-and post-intervention study *Med. Phys.* **37** 3633–47

[4] Chandrana C, Kharin N, Vince G, Roy S and Fleischman A 2010 Demonstration of second-harmonic IVUS feasibility with focused broadband miniature transducers *IEEE Trans. Ultrason. Ferroelectr. Freq. Control* **57** 1077–85

[5] Chen F, Eriksson P, Kimura T, Herzfeld I and Valen G 2005 Apoptosis and angiogenesis are induced in the unstable coronary atherosclerotic plaque *Coronary Artery Dis.* **16** 191–7

[6] Ciompi F, Pujol O, Fernandez-Nofrerias E, Mauri J and Radeva P 2009 ECOC random fields for lumen segmentation in radial artery IVUS sequences *Proc. 12th Int. Conf. on Medical Image Computing and Computer Assisted Intervention* (*London, UK*) pp 869–876

[7] Constantinides P 1990 Cause of thrombosis in human atherosclerotic arteries *Am. J. Cardiol.* **66** 37G–40G

[8] Fabry M E, Kaul D K, Raventos C, Baez S, Rieder R and Nagel R L 1981 Some aspects of the pathophysiology of homozygous Hb CC erythrocytes *J. Clin. Invest.* **67** 1284–91

[9] Fleiner M, Kummer M, Mirlacher M, Sauter G, Cathomas G, Krapf R and Biedermann B C 2004 Arterial neovascularization and inflammation in vulnerable patients *Circulation* **110** 2843–50

[10] Friedberg C K 1949 Coronary arteriosclerosis *Diseases of the Heart* (Philadelphia, PA: Saunders) pp 336–52

[11] Frijlink M E, Goertz D E, Vos H J, Tesselaar E, Blacquiere G, Gisolf A, Krams R and van der Steen A F 2006 Harmonic intravascular ultrasound imaging with a dual-frequency catheter *Ultrasound Med. Biol.* **32** 1649–54

[12] Frijlink M, Goertz D, van Damme L, Krams R and van der Steen A 2006 Intravascular ultrasound tissue harmonic imaging *in vivo IEEE Ultrason. Ferroelectr. Freq. Control* **53** 1844–52

[13] Galis Z and Lessner S 2009 Will the real plaque vasculature please stand up? Why we need to distinguish the vasa plaquorum from the vasa vasorum *Trends Cardiovasc. Med.* **19** 87–94

[14] Gatta C, Balocco S, Ciompi F, Hemetsberger R, Rodriguez-Leor O and Radeva P 2010 Real-time gating of IVUS sequences based on motion blur analysis: method and quantitative validation *Proc. 13th Int. Conf. on Medical Image Computing and Computer Assisted Intervention* (*Beijing, China*) **vol 6362** pp 59–67

[15] Gatta C, Pujol O, Leor O, Ferre J and Radeva P 2008 Robust image-based IVUS pullbacks gating *Proc. 11th Int. Conf. on Medical Image Computing and Computer Assisted Intervention* ed G Fichtinger, G Szekely, D Metaxas and L Axel (New York: Springer) pp 518–25

[16] Goertz D E, Frijlink M E, de Jong N and van der Steen A F 2006 Nonlinear intravascular ultrasound contrast imaging *Ultrasound Med. Biol.* **32** 491–502

[17] Goertz D E, Frijlink M E, Tempel D, Bhagwandas V, Gisolf A, Krams R, de Jong N and van der Steen A 2007 Subharmonic contrast intravascular ultrasound for vasa vasorum imaging *Ultrasound Med. Biol.* **33** 1859–72

[18] Goertz D E *et al* 2006 Contrast harmonic intravascular ultrasound: a feasibility study for vasa vasorum imaging *Invest. Radiol.* **41** 631–8

[19] Gossl M, Malyar N, Rosol M, Beighley P and Ritman E 2003 Impact of coronary vasa vasorum functional structure on coronary vessel wall perfusion distribution *Am. J. Physiol. Heart Circ. Physiol.* **285** H2019–26

[20] Granada J and Feinstein S 2008 Imaging of the vasa vasorum *Nat. Rev. Cardiol.* **5** S18–25

[21] Hayden M and Tyagi S 2004 Vasa vasorum in plaque angiogenesis, metabolic syndrome, type 2 diabetes mellitus, and atheroscleropathy: a malignant transformation *Cardiovasc. Diabetol.* **3** 1

[22] Katouzian A, Baseri B, Konofagou E and Laine A 2008 Automatic detection of blood versus non-blood regions on intravascular ultrasound (IVUS) images using wavelet packet signatures *Proc. SPIE Medical Imaging: Ultrasonic Imaging and Signal Processing* (*San Diego, CA*) pp 1–8

[23] Kolodgie F *et al* 2003 Intraplaque hemorrhage and progression of coronary atheroma *N. Engl. J. Med.* **349** 2316–25
[24] Lametschwandtner A, Kachlik D, Stingl J and Setina M 2007 Spatial analysis of vascular corrosion casts to investigate the architectonic arrangement of vasa vasorum of the human great saphenous vein in normal and pathological conditions *Microsc. Microanal.* **13** 488–9
[25] Langheinrich A C, Michniewicz A, Sedding D G, Walker G, Beighley P E, Rau W S, Bohle R M and Ritman E L 2006 Correlation of vasa vasorum neovascularization and plaque progression in aortas of apolipoprotein E(-/-)/low-density lipoprotein(-/-) double knockout mice' *Arterioscler. Thromb. Vasc. Biol.* **26** 347–52
[26] Maton A 1993 *Human Biology and Health* (Englewood Cliffs, NJ: Prentice Hall)
[27] Mendizabal-Ruiz E G, Rivera M and Kakadiaris I A 2008 A probabilistic segmentation method for the identification of luminal borders in intravascular ultrasound images *Proc. IEEE Computer Society Conf. on Computer Vision and Pattern Recognition* (*Anchorage, AK* (Piscataway, NJ: IEEE)) pp 1–8
[28] Mendizabal-Ruiz E and Kakadiaris I 2012 Probabilistic segmentation of the lumen from intravascular ultrasound radio frequency data *Proc. 15th Int. Conf. on Medical Image Computing and Computer Assisted Intervention* (*Nice, France*) https://doi.org/10.1007/978-3-642-33418-4_56
[29] Mitra A K, Dhume A S and Agrawal D K 2004 Vulnerable plaques—ticking of the time bomb *Can. J. Physiol. Pharmacol.* **82** 860–71
[30] Moraes M and Furuie S 2011 Automatic coronary wall segmentation in intravascular ultrasound images using binary morphological reconstruction *Ultrasound Med. Biol.* **37** 1486–99
[31] Moran C, Watson R, Fox K and McDicken W 2002 *In vitro* acoustic characterisation of four intravenous ultrasonic contrast agents at 30 MHz *Ultrasound Med. Biol.* **28** 785–91
[32] Moreno P R, Purushothaman R, Fuster V, Echeverri D, Truszczynska H, Sharma S K, Badimon J J and O'Connor W N 2004 Plaque neovascularization is increased in ruptured atherosclerotic lesions of human aorta: implications for plaque vulnerability *Circulation* **110** 2032–8
[33] Naghavi M *et al* 2006 From vulnerable plaque to vulnerable patient—Part III: executive summary of the Screening for Heart Attack Prevention and Education (SHAPE) task force report *Am. J. Cardiol.* **98** 2H–15H
[34] Naghavi M *et al* 2003 From vulnerable plaque to vulnerable patient: a call for new definitions and risk assessment strategies: Part I *Circulation* **108** 1664–72
[35] Naghavi M *et al* 2003 From vulnerable plaque to vulnerable patient: a call for new definitions and risk assessment strategies: Part II *Circulation* **108** 1772–8
[36] O'Malley S, Carlier S, Naghavi M and Kakadiaris I 2007 Image-based frame gating of IVUS pullbacks: a surrogate for ECG *Proc. IEEE Int. Conf. on Acoustics, Speech, and Signal Processing* (*Honolulu, HI* (Piscataway, NJ: IEEE)) pp 433–6
[37] O'Malley S, Granada J, Carlier S, Naghavi M and Kakadiaris I 2008 Image-based gating of intravascular ultrasound pullback sequences *IEEE Trans. Inf. Technol. Biomed.* **12** 299–306
[38] O'Malley S, Naghavi M and Kakadiaris I 2006 Image-based frame gating for stationary-catheter IVUS sequences *Proc. Int. Workshop on Computer Vision for Intravascular and Intracardiac Imaging* (*Copenhagen, Denmark*) pp 14–21

[39] Papadogiorgaki M, Mezaris V, Chatzizisis Y S, Giannoglou G D and Kompatsiaris I 2008 Image analysis techniques for automated IVUS contour detection *Ultrasound Med. Biol.* **34** 1482–98

[40] Ross R 1993 The pathogenesis of atherosclerosis: a perspective for the 1990s *Nature* **362** 801–9

[41] Rueckert D, Sonoda L, Hayes C, Hill D, Leach M and Hawkes D 1999 Non-rigid registration using free-form deformations: application to breast MR images *IEEE Trans. Med. Imaging* **18** 712–21

[42] Unal G, Bucher S, Carlier S, Slabaugh G, Fang T and Tanaka K 2008 Shape-driven segmentation of the arterial wall in intravascular ultrasound images *IEEE Trans. Inf. Technol. Biomed.* **12** 335–47

[43] Virmani R, Burke A P, Farb A and Kolodgie F D 2006 Pathology of the vulnerable plaque *J. Am. Coll. Cardiol.* **47** 13–8

[44] Virmani R, Kolodgie F D, Burke A P, Finn A V, Gold H K, Tulenko T N, Wrenn S P and Narula J 2005 Atherosclerotic plaque progression and vulnerability to rupture: angiogenesis as a source of intraplaque hemorrhage *Arterioscler. Thromb. Vasc. Biol.* **25** 2054–61

[45] Zhu X, Zhangc P, Shaoa J, Chenga Y, Zhangc Y and Bai J 2011 A snake-based method for segmentation of intravascular ultrasound images and its *in vivo* validation *Ultrasonics* **51** 181–9

IOP Publishing

Vascular and Intravascular Imaging Trends, Analysis, and Challenges, Volume 1

Stent applications

Petia Radeva and Jasjit S Suri

Chapter 9

Assessment of atherosclerosis in large arteries from PET images

M'hamed Bentourkia

Atherosclerosis is a systemic process mainly occurring in the vessel wall of the medium and large arteries such as the carotid, the aorta, the iliac and the femoral arteries. This process is characterized by the formation of atheroma or plaque, a deposit of cells, connective-tissue elements and lipids, resulting in an asymmetric thickening of the intima, the innermost layer of the artery. The plaque may grow slowly and silently over decades until it obstructs the lumen or it ruptures and provokes a thrombosis and may cause myocardial infarction, stroke and peripheral vascular disease. Atherosclerosis can be asymptomatic as it can affect young individuals, but its manifestation is more impairing in the elderly. In this chapter, we present an overview of the formation of the plaque, its detection and current management, and its imaging with positron emission tomography (PET).

9.1 Introduction

Atherosclerosis is a process causing hardening and narrowing of blood vessels. The disease occurs in the vessel wall of the medium and large arteries of the carotid, the aorta, the iliac and the femoral arteries. The wall thickening, called atheroma, generally referred to as an atheromatous plaque or simply plaque, is formed by a deposit of cells, connective-tissue elements, lipids and debris [1, 2]. In aging, endothelial dysfunction in conjunction with reactive oxygen species are recognized to provoke vascular inflammation which initiates or contributes to particle migration and accumulation in the sub-endothelial space [3, 4]. The resultant plaque progressively and silently develops over several years to generate calcifications or to rupture and provoke a thrombosis. Atherosclerosis can be found in young individuals without provoking symptoms, but its effect is more pronounced in the

doi:10.1088/2053-2563/ab01fach9

elderly and it is often accompanied by persistent inflammation making it a chronic inflammatory disease of the arterial walls.

The degree of inflammation is thought to be related to the risk of plaque rupture, thus the possibility of measuring the inflammation at a certain threshold could be a good indicator of plaque complexity. Plaque rupture is responsible for a large proportion of cardiovascular diseases (CVDs). The external causes of atherosclerosis are numerous and include aging, fat-rich diets, smoking and sedentariness.

The diagnosis of atherosclerosis is usually assessed through blood-based biomarkers [5]. Commonly used biomarkers are C-reactive protein, low- and high-density lipoprotein cholesterol, triglycerides, serum creatinine and several others [6–8]. Imaging has been used recently to mainly study the plaque characteristics and inflammation, and in attempts to develop a measure of plaque vulnerability.

The treatment of atherosclerosis, if diagnosed before complications, is usually based on the intake of statins [9]. The inflammatory cells have been associated with plaque rupture and the inflammation is used as a target for therapy [10]. Some studies have reported diet-based therapies involving canola and olive oil [11–13].

9.2 The formation of atherosclerosis

Retrospective analyses of medical images from patients imaged for cancer diagnoses or for other diseases revealed the presence of atherosclerosis at ages as early as the twenties. Also, post-mortem examinations provided evidence of atherosclerosis as early as the second decade in life. In the elderly, atherosclerosis is nearly always present in different parts of the arteries. Note that most individuals live with atherosclerosis as it does not always present any symptoms and specifically no inflammation. Unfortunately, many patients ignore this disease until they have complications.

The arteries are made of active muscular tubes comprised of three main layers: the intima, which is the inner layer and is lined by a smooth tissue called the endothelium; the smooth muscle, which is the media that handles the high pressure of blood; and the adventitia, which is the outer layer, acts as a supportive element and serves to anchor the artery in nearby tissues. The endothelium is a metabolically active system. It acts as an anatomical barrier to separate circulating blood components and the vessel wall. Among other functions, it regulates the deposition of extracellular matrix (molecules secreted by the cells and permitting communication between cells and providing support, binding cells together or separating one tissue from another), protects the vessel from potentially toxic substances and cells circulating in the blood, and regulates hemostasis (arrest of bleeding by vasoconstriction and coagulation), vasculogenesis (creation or development of new blood vessels), vascular tone (contraction of smooth muscle) [14], leukocyte and platelet adhesion, and inflammatory and reparative responses to local injury [15].

The leukocytes are cells produced from multipotent cells in the bone morrow. They are transported in blood to the site of injury and their function is to neutralize invading micro-organisms or to act on inflammation. When an infection is declared, the number of the leukocytes increases and they become more mobile and move through blood and tissue. There are two types of leukocytes, depending on whether or not they have granules in their cytoplasm: the agranulocytes are lymphocytes and monocytes; the granulocytes are neutrophils, basophils and eosinophils. It is important to briefly define here the cells that are involved in the plaque formation and in the inflammation, and all the defense processes. The plaque is not a deposit of inert lipids or other aggregates, indeed, at early stages, the plaque is a meeting point of several active cells. The lymphocytes are subdivided into three types of cells: the natural killer cells (NK), the T cells and the B cells. NK cells play a major role in the defense of the cells from both tumors and virally infected cells. They attack cells which do not express major histocompatibility complex class I antigens [16, 17]. The T cells are lymphocytes that differentiate in the thymus gland. When exposed to an antigen, the T cells divide rapidly and produce new T cells sensitized to that antigen and combat pathogen-infected cells [18]. The B cells produce large amounts of antibodies in response to pathogens such as bacteria and viruses in order to destroy them. After being activated, both T cells and B cells produce cells called memory cells of the antigens they have been sensitized to, in order to rapidly respond in the future if the same antigens are detected. The monocytes develop into different types of macrophages in the tissue, to subsequently phagocyte invading substances by producing antibodies or by engulfing the pathogens. They can also kill infected cells via antibodies. The macrophages encode on their plasma membrane the antigens they encounter in order to be recognized by the T cells that are sensitized for these same antigens. The antibodies are proteins that binds to antigens, and this labeling allows their recognition and their phagocytosis.

The neutrophils, upon detection of an infection, migrate from the blood stream through the endothelium to the infected region by means of processes collectively called the leukocyte adhesion cascade. The neutrophils are first captured from the blood by endothelial surface selectin molecules including intercellular adhesion molecule 1 (ICAM-1) and vascular cell adhesion molecule 1 (VCAM-1) [19, 20]. These cells have the ability to destroy cell debris and foreign material by oxidative and non-oxidative processes [20]. The basophils release the contents of their granules including histamine, cytokines and lipid inflammatory mediators, responsible for allergic reactions [21–23]. The eosinophils have also been reported to be involved in allergic reactions [24, 25].

In normal conditions, the endothelium does not allow the adhesion of leukocytes and platelets, and inflammatory and reparative cells. This is not the case under some favorable circumstances. The endothelium then provokes the expression of adhesion molecules that induce the fixation of the leukocytes in the arterial wall when exposed to atherogenic diets, which favor the ingestion of high saturated fats, or when the person has hypertension or hyperglycemia, is overweight or is a smoker, or is above 60 years of age (note that the plaque can be formed even in the twenties) [26, 27]. This anomaly allows the build-up of the plaque, generally and initially made of immune cells, vascular and smooth muscle cells, and lipid-laden cells. With time, the plaque becomes predominantly made of macrophages, T cells, foam cells and lipids, and is surrounded by a cap made of smooth muscle cells and collagen-rich matrix [1, 26]. The immune cells become active and produce inflammatory cytokines which are important in cell signaling. T cells also produce cytokines which inhibit the production of collagen by the smooth muscle cells, which in turn stimulates macrophages to express collagen-degrading enzymes. The result of this action is the weakening of the fibrous cap. At this stage of the development of atherosclerosis, the plaque might become vulnerable by a thinning of the shoulders of the cap (the region of attachment of the fibrous cap to the artery wall) and then it can rupture [2, 28, 29]. Before the plaque is ruptured, noticeable activity of the macrophage can be measured as they have high metabolic rates related to inflammation. In other words, the plaque rupture can be due to a highly inflamed artery but not to the volume of the plaque itself or to the thickness of the fibrous cap. When the plaque ruptures, a blood clot (thrombus) is formed in the blood vessels and provokes the acute complications of atherosclerosis. Figure 1 in [30] summarizes the different stages in the development of the plaque.

The plaque can remain intact for the whole life of an individual, as it can rupture and provoke a CVD, or it can harden and calcify. In some cases, especially in young individuals, the plaque can disappear without any treatment [1]. Calcification of the arteries resembles bone formation and occurs via active processes. Bone-forming cells (osteoblasts), cytokines, transcription factors and bone morphogenetic proteins are involved in artery calcification [31]. It was suggested that the smooth muscle cells in the lesion undergo apoptosis and initiate lipoprotein and phospholipid accumulation and hydroxyapatite deposition. The macrophages are also involved in the synthesis and deposition of collagenous proteins that favors hydroxyapatite deposition [31, 32]. Plaques can be found in three structured types: non-calcified, calcified, and a mixture of calcification and non-calcification in the same lesion. Some authors reported that the most calcified plaques may be more stable, and the vulnerable plaques may be those with calcified and non-calcified tissue [17, 33]. It was considered that the calcification contributes to the stiffening of the artery which is a protection against biomechanical stress [34]. Other authors reported, however, that the calcification causes some fragility of the blood vessel where the plaque can fracture near the shoulders of the cap, in comparison to a large calcification of the plaque [35].

Atherosclerosis is often linked to aging. As explained above, plaques are made of vascular smooth muscle cells, blood-derived inflammatory cells, lipids and extracellular matrix proteins, all coated by a fibrous cap. With age, the cap becomes thin and tends to rupture [2]. Moreover, the number of vascular smooth muscle cells in the media layer decreases due to apoptosis, the elastin (a protein constituent of elastic fibers) is degraded in the media and the space is replaced by collagen accumulation and calcification. Elastin degradation is a major cause of artery stiffening with aging [4].

9.3 Management of atherosclerosis

It is not usual at the moment to screen suspected individuals for atherosclerosis and to decide their orientation for a specific treatment before the appearance of symptoms. The detection of plaques, calcifications or even arterial inflammation does not mean that the individual will certainly have a complication with CVD consequences. In fact, the most important diagnosis is to be able to detect vulnerable plaques. When symptoms are present or in the presence of acute complications, the patient is then directed for more investigations to prescribe appropriate treatment.

Having an idea of the triggers of atherosclerosis, although some causes are purely innate genetic predispositions, the first suggested therapy for patients is to change some habits, such as cessation of smoking, reducing fat in diets and regularly practicing physical activity. Aging, however, remains a natural contributor to atherosclerosis. We enumerate hereafter some therapies and lifestyle behaviors that can help prevent plaque formation, reduce inflammation or strengthen the cap.

The release of nitric oxide, a vasodilator substance used in the vascular smooth muscle, by the endothelium cells can be up-regulated by estrogens, physical exercise and diet. It can be down-regulated by oxidative stress, smoking and low-density lipoproteins (LDL) [27]. LDL can be bound to proteoglycan and retained in the intima and undergoes oxidative modification inducing the expression of adhesion molecules, chemokines and pro-inflammatory cytokines. The high-density lipoprotein (HDL) reverses cholesterol transport and can also transport antioxidant enzymes such as platelet-activating factor acetylhydrolase and paraoxonase, which can break down oxidized lipids and neutralize their pro-inflammatory effects [36–38]. Angiotensin II, a peptide hormone related to hypertension that causes vasoconstriction and a subsequent increase in blood pressure, contributes to the regulation of vascular tone, salt and water balance, and blood pressure, and it promotes vascular smooth muscle cell migration [39]. Angiotensin II also provokes the production of superoxide anion O_2^-, a reactive oxygen species, from the endothelial cells and smooth muscle cells, and increases the expression of pro-inflammatory cytokines such as interleukin (IL)-6 and MCP-1 and the vascular cell adhesion molecule VCAM-1 on endothelial cells. Angiotensin-converting enzyme inhibitor therapy may interrupt such pro-inflammatory pathways [36]. In obese individuals, the synthesis of very low-density lipoprotein (VLDL) can lower HDL cholesterol. Adipose tissue can also synthesize cytokines such as tumor necrosis factor-alpha (TNF-α) and IL-6, thus promoting inflammation [36].

Cholesterol is an organic molecule that is an essential component of cell membranes. It functions also as the immediate precursor in various metabolic pathways and as a constituent of LDL which may cause atherosclerosis [40]. Cholesterol is ingested with daily meals and more than two thirds of the body's cholesterol is synthesized in the liver through the HMGCoA-reductase pathway. Therefore, inhibition of the hepatic biosynthesis of cholesterol could help in reducing its levels. To reduce cholesterol biosynthesis in the liver and consequently lower cholesterol levels, the enzyme HMGCoA-reductase is inhibited by statins [40, 41]. Statins lower LDL levels and also attenuate plaque inflammation. Statins are found under several classes: pravastatin, cerivastatin, simvastatin, fluvastatin, atorvastatin and rosuvastatin. Pravastatin and cerivastatin can reduce macrophage content in atherosclerotic plaques, whereas simvastatin, fluvastatin and atorvastatin appear to reduce intimal inflammation and suppress the expression of tissue factor and matrix metalloproteinases (MMP) [36]. Atorvastatin and rosuvastatin have been shown to reduce LDL to 50% and to increase HDL [9, 33, 42].

It has been reported that vitamin D has a protective effect on the endothelium, on the vascular smooth muscle cells and on arterial inflammation [43, 44]. Also, vascular calcifications have been targeted for therapies to prevent or regress the calcifications [17]. The effects of day-to-day diets also have an impact on atherosclerosis. It has been reported that olive oil [45], canola oil [13] and soya bean oil [46] have a positive impact in reducing the incidence of cardiovascular events. The diets mainly focused on reducing saturated fatty acid in daily meals [46].

9.4 Detection of atherosclerosis

It is known that atherosclerosis is present in most individuals, even at the age of about twenty, and that most people do not develop any CVD during their life. Others, however, and mostly those who are predisposed to this disease and those who are overweight, tobacco smokers or fatty diet consumers are more exposed to the disease. Generally, atherosclerosis is diagnosed after a cardiac complication or during a medical check-up.

9.4.1 Biomarkers

Atherosclerosis risk prediction models include traditional risks such as hypertension, cholesterol levels, diabetes, smoking, diet, age, gender and family history. In addition to these risk prediction factors, numerous biomarkers are actually used to predict atherosclerosis complications and to improve clinical decisions. Biomarkers of inflammation include: adhesion molecules VCAM-1; cytokines TNF-α, IL-1 and IL-18; proteases MMP-9; the messenger cytokine IL-6; platelet products CD40L and myeloid-related protein (MRP) 8/14; adipokines such as adiponectin; and acute phase reactants such as C-reactive protein (CRP), PAI-1 and fibrinogen [7]. The CRP is an inflammatory marker primarily produced by the liver in response to interleukin-1, interleukin-6 and TNF-α [5]. CRP can also be produced in the atherosclerotic plaques. A high-sensitivity CRP (hsCRP) assay has been demonstrated to predict myocardial infarction, ischemic stroke, cardiovascular death, incident diabetes and incident hypertension [5]. CRP is an excellent biomarker which does not depend on food intake and has a long half-life, in addition to its remarkable dynamic range [7]. Clinically, CRP remains the most independent marker and powerful predictor of coronary events and in detecting vulnerable plaques.

9.4.2 Imaging

The other means of atherosclerosis detection is by imaging. The advantage of imaging on biomarkers is that biomarkers are systemic detectors of the disease while imaging can precisely locate the part of the arteries with plaques. Imaging cannot, however, at least at the moment in clinics, assess the vulnerability of the plaque. The other hindrances in using imagery are its high cost and the difficulty in repeating the measurements. Within imaging technology, there are different types: invasive, anatomic, molecular or functional. The ultimate targets of the measurements can be plaque composition and morphology, plaque volume and thickness of the fibrous cap, plaque constituent metabolism and the degree of inflammation. These imaging techniques have not been demonstrated to correlate with the clinical histopathological parameters [47]. We outline below some of the imaging techniques used in the assessment of atherosclerosis, namely ultrasound, x-rays, magnetic resonance imaging, optical coherence tomography (OCT) and radionuclide imaging. The description of these and other techniques, such as intravascular angioscopy and colorimetry, thermography, optical coherence tomography, near infrared spectroscopy, Raman spectroscopy, fluorescence emission spectroscopy, elastography, magnetic resonance spectroscopy, nuclear immunoscintigraphy, electrical impedance imaging, vascular tissue Doppler, shear stress imaging, contrast-enhanced MRI with and without immunolabeled agents, electron beam computed tomography, and multi-slice spiral/helical computed tomography, can be found in [48–51].

9.4.2.1 Diagnostic intravascular ultrasound

Diagnostic intravascular ultrasound (IVUS) uses catheters with a transducer ranging in size from 0.96 to 1.17 mm and provides a very high axial resolution of about 80 μm and a lateral resolution of about 200 μm. Using this information the plaque can be qualified as soft, fibrous or calcified. In normal individuals, the thickness of the intima is about 0.15 mm [47, 48]. IVUS permits direct and real-time measurements of the atheroma and provides tomographic sections of the artery. Wall thickness and quantitative analysis of plaque mass and area can be determined. Because it is invasive, its usage is lengthy in time and limited to accessible arteries. However, carotid and femoral arteries (in particular the carotids) can be easily and non-invasively imaged in longitudinal or transverse views. Contrast-enhanced ultrasound has the potential to provide information about carotid plaque composition, in addition to identifying micro-vasculatures within the carotid plaque, which is a sign of plaque vulnerability [52]. Figure 3 in [53] shows two images of coronary artery intravascular ultrasound before and after treatment with atorvastatin, 18 mg day^{-1} for 18 months, which is seen to have reduced the atheroma area from 13 mm^2 to 7.4 mm^2 [53].

9.4.2.2 Tomographic x-rays

Tomographic x-ray imaging (or computed tomography, CT) mainly allows one to locate the extent of the plaque and the calcifications. Because CT is non-invasive and fast, it can scan the whole body and provides a map of the arteries. By assessing the density of tissue at the plaque level, this technique can discriminate plaque stages. For the calcification, the thresholds for the densities in the images can be set to estimate the degree of calcification. The scores were established by Agatston *et al* as 1 for 130 to 199, 2 for 200 to 299, 3 for 300 to 399 and 4 for more than 400 Hounsfield units [34, 54]. By using contrast agents injected through the arm vein, CT angiography can detect the narrowing of the arteries but cannot detect the plaque or its composition. Similar to CT angiography but more invasive, coronarography, also called invasive coronary angiography, is based on the introduction of a catheter through the radial or femoral artery, which is then conducted to the coronary artery where a contrast agent is injected followed by x-ray imaging (see figure 2 in [55]). Electron beam computed tomography (EBCT), having a fast acquisition time (100 ms/slice) and a low dose (0.7 mSv), is used to non-invasively image coronary arteries. EBCT is generally used in assessing the coronary artery calcification scores and volumes with electrocardiographic gating, where it was observed to reduce the variability in the images and to monitor atherosclerosis progression and the effects of medications.

9.4.2.3 Magnetic resonance

Magnetic resonance imaging (MRI) allows the imaging of both plaque volume and composition. It has the potential to characterize the plaque through different imaging techniques (T1, T2 and proton-density weighting, perfusion, diffusion and biochemical contrasts) providing their composition: fibrous cap, lipids and calcifications [56–58]. MRI can be used to assess the effect of a treatment by measuring the extent of the plaque and its constituents (see figure 5 in [59]). The interest in using conventional gadolinium-based contrast agents is useful for fibrous cap delimitation, plaque vascularization and inflammation which could contribute to detect plaque vulnerability. Magnetic resonance angiography allows generating images of flowing blood in the arteries, similar to x-ray angiography, providing information on stenosis. With 1.5 T MRI scanners, the spatial resolution in image slices approximates 0.25×0.25 mm^2 in the carotid and 0.46×0.46 mm^2 in the coronary artery [60]. With 3 T scanners, the signal-to-noise ratio and contrast-to-noise ratio jump to 223% and 255%, respectively, and the images are acquired at a spatial resolution of $0.31 \times 0.31 \times 3$ mm^3 in the carotid wall [61]. There is a compromise between signal-to-noise ratio, acquisition time and spatial resolution. The time usually needed to image a carotid artery is about 45 min [62].

9.4.2.4 Optical coherence tomography

OCT is an intravascular imaging modality, based on infrared light emission at wavelengths of 1280–1350 nm. It is like ultrasound imaging but uses light instead of sound and the reflected light on the tissue borders is analyzed with interferometers. It is a very fast imaging method that can be processed in the time or frequency domains. The light is delivered through an optical fiber and the beam is directed by a microprism. The images are obtained at 20 frames/sec at axial and lateral spatial resolutions of 10–15 μm and 94 μm, respectively, with a maximal depth in tissue of 3 mm (see figure 8 in [63]). OCT has some limitations. For example, it cannot provide measurements of arteries in the presence of blood; blood flow has to be stopped by inflating a proximal occlusion balloon. OCT provides better arterial wall images than IVUS and can detect early construction of the plaques, while it does not allow enough penetration to visualize thick plaques.

9.4.2.5 Radionuclide imaging

Radionuclide imaging has the advantage of providing information on a given physiological phenomenon in diverse ways. However, because it is based on radiation emission that could be risky to the patient, small amounts of the radiotracer are injected into the patient, and consequently, the scanners are made of larger detectors to count more radiations. At the end, the images present reduced contrast and spatial resolution. The two main devices used in tomographic radionuclide imaging are PET and single photon emission computed tomography (SPECT). PET relies on the detection of two coincident gamma rays of the same energy, while SPECT detects single photons of different energies depending on the isotopes used for imaging. PET imaging coupled to CT imaging will be covered in the next section. We provide an overview in the rest of this section of some studies performed with SPECT using different radioisotopes and radiotracers.

LDL is recognized to be involved in the formation and vulnerability of the plaque, thus it was labeled with the isotopes ^{99m}Tc ($t_{1/2} = 6$ h, $E\gamma = 141$ keV) [47, 64], ^{111}In ($t_{1/2} = 2.8$ day, $E\gamma = 245$ keV) [65], ^{123}I ($t_{1/2} = 13.2$ h, $E\gamma = 159$ keV) and ^{131}I ($t_{1/2} = 8$ day, $E\gamma = 364$ keV) [66–68]. ^{99m}Tc-LDL was found to be located in lesions rich in macrophages, however, it was found not to be suitable in coronary arteries as its specific uptake was very low and its washout was found to be very slow, making the blood activity very high and resulting in a poor lesion-to-background ratio [47]. Radiotracers with iodinated LDL were found to be inefficient as they were found to rapidly deiodinate in the tissues [66].

Several studies reported imaging of atherosclerosis in animal models using different radiotracers, among them ^{111}In-LDL, which was evaluated in the aorta of hypercholesterolemic rabbits and showed an uptake 2.5 times higher than in normal rabbits [65]. Oxidized LDL was shown to be present in atherosclerotic arteries but not in normal arteries [69, 70]. Endothelial cells, smooth muscle cells and monocyte macrophages have been reported to oxidize LDL [71]. Labeled antibodies against oxidized LDL with ^{125}I ($t_{1/2} = 59$ day, $E\gamma = 35$ keV) was used in rabbit imaging (^{125}I-MDA2, a monoclonal antibody against malondialdehyde-lysine epitopes) [69]. The authors concluded that ^{125}I-MDA2 has excellent uptake and specificity for atherosclerosis lesions. However, its application in humans should take into account the low energy of the isotope and other parameters related to imaging.

Several other techniques reported imaging in atherosclerosis based on markers, we refer here to some of them [72–84].

9.5 Imaging of atherosclerosis with PET/CT

CT imaging is not only coupled to PET to seek compensation for the low spatial resolution of PET, but also as a complement for better assessment of atherosclerosis, such as the grading of the calcification. Of course, images acquired with CT and those acquired with PET in the same patient and in the same session have different sizes. Either axially or transaxially, CT images have smaller voxels than PET images. In order to match the two sets of images for image fusion or registration, an interpolation is mandatory. This interpolation generally introduces uncertainties in voxel values. Since the atheromatous plaques and the calcifications have small sizes in comparison to the PET spatial resolution, these uncertainties drastically affect the artery images. Most PET scanners are now equipped as bimodality PET/CT scanners. Note that several works on atherosclerosis have been reported using dual modality PET and MRI [48, 85–87].

Imaging is *a priori* intended to visualize structures such as stenosis, wall thickness and plaque volume, and consequently to be able to measure their extent. However, PET imaging, in addition to its higher sensitivity to the picomolar [88], can also report measurements of metabolism and other physiological parameters. In fact, it is not the size of the plaque which is of importance, but its inflammation, which is of crucial importance as an indication of its vulnerability. The degree of inflammation can be assessed by the metabolism of the cells within the plaque. During the measurement with PET, the acquisition can be reconstructed in a sequence of images as a function of time. This dynamic imaging is very useful as it can help in discriminating tissue activity from blood activity and two or more tissue types. Moreover, within a single tissue, dynamic imaging can help in determining the state of the radiotracer as compartments which add more precision in the quantitative analysis. This type of measurement is more appropriate in research than in the clinic as the patient is injected with the radiotracer when lying within the scanner and the measurement takes a longer time than in the clinic. In the clinic, the patient is injected with the radiotracer and remains for some time before being imaged for a short time. In this way more patients can be imaged in the clinic.

9.5.1 Fast quantitative assessment

Several studies on atherosclerosis have been reported using PET. However, most of these studies have been carried out retrospectively. Patients referred to PET imaging by their practitioners for a given disease such as cancer or cardiovascular problems generate considerable data to be exploited for other analyses. These data are generally composed of static images, thus the only way to quantitatively extract useful information from these data is by using simplified models. The two most commonly used models are the standardized uptake value (SUV) and the target-to-background ratio (TBR).

Based on the images, SUV is either calculated from a region of interest (ROI) or from image voxels. Its value, which is unitless, depends on image intensity C_{PET}, the injected activity A and patient weight w:

$$\mathrm{SUV} = \frac{C_{\mathrm{PET}}[\mathrm{Bq\ kg^{-1}}]}{A[\mathrm{Bq}]/w[\mathrm{kg}]}, \tag{9.1}$$

where C_{PET} in Bq kg^{-1} is the mean intensity in an ROI or in a voxel and is measured in a given interval of time in a steady state with minimal variation. Activity A in Bq is the injected activity of the radiotracer, and w in kg is the body weight of the subject. SUV is a simple and rapid quantitative technique, sometimes it is called semi-quantitative. By using the same PET measurement protocol in two or more measurements, SUV can be used, for example, to compare inflammation progress or the effect of treatments. SUV is very helpful for cancer diagnoses. However, it is not robust and this is a function of several factors: (1) the radiotracer is not equally distributed in the body in tissues compared to fat and hence the division by the weight is not certain; (2) the time of image acquisition affects the radiotracer uptake in the tissues which directly affects SUV; (3) the ROI or the voxel grouping are very subjective due to uncertainty introduced by the operator and the ROI can be affected by partial volume effect and spillover; and (4) C_{PET} is a measure of the whole radiotracer without distinction of blood and tissue in the ROI and thus SUV cannot discriminate between perfused and necrosed tumors or inflamed tissues. Other factors influencing SUV can be found in [89–92].

To correct for the uncertainty on body weight by taking the fat into consideration, it is usual to replace the subject's weight by the subject's body surface area (BSA) given by [90]

$$\mathrm{BSA}[\mathrm{m}^2] = w^{0.425}[\mathrm{kg}] \times \mathrm{height}^{0.725}[\mathrm{cm}] \times 0.007184. \quad (9.2)$$

Another form of BSA is given by [93]

$$\mathrm{BSA}[\mathrm{m}^2] = [w[\mathrm{kg}] \times \mathrm{height}[\mathrm{cm}]/3600]^{1/2}. \quad (9.3)$$

Let us see the difference between equations (9.2) and (9.3). We calculated BSA1 according to equation (9.2) and BSA2 according to equation (9.3) for the values of the weights w and the heights h: w = [10 20 30 40 50 60 70 80 90 100 110 120 130]; h = [100 160 170 175 180 160 185 165 160 178 182 158 173]. The plot of BSA2 as a function of BSA1 is shown in figure 9.1 together with the regression line which has a slope of 1.09 and an intercept of −0.15. Also they were correlated (99%) and not significantly different (p = 0.95 at 5%). The two definitions of BSA could then be considered to be equivalent.

TBR was used in several publications to account for radiotracer uptake in artery tissue in comparison to an ROI drawn on a venous blood image, thus TBR accounts for artery plaque SUV divided by venous blood SUV [94, 95]:

$$\mathrm{TBR} = \mathrm{SUV}_{\mathrm{artery}}/\mathrm{SUV}_{\mathrm{vein}}. \quad (9.4)$$

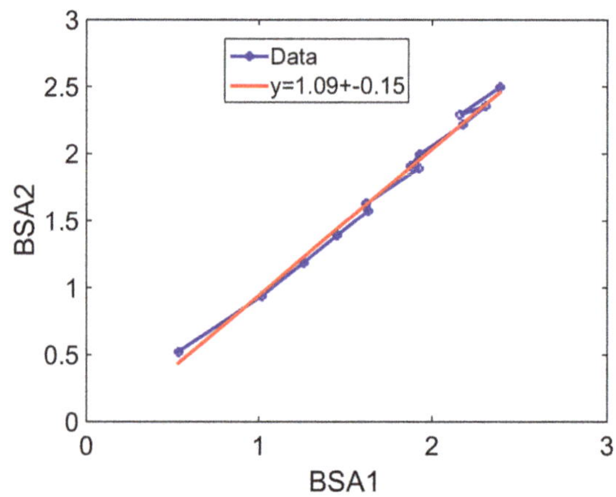

Figure 9.1. Comparison of BSA1 and BSA2 as defined in equations (9.2) and (9.3).

9.5.2 Kinetic modeling

In research, the subjects, either animals or humans, are selected based on predetermined criteria, and the imaging is performed according to a predefined protocol. In order to extract maximal information from the images, the subjects are directly measured at the start of the radiotracer injection. The data are then collected in list mode which can be reconstructed later in any time framing. This dynamic acquisition can be used with SUV and TBR by considering the optimal interval of time of the images. Moreover, uptake of the radiotracer in an artery can be evaluated as a curve instead of a single data point. Any image voxel is made of the contribution of the radiotracer in blood and tissue, and this is more justified in the artery images, adding the fact that artery tissue forms a thin layer in the image even on CT images, and it cannot be discriminated. The mixture of blood and tissue responses is mainly due to the limited spatial resolution of the scanner (about 3 mm) and to the subject's organ movement. There are, however, mathematical tools to allow decomposing a sequence of dynamic images into two components in order to isolate uptake of the radiotracer in artery tissue. Because the dynamic behavior of the radiotracer concentration in tissue and in blood is different as a function of time (two curves of different shapes), the mathematics can thus split the intensity of a voxel into two fractions of intensities representing the two components. This operation can be achieved by algorithms such as factor analysis of dynamic structures (FADS) [96] and independent component analysis (ICA) [97]. The extraction of the blood component from PET images is crucial in kinetic modeling. Instead of sampling blood from the patient, which subsequently needs centrifugation to extract blood plasma, measurement of the radioactivity in the samples and calibration and timing with the PET images, the mathematically obtained image of the blood component can be used in a straightforward manner.

We briefly describe two approaches of kinetic modeling which are more accurate then SUV. More details can be found in [98]. The first one is compartmental modeling and here it is expressed based on 18F-fluorodeoxyglucose (18F-FDG), an analogue of glucose, which is limited at the phosphorylation step [99]. 18F-FDG provides high contrast images in tissues metabolizing glucose. The second approach is an approximation of the first one, assuming no dephosphorylation of 18F-FDG. This approach is the graphical analysis method or, as it is commonly called, the Patlak method [100].

The 18F-FDG compartmental model is shown in figure 9.2 from which a set of differential equations are deduced.

$$\frac{dC_f(t)}{dt} = K_1 C_b(t) - (k_2 + k_3)C_f(t) + k_4 C_m(t) \tag{9.5}$$

$$\frac{dC_m(t)}{dt} = k_3 C_f(t) - k_4 C_m(t).$$

These two equations can be directly used in an algorithm to compute the rate

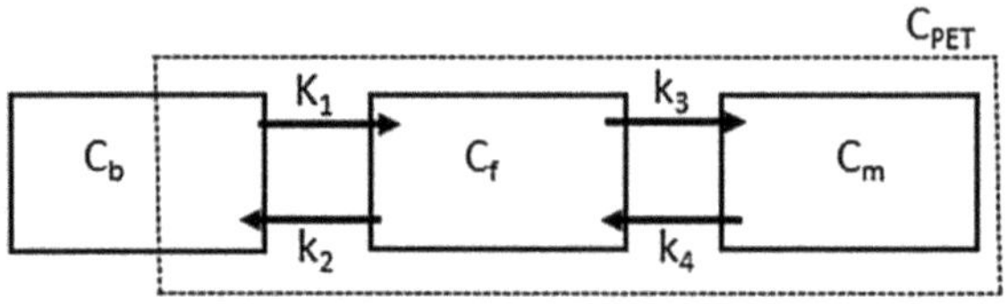

Figure 9.2. Three-compartment 18F-FDG model. C_b, C_f and C_m are the compartments for blood, free and metabolized 18F-FDG. C_{PET} represents what the scanner measures in a voxel or in an ROI. The radiotracer is exchanged between the compartments by means of the rate constants $K_1 - k_4$. Note that K_1 is the perfusion and has units in ml g^{-1} min^{-1} while $k_2 - k_4$ have units in min^{-1}.

constants $K_1 - k_4$, or they can be analytically solved to isolate each compartment and used to output the four rate constants.

The measured radioactivity $C_{\text{PET}}(t)$ is the sum of the radioactivity emitted from the three compartments: blood (C_b), free 18F-FDG (C_f) and metabolized 18F-FDG (C_m). In terms of equations, $C_{\text{PET}}(t)$ is expressed as

$$C_{\text{PET}}(t) = \frac{K_1}{\alpha_2 - \alpha_1}[(k_3 + k_4 - \alpha_1)e^{-\alpha_1 t} + (\alpha_2 - k_3 - k_4)e^{-\alpha_2 t}] \otimes C_p(t) + \upsilon C_b(t), \quad (9.6)$$

where α_1 and α_2 are combinations of the rate constants [99]; $C_p(t)$ is the concentration of the radiotracer in the plasma. $C_p(t)$ can be determined from blood samples or simply from the blood component image obtained from the decomposed images with FADS or ICA or with other algorithms. The fourth parameter ν accounts for the fraction of blood measured in tissue with PET. The symbol $\otimes$ represents the operation of convolution.

Generally the algorithm of Levenberg–Marquardt is used to adjust the model in the right member of (9.6) to the PET data in the left member [101].

From the calculated rate constants, the metabolic rates for glucose (MRG) are deduced:

$$\text{MRG}(\mu\text{moles}/100\ \text{g/min}) = \frac{gl(\text{mg of glucose}/100\ \text{ml of plasma})}{\text{LC} \times 0.182(\text{mg}\ \mu\text{moles}^{-1})} \times \frac{K_1(\text{ml g}^{-1}\text{min}^{-1}) \times k_3(\text{min}^{-1})}{k_2(\text{min}^{-1}) + k_3(\text{min}^{-1})}, \quad (9.7)$$

where gl is the concentration of glucose in plasma, and LC is the lumped constant. LC could be considered as unity to obtain relative values of MRG. The factor 0.182 in the denominator accounts for the molecular mass of glucose which is 182 g mole^{-1}.

In some tissues such as the heart and tumors, there is no dephosphorylation back to 18F-FDG which means there is no k_4 in the model. The model then reduces to the graphical analysis model [98, 100]:

$$\frac{C_{\text{PET}}(t)}{C_p(t)} = \frac{K_1 k_3}{k_2 + k_3} \frac{\int_0^t C_p(u)du}{C_p(t)} + \frac{K_1 k_2}{k_2 + k_3}. \quad (9.8)$$

In this case, equation (9.8) appears as a linear regression with slope $\frac{K_1 k_3}{k_2 + k_3}$. This is the same ratio as in equation (9.7). The slope is evaluated on the last few data points where the plot is linear.

The complexity of kinetic modeling resides in the determination of the plasma function (or as it is usually called, the input function). The other difficulty is the uncertainty on the region to consider for kinetic modeling. Since the artery plaque is small and contains a few voxels, the time–activity curve ($C_{PET}(t)$) is noisy and, consequently, the values of MRG are obtained with high variations, which affects the difference between the normal and inflamed artery.

9.5.3 Multiple approaches in atherosclerosis quantitation with PET

Until now, the most commonly used radiotracer to assess the vulnerability of plaque is 18F-FDG, because the inflammation, including the aggregated cells in the plaque, metabolize glucose. It is expected that the more the plaque uses glucose, the more it is vulnerable. Another reason for the use of glucose is its production and availability in every PET center. Wu *et al* reported that 18F-FDG uptake is a function of the availability of MMP in the plaque, which is an indicator of advanced atherosclerosis and plaque rupture [102]. However, although PET-18F-FDG has the potential to measure the progress of the disease, it was shown to be in discrepancy with CT. Uptake of 18F-FDG could be present with the presence or absence of calcification, as seen on CT images, and the opposite is also true, i.e. the presence of calcification on CT images with no uptake of 18F-FDG [103]. Davies *et al* combined PET-18F-FDG with MRI in a dynamic PET acquisition of 120 min. However, the authors calculated the ratio of radiotracer uptake in the lesions with respect to uptake in a normal artery and they established a classification of inflammation depending on the deviation from the mean values [85]. Instead of taking advantage of the dynamic measurements and computing MRG values, they only used the last 30 min of the acquisition where the radioactivity in the blood is expected to be reduced and they averaged voxel intensity in ROIs based on MRI images.

It has been shown that 18F-FDG uptake in the arteries correlates with some cardiovascular risk factors. Therapies with either medication or lifestyle could decrease 18F-FDG uptake, but it has not been demonstrated to be translated to lowering the impact of the disease or even coupled to systemic biomarkers [88, 104, 105]. Repeated measurements with 18F-FDG showed up to 50% variability between 6 months and 26 months, and it was reported that 18F-FDG uptake could remain constant for a period of 6 months [88]. Atherosclerosis can be diagnosed in young individuals, and it is recognized that healthy elderly people are also affected by atherosclerosis, and the disease may progress within a year [106]. In this study, the authors demonstrated different mean 18F-FDG SUVs in three groups of patients: healthy, with hypercholesterolemia and with chest angina, all of them above 65 years of age. The hypercholesterolemia subjects were prescribed Rosuvastatin and the group with angina were taking their own medication, and the measurements were repeated 12 months later [106] (figure 9.3). Their results showed on average a

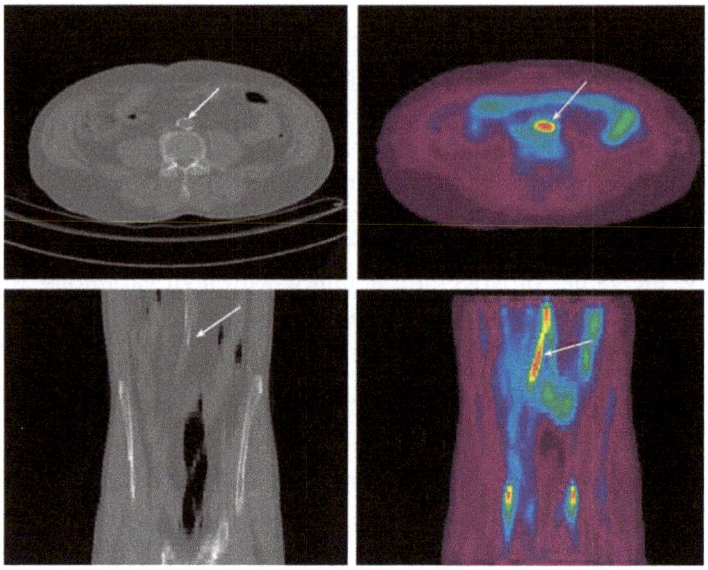

Figure 9.3. CT (left) and PET-18F-FDG (right) images of calcified aorta (arrows) in transaxial (top) and coronal (bottom) slices.

high 18F-FDG uptake in groups 2 and 3 at first scans with respect to group 1, and the increase of 18F-FDG uptake 12 months later was less in group 3 than in the other two groups.

Instead of estimating glucose metabolism which *a priori* was not specific enough to prevent plaque rupture, some researchers based their works on the presence of some proteins or other substrates indicating plaque vulnerability. They investigated, among other attempts, in particular in animal imaging, the mechanisms by which the plaque becomes vulnerable. Several radiotracers have been utilized, among them 18F-NaF [107–109], 11C-PK11195 [110], 11C-choline, 68Ga-[1,4,7,10-tetraa-zacy-clododecane-*N*,*N*′,*N*″,*N*‴-tetraacetic acid]-D-Phe1, Tyr3-octreotate (DOTATATE) [88, 111] and 18F-VCAM-1 [112]. Joshi *et al* reported that 18F-NaF binds to regions with necrosis, macrophages, apoptosis and micro-calcification [109]. 18F-NaF is recognized to bind to bones and produces excellent images without uptake in most tissues. Then, what is the difference between imaging with 18F-NaF and CT as both of them can show the calcifications? Considering their advantages, CT provides high resolution images while 18F-NaF produces a low dose to the patient, but this is not crucial. The response to this question was given by Joshi *et al* where they specified that CT provides images of calcified arteries at the final stage of calcification, while 18F-NaF can detect the slowly developing and metabolically active calcifications that are not apparent on CT images and in some cases not on 18F-FDG images (see figure 1 in [109]). Other works reported the specificity of 18F-NaF to detect active plaques (see figure 2 in [108]). They noticed large calcified structures on CT images but with low uptake of 18F-NaF and, in other regions, they observed intense uptake of 18F-NaF with minimal or no CT calcification. However, the potential of 18F-NaF to prevent plaque rupture remains to be confirmed.

9.6 Discussion

Imaging technologies have evolved signficantly despite their high cost and the need to form multidisciplinary research or clinical teams. The dual modality imaging devices, PET/CT, PET/MRI and SPECT/CT, combine inputs from the departments of radiology and nuclear medicine, if the latter includes PET imaging. The specifically missing contribution is not on the hardware side, it is more methodological, where some techniques need to be implemented and analyses need to be carried on quantitatively. Most of the studies relied on SUV for their statistics. The other crucially missing contribution is that related to the production of radiotracers. It is in fact costly in resources and time to produce and validate a radiotracer.

From the PET imaging side, it is possible to label a molecule to measure the concentration, perfusion, metabolism or receptors, but the focus should be on the atheromatous plaque if the mechanisms are understood. This means that we know what is happening in the plaque, and we want to measure it through imaging (the bottom-up approach). Alternatively, we do not know what exactly is happening there, and we are trying to understand the phenomenon by imaging (a top-down approach). Researchers are yet at the exploration stage, trying to design an appropriate radiotracer to potentially provide accurate measurements of disease progression.

Following these ideas, several researchers are intensively developing radiotracers targeting LDL, antibodies, MMPs, nanoparticles, monocytes and other cells. At present, the variability in quantitative imaging is large [86], which is more drastic in radionuclide imaging. If a molecule specific to the vulnerable plaque is identified and labeled with an isotope, the low spatial resolution of PET will not be a hindrance. The imaging tools are not used for diagnoses and follow-up of atherosclerosis, they are mostly used for research to understand the development of the disease and to prevent cardiovascular complications.

9.7 Conclusions

The techniques reported to date are largely based on simple approaches of analyses such as SUV and uptake of the radiotracer. This is partly because of the high variability in such small regions of the developing plaque, even when imaged with multimodalities. To overcome the low spatial resolution of PET, specific radiotracers to prevent plaque rupture should be designed. It is not expected that the plaque vulnerability will be assessed as present or absent, but it is expected that this vulnerability will be determined in grades.

References

[1] Hansson G K 2005 Inflammation, atherosclerosis, and coronary artery disease *N. Engl. J. Med.* **352** 1685–95

[2] Costopoulos C, Liew T V and Bennett M 2008 Ageing and atherosclerosis: mechanisms and therapeutic options *Biochem. Pharmacol.* **75** 1251–61

[3] Cai H and Harrison D G 2000 Endothelial dysfunction in cardiovascular diseases: the role of oxidant stress *Circ. Res.* **87** 840–4

[4] Lee S J and Park S H 2013 Arterial ageing *Korean Circ. J.* **43** 73–9

[5] Brown T M and Bittner V 2008 Biomarkers of atherosclerosis: clinical applications *Curr. Cardiol. Rep.* **10** 497–504

[6] Revkin J H, Shear C L, Pouleur H G, Ryder S W and Orloff D G 2007 Biomarkers in the prevention and treatment of atherosclerosis: need, validation, and future *Pharmacol. Rev.* **59** 40–53

[7] Packard R R and Libby P 2008 Inflammation in atherosclerosis: from vascular biology to biomarker discovery and risk prediction *Clin. Chem.* **54** 24–38

[8] Fischer K *et al* 2014 Biomarker profiling by nuclear magnetic resonance spectroscopy for the prediction of all-cause mortality: an observational study of 17,345 persons *PLoS Med.* **11** e1001606

[9] Jones P H *et al* 2003 Comparison of the efficacy and safety of rosuvastatin versus atorvastatin, simvastatin, and pravastatin across doses (STELLAR* Trial) *Am. J. Cardiol.* **92** 152–60

[10] Duivenvoorden R *et al* 2013 Relationship of serum inflammatory biomarkers with plaque inflammation assessed by FDG PET/CT: the dal-PLAQUE study *JACC Cardiovasc. Imaging* **6** 1087–94

[11] Berrougui H, Cloutier M, Isabelle M and Khalil A 2006 Phenolic-extract from argan oil (*Argania spinosa* L.) inhibits human low-density lipoprotein (LDL) oxidation and enhances cholesterol efflux from human THP-1 macrophages *Atherosclerosis* **184** 389–96

[12] Loued S, Berrougui H, Componova P, Ikhlef S, Helal O and Khalil A 2013 Extra-virgin olive oil consumption reduces the age-related decrease in HDL and paraoxonase 1 anti-inflammatory activities *Br. J. Nutr.* **110** 1272–84

[13] Jones P J *et al* 2015 High-oleic canola oil consumption enriches LDL particle cholesteryl oleate content and reduces LDL proteoglycan binding in humans *Atherosclerosis* **238** 231–8

[14] Webb R C and Bohr D F 1981 Regulation of vascular tone, molecular mechanisms *Prog. Cardiovasc. Dis.* **24** 213–42

[15] Farouque H M and Meredith I T 2001 The assessment of endothelial function in humans *Coronary Artery Dis.* **12** 445–54

[16] Zamai L *et al* 2007 NK cells and cancer *J. Immunol.* **178** 4011–6

[17] Wu M, Rementer C and Giachelli C M 2013 Vascular calcification: an update on mechanisms and challenges in treatment *Calcif. Tissue Int.* **93** 365–73

[18] Tse K, Tse H, Sidney J, Sette A and Ley K 2013 T cells in atherosclerosis *Int. Immunol.* **25** 615–22

[19] Lawson C and Wolf S 2009 ICAM-1 signaling in endothelial cells *Pharmacol. Rep.* **61** 22–32

[20] Padmanabhan J and Gonzalez A L 2012 The effects of extracellular matrix proteins on neutrophil-endothelial interaction--a roadway to multiple therapeutic opportunities *Yale J. Biol. Med.* **85** 167–85

[21] Bischoff S C, Krieger M, Brunner T and Dahinden C A 1992 Monocyte chemotactic protein 1 is a potent activator of human basophils *J. Exp. Med.* **175** 1271–5

[22] Siracusa M C, Kim B S, Spergel J M and Artis D 2013 Basophils and allergic inflammation *J. Allergy Clin. Immunol.* **132** 789–801 quiz 788

[23] Merluzzi S, Betto E, Ceccaroni A A, Magris R, Giunta M and Mion F 2015 Mast cells, basophils and B cell connection network *Mol. Immunol.* **63** 94–103

[24] Isobe Y, Kato T and Arita M 2012 Emerging roles of eosinophils and eosinophil-derived lipid mediators in the resolution of inflammation *Front. Immunol.* **3** 270

[25] Furuta G T, Atkins F D, Lee N A and Lee J J 2014 Changing roles of eosinophils in health and disease *Ann. Allergy Asthma Immunol.* **113** 3–8

[26] Libby P 2006 Inflammation and cardiovascular disease mechanisms *Am. J. Clin. Nutr.* **83** 456s–60s

[27] Vanhoutte P M, Shimokawa H, Tang E H and Feletou M 2009 Endothelial dysfunction and vascular disease *Acta Physiol.* **196** 193–222

[28] Veress A I, Cornhill J F, Herderick E E and Thomas J D 1998 Age-related development of atherosclerotic plaque stress: a population-based finite-element analysis *Coronary Artery Dis.* **9** 13–9

[29] Pugliese G, Iacobini C, Fantauzzi C B and Menini S 2015 The dark and bright side of atherosclerotic calcification *Atherosclerosis* **238** 220–30

[30] Sanz J and Fayad Z A 2008 Imaging of atherosclerotic cardiovascular disease *Nature* **451** 953–7

[31] Alexopoulos N and Raggi P 2009 Calcification in atherosclerosis *Nat. Rev. Cardiol.* **6** 681–8

[32] Leopold J A 2014 Vascular calcification: mechanisms of vascular smooth muscle cell calcification *Trends Cardiovasc. Med.* **25** 267–74

[33] Nicoll R and Henein M Y 2013 Arterial calcification: friend or foe? *Int. J. Cardiol.* **167** 322–7

[34] Nandalur K R, Baskurt E, Hagspiel K D, Phillips C D and Kramer C M 2005 Calcified carotid atherosclerotic plaque is associated less with ischemic symptoms than is noncalcified plaque on MDCT *Am. J. Roentgenol.* **184** 295–8

[35] Schmermund A and Erbel R 2001 Unstable coronary plaque and its relation to coronary calcium *Circulation* **104** 1682–7

[36] Libby P 2002 Inflammation in atherosclerosis *Nature* **420** 868–74

[37] Benowitz N L 2003 Cigarette smoking and cardiovascular disease: pathophysiology and implications for treatment *Prog. Cardiovasc. Dis.* **46** 91–111

[38] Gaziano T A, Bitton A, Anand S, Abrahams-Gessel S and Murphy A 2010 Growing epidemic of coronary heart disease in low- and middle-income countries *Curr. Probl. Cardiol.* **35** 72–115

[39] Muthalif M M *et al* 2000 Angiotensin II-induced hypertension: contribution of Ras GTPase/Mitogen-activated protein kinase and cytochrome P450 metabolites *Hypertension* **36** 604–9

[40] Tomkin G H and Owens D 2012 LDL as a cause of atherosclerosis *Open Atheroscler. Thromb. J.* **5** 13–21

[41] Liao J K and Laufs U 2005 Pleiotropic effects of statins *Annu. Rev. Pharmacol. Toxicol.* **45** 89–118

[42] Rosenson R S 2004 Statins in atherosclerosis: lipid-lowering agents with antioxidant capabilities *Atherosclerosis* **173** 1–12

[43] Kassi E, Adamopoulos C, Basdra E K and Papavassiliou A G 2013 Role of vitamin D in atherosclerosis *Circulation* **128** 2517–31

[44] Lutsey P L and Michos E D 2013 Vitamin D, calcium, and atherosclerotic risk: evidence from serum levels and supplementation studies *Curr. Atheroscler. Rep.* **15** 293
[45] Helal O, Berrougui H, Loued S and Khalil A 2013 Extra-virgin olive oil consumption improves the capacity of HDL to mediate cholesterol efflux and increases ABCA1 and ABCG1 expression in human macrophages *Br. J. Nutr.* **109** 1844–55
[46] Uusitalo U *et al* 1996 Fall in total cholesterol concentration over five years in association with changes in fatty acid composition of cooking oil in Mauritius: cross sectional survey *Brit. Med. J.* **313** 1044–6
[47] Vallabhajosula S and Fuster V 1997 Atherosclerosis: imaging techniques and the evolving role of nuclear medicine *J. Nucl. Med.* **38** 1788–96
[48] Fayad Z A and Fuster V 2001 Clinical imaging of the high-risk or vulnerable atherosclerotic plaque *Circ. Res.* **89** 305–16
[49] Naghavi M, Madjid M, Khan M, Mohammadi R, Willerson J and Casscells S W 2001 New developments in the detection of vulnerable plaque *Curr. Atheroscler. Rep.* **3** 125–35
[50] Davies J R, Rudd J H and Weissberg P L 2004 Molecular and metabolic imaging of atherosclerosis *J. Nucl. Med.* **45** 1898–907
[51] Jaffer F A, Libby P and Weissleder R 2006 Molecular and cellular imaging of atherosclerosis: emerging applications *J. Am. Coll. Cardiol.* **47** 1328–38
[52] Owen D R, Lindsay A C, Choudhury R P and Fayad Z A 2011 Imaging of atherosclerosis *Annu. Rev. Med.* **62** 25–40
[53] Choudhury R P, Fuster V and Fayad Z A 2004 Molecular, cellular and functional imaging of atherothrombosis *Nat. Rev. Drug Discov.* **3** 913–25
[54] Agatston A S, Janowitz W R, Hildner F J, Zusmer N R, Viamonte M Jr and Detrano R 1990 Quantification of coronary artery calcium using ultrafast computed tomography *J. Am. Coll. Cardiol.* **15** 827–32
[55] Achenbach S and Raggi P 2010 Imaging of coronary atherosclerosis by computed tomography *Eur. Heart J.* **31** 1442–8
[56] Nighoghossian N, Derex L and Douek P 2005 The vulnerable carotid artery plaque: current imaging methods and new perspectives *Stroke* **36** 2764–72
[57] Corti R and Fuster V 2011 Imaging of atherosclerosis: magnetic resonance imaging *Eur. Heart J.* **32** 1709–19b
[58] Zhu X J *et al* 2013 Morphologic characteristics of atherosclerotic middle cerebral arteries on 3T high-resolution MRI *Am. J. Neuroradiol.* **34** 1717–22
[59] Yuan C, Oikawa M, Miller Z and Hatsukami T 2008 MRI of carotid atherosclerosis *J. Nucl. Cardiol.* **15** 266–75
[60] Yuan C and Kerwin W S 2004 MRI of atherosclerosis *J. Magn. Reson. Imaging* **19** 710–9
[61] Koktzoglou I *et al* 2006 Multislice dark-blood carotid artery wall imaging: a 1.5 T and 3.0 T comparison *J. Magn. Reson. Imaging* **23** 699–705
[62] Saam T *et al* 2007 The vulnerable, or high-risk, atherosclerotic plaque: noninvasive MR imaging for characterization and assessment *Radiology* **244** 64–77
[63] Prati F *et al* 2010 Expert review document on methodology, terminology, and clinical applications of optical coherence tomography: physical principles, methodology of image acquisition, and clinical application for assessment of coronary arteries and atherosclerosis *Eur. Heart J.* **31** 401–15
[64] Lees A M *et al* 1988 Imaging human atherosclerosis with 99mTc-labeled low density lipoproteins *Arterioscler. Thromb. Vasc. Biol.* **8** 461–70

[65] Rosen J M *et al* 1990 Indium-111-labeled LDL: a potential agent for imaging atherosclerotic disease and lipoprotein biodistribution *J. Nucl. Med.* **31** 343–50
[66] Vallabhajosula S *et al* 1988 Radiotracers for low density lipoprotein biodistribution studies *in vivo*: technetium-99m low density lipoprotein versus radioiodinated low density lipoprotein preparations *J. Nucl. Med.* **29** 1237–45
[67] Virgolini I *et al* 1991 Indium-111-labeled low-density lipoprotein binds with higher affinity to the human liver as compared to iodine-123-low-density-labeled lipoprotein *J. Nucl. Med.* **32** 2132–8
[68] Pirich C and Sinzinger H 1995 Evidence for lipid regression in humans *in vivo* performed by 123iodine-low-density lipoprotein scintiscanning *Ann. New York Acad. Sci.* **748** 613–21
[69] Tsimikas S, Shortal B P, Witztum J L and Palinski W 2000 *In vivo* uptake of radiolabeled MDA2, an oxidation-specific monoclonal antibody, provides an accurate measure of atherosclerotic lesions rich in oxidized LDL and is highly sensitive to their regression *Arterioscler. Thromb. Vasc. Biol.* **20** 689–97
[70] Briley-Saebo K, Yeang C, Witztum J L and Tsimikas S 2014 Imaging of oxidation-specific epitopes with targeted nanoparticles to detect high-risk atherosclerotic lesions: progress and future directions *J. Cardiovasc. Transl. Res.* **7** 719–36
[71] Palinski W *et al* 1990 Antisera and monoclonal antibodies specific for epitopes generated during oxidative modification of low density lipoprotein *Arteriosclerosis* **10** 325–35
[72] Davis H H *et al* 1978 Scintigraphic detection of atherosclerotic lesions and venous thrombi in man by indium-111-labelled autologous platelets *Lancet* **1** 1185–7
[73] Minar E *et al* 1989 Indium-111-labeled platelet scintigraphy in carotid atherosclerosis *Stroke* **20** 27–33
[74] Palac R T, Gray L L, Turner F E, Brown P H, Malinow M R and Demots H 1989 Detection of experimental atherosclerosis with indium-111 radiolabelled hematoporphyrin derivative *Nucl. Med. Commun.* **10** 841–50
[75] Miller D D *et al* 1991 *In vivo* technetium-99m S12 antibody imaging of platelet alpha-granules in rabbit endothelial neointimal proliferation after angioplasty *Circulation* **83** 224–36
[76] Demacker P N, Dormans T P, Koenders E B and Corstens F H 1993 Evaluation of indium-111-polyclonal immunoglobulin G to quantitate atherosclerosis in Watanabe heritable hyperlipidemic rabbits with scintigraphy: effect of age and treatment with antioxidants or ethinylestradiol *J. Nucl. Med.* **34** 1316–21
[77] Hardoff R *et al* 1993 External imaging of atherosclerosis in rabbits using an 123I-labeled synthetic peptide fragment *J. Clin. Pharmacol.* **33** 1039–47
[78] Stratton J R, Cerqueira M D, Dewhurst T A and Kohler T R 1994 Imaging arterial thrombosis: comparison of technetium-99m-labeled monoclonal antifibrin antibodies and indium-111-platelets *J. Nucl. Med.* **35** 1731–7
[79] Chakrabarti M *et al* 1995 Biodistribution and radioimmunopharmacokinetics of 131I-Ama monoclonal antibody in atherosclerotic rabbits *Nucl. Med. Biol.* **22** 693–7
[80] Moriwaki H *et al* 1995 Functional and anatomic evaluation of carotid atherothrombosis. A combined study of indium 111 platelet scintigraphy and B-mode ultrasonography *Arterioscler. Thromb. Vasc. Biol.* **15** 2234–40
[81] Narula J *et al* 1995 Noninvasive localization of experimental atherosclerotic lesions with mouse/human chimeric Z2D3 F(ab′)2 specific for the proliferating smooth muscle cells of

human atheroma. Imaging with conventional and negative charge-modified antibody fragments *Circulation* **92** 474–84
[82] Matter C M *et al* 2004 Molecular imaging of atherosclerotic plaques using a human antibody against the extra-domain B of fibronectin *Circ. Res.* **95** 1225–33
[83] Weissleder R, Kelly K, Sun E Y, Shtatland T and Josephson L 2005 Cell-specific targeting of nanoparticles by multivalent attachment of small molecules *Nat. Biotechnol.* **23** 1418–23
[84] Danila D, Partha R, Elrod D B, Lackey M, Casscells S W and Conyers J L 2009 Antibody-labeled liposomes for CT imaging of atherosclerotic plaques: *in vitro* investigation of an anti-ICAM antibody-labeled liposome containing iohexol for molecular imaging of atherosclerotic plaques via computed tomography *Tex. Heart Inst. J.* **36** 393–403
[85] Davies J R *et al* 2005 Identification of culprit lesions after transient ischemic attack by combined 18F fluorodeoxyglucose positron-emission tomography and high-resolution magnetic resonance imaging *Stroke* **36** 2642–7
[86] Kwee R M *et al* 2009 Multimodality imaging of carotid artery plaques: 18F-fluoro-2-deoxyglucose positron emission tomography, computed tomography, and magnetic resonance imaging *Stroke* **40** 3718–24
[87] Calcagno C *et al* 2013 The complementary roles of dynamic contrast-enhanced MRI and 18F-fluorodeoxyglucose PET/CT for imaging of carotid atherosclerosis *Eur. J. Nucl. Med. Mol. Imaging* **40** 1884–93
[88] Tarkin J M, Joshi F R and Rudd J H 2014 PET imaging of inflammation in atherosclerosis *Nat. Rev. Cardiol.* **11** 443–57
[89] Zasadny K R and Wahl R L 1993 Standardized uptake values of normal tissues at PET with 2-[fluorine-18]-fluoro-2-deoxy-D-glucose: variations with body weight and a method for correction *Radiology* **189** 847–50
[90] Kim C K, Gupta N C, Chandramouli B and Alavi A 1994 Standardized uptake values of FDG: body surface area correction is preferable to body weight correction *J. Nucl. Med.* **35** 164–7
[91] Keyes J W Jr 1995 SUV: standard uptake or silly useless value? *J. Nucl. Med.* **36** 1836–9 .
[92] Thie J A 2004 Understanding the standardized uptake value, its methods, and implications for usage *J. Nucl. Med.* **45** 1431–4
[93] Verbraecken J, Van de Heyning P, De Backer W and Van Gaal L 2006 Body surface area in normal-weight, overweight, and obese adults. a comparison study *Metab. Clin. Exp.* **55** 515–24
[94] Tawakol A *et al* 2006 *In vivo* 18F-fluorodeoxyglucose positron emission tomography imaging provides a noninvasive measure of carotid plaque inflammation in patients *J. Am. Coll. Cardiol.* **48** 1818–24
[95] Rudd J H *et al* 2007 (18)Fluorodeoxyglucose positron emission tomography imaging of atherosclerotic plaque inflammation is highly reproducible: implications for atherosclerosis therapy trials *J. Am. Coll. Cardiol.* **50** 892–6
[96] Hermansen F, Ashburner J, Spinks T J, Kooner J S, Camici P G and Lammertsma A A 1998 Generation of myocardial factor images directly from the dynamic oxygen-15-water scan without use of an oxygen-15-carbon monoxide blood-pool scan *J. Nucl. Med.* **39** 1696–702
[97] Hyvarinen A and Oja E 2000 Independent component analysis: algorithms and applications *Neural Netw.* **13** 411–30

[98] Bentourkia M 2011 Tracer kinetic modeling: methodology and applications *Basic Sciences of Nuclear Medicine* ed M M Khalil (Berlin: Springer) pp 353–76
[99] Phelps M E, Huang S C, Hoffman E J, Selin C, Sokoloff L and Kuhl D E 1979 Tomographic measurement of local cerebral glucose metabolic rate in humans with (F-18)2-fluoro-2-deoxy-D-glucose: validation of method *Ann. Neurol.* **6** 371–88
[100] Patlak C S and Blasberg R G 1985 Graphical evaluation of blood-to-brain transfer constants from multiple-time uptake data. Generalizations *J. Cereb. Blood Flow Metab.* **5** 584–90
[101] Press W H, Teukolsky S A, Vetterling W T and Flannery B P 1988 *Numerical Recipes in C: The Art of Scientific Computing* (Cambridge: Cambridge University Press)
[102] Wu Y-W *et al* 2007 Characterization of plaques using 18F-FDG PET/CT in patients with carotid atherosclerosis and correlation with matrix metalloproteinase-1 *J. Nucl. Med.* **48** 227–33
[103] Chen W, Bural G G, Torigian D A, Rader D J and Alavi A 2009 Emerging role of FDG-PET/CT in assessing atherosclerosis in large arteries *Eur. J. Nucl. Med. Mol. Imaging* **36** 144–51
[104] Tahara N *et al* 2006 Simvastatin attenuates plaque inflammation: evaluation by fluorodeoxyglucose positron emission tomography *J. Am. Coll. Cardiol.* **48** 1825–31
[105] Sheikine Y and Akram K 2010 FDG-PET imaging of atherosclerosis: do we know what we see? *Atherosclerosis* **211** 371–80
[106] Orellana M R *et al* 2013 Assessment of inflammation in large arteries with 18F-FDG-PET in elderly *Comput. Med. Imaging Graph.* **37** 459–65
[107] Derlin T *et al* 2010 Feasibility of 18F-sodium fluoride PET/CT for imaging of atherosclerotic plaque *J. Nucl. Med.* **51** 862–5
[108] Dweck M R *et al* 2012 Coronary arterial 18F-sodium fluoride uptake: a novel marker of plaque biology *J. Am. Coll. Cardiol.* **59** 1539–48
[109] Joshi N V *et al* 2014 18 F-fluoride positron emission tomography for identification of ruptured and high-risk coronary atherosclerotic plaques: a prospective clinical trial *Lancet* **383** 705–13
[110] Gaemperli O *et al* 2012 Imaging intraplaque inflammation in carotid atherosclerosis with 11C-PK11195 positron emission tomography/computed tomography *Eur. Heart J.* **33** 1902–10
[111] Cocker M S *et al* 2012 Imaging atherosclerosis with hybrid [18F]fluorodeoxyglucose positron emission tomography/computed tomography imaging: what Leonardo da Vinci could not see *J. Nucl. Cardiol.* **19** 1211–25
[112] Nahrendorf M *et al* 2009 18 F-4V for PET-CT imaging of VCAM-1 expression in atherosclerosis *JACC Cardiovasc. Imaging* **2** 1213–22

IOP Publishing

Vascular and Intravascular Imaging Trends, Analysis, and Challenges, Volume 1
Stent applications
Petia Radeva and Jasjit S Suri

Chapter 10

3D–2D registration of vascular structures

Timur Aksoy, Gozde Unal, Franjo Pernuš and Žiga Špiclin

10.1 Clinical interventions and 3D–2D registration

Clinical interventions on vascular structures are currently performed using advanced imaging and image-guidance technologies. Angiography is a general term for medical imaging techniques, such as contrast enhanced fluoroscopy or x-rays, digitally subtracted angiography (DSA), computed tomography (CTA) and magnetic resonance angiography (MRA), etc, that are used to visualize blood vessels and other vascular structures and pathologies for diagnostic and guidance purposes. To acquire an angiographic image, with the exception of phase contrast and time-of-flight MRA, a needle or catheter is inserted into a blood vessel. Through the needle a contrast agent is injected into the blood vessel to highlight and inspect the vascular structures, while a catheter is carefully advanced towards the site of pathology to be treated. As catheterization delivers the contrast agent directly into the vasculature of interest, the vascular structures are better enhanced in the images. If a condition that requires further treatment such as aneurysm, arteriovenous malformation, vessel clotting, occlusion or dilation is detected, a minimally invasive endovascular intervention is usually performed immediately. In such cases a device such as coil, stent, balloon or embolization material is inserted through the catheter to treat the condition [1]. Atherosclerosis, for example, is a vascular disease, in which arteries are blocked due to build-up of plaques on the vessel walls. The minimally invasive intervention for treatment of this disease is carried out by first performing a balloon angioplasty, in which a collapsed balloon is inserted into the vessel, advanced to the stenotic region and then inflated at the site to widen the narrowed section of artery [1]. Afterwards, a stent is inserted through the catheter at the vessel section to allow the blood to flow normally. To carry out such a complex procedure, accurate image-guidance during endovascular procedures is of utmost importance.

doi:10.1088/2053-2563/ab01fach10

Performing minimally invasive endovascular interventions on vascular pathologies that may affect different anatomical regions, e.g. coronary arteries, cerebral vessels, and vessels in the organs of abdomen or thorax, also requires accurate guidance through a probably complex vessel network to reach the site of pathology. Guidance during the intervention is limited to 2D x-ray imaging, because of the high temporal and spatial resolution of this modality. However, navigation to the site and execution of the treatment may be difficult due to lack of depth information and possible occlusion of the structures of interest in 2D projections. Intra-interventional imaging can be enhanced by bringing the information in 3D pre-interventional images into the patient space during the intervention. 3D–2D image registration is the key enabling technology of enhanced image-guided interventions (IGIs), and establishes the spatial alignment of pre-interventional 3D volume to intra-interventional 2D images.

Medical 3D–2D registration is concerned with bringing the corresponding anatomical structures in a 3D volume and 2D image(s) into spatial alignment. For instance, the 3D–2D registration can be performed during IGI to co-locate the arteries and veins visualized by different angiographic imaging techniques, such as contrast enhanced x-ray, DSA, CTA, MRA, etc. Furthermore, valuable depth information can be provided to the surgeon during IGI in the form of enhanced visualization and navigation aids, with the purpose to resolve occluded structures embedded in complex vessel networks, and for a precise localization and assessment of potentially fatal pathological conditions such as aneurysms, stenoses, atherosclerotic plaques and clotting (figure 10.1). The main benefits of enhancing IGIs through 3D–2D image registration are faster treatment execution and prevention of tissue damage that may otherwise result from misplaced catheters, wires and stents.

The organization of this chapter on 3D–2D registration of vascular structures is as follows: in section 10.2 a mathematical definition of the 3D–2D registration problem is given and, in section 10.3, 3D–2D methods are classified with respect to five criteria: type of image modality, spatial transformation, dimensional correspondence, number of 2D views and registration basis. In section 10.4 a detailed review of registration bases that define how similarity is assessed between the images

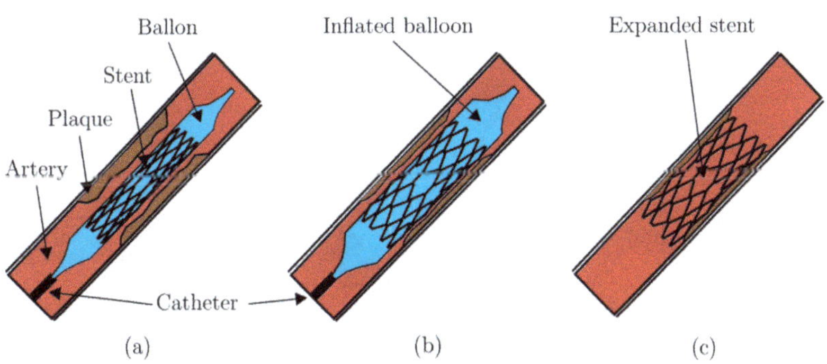

Figure 10.1. Treatment of atherosclerosis performed through a catheter under image-guidance involves three steps: (a) insert a balloon and a stent through the catheter, (b) inflate the balloon to widen the narrowed vessel segment and (c) position the stent to reinforce the vessel segment.

is performed, followed by a detailed classification and review of techniques for estimating the spatial transformation via optimization of the similarity measure in section 10.5. The validation procedures presented in section 10.6 constitute an important phase of the development of the registration method and are used to determine the potential of a method for clinical application. This chapter concludes by showcasing the results of state-of-the-art methods on clinical data in section 10.7 and discussion of the open challenges in the translation of 3D–2D registration technology into clinical applications in section 10.8.

10.2 Mathematical definition of 3D–2D registration

The goal of medical 3D–2D registration can be defined as finding an optimal spatial transformation $\mathcal{T}$ of a structure and/or a 2D imaging detector plane in 3D space such that projections of the structure are matched with the projections captured in the 2D imaging plane. 3D–2D registration is difficult due to dimensional inconsistency between the images being brought into alignment. There are two main approaches to address this inconsistency. The first one involves projection of the 3D structure onto the 2D imaging plane and maximization of the similarity (S) of image information in 2D (figure 10.2(a)). This process can be expressed as a minimization of the following cost function $C(\mathcal{T})$:

$$\underset{\mathcal{T}}{\operatorname{argmin}} C(\mathcal{T}) = -S_2(I(\mathbf{x}), \mathbf{P}_F(V(\mathcal{T}(\mathbf{x})))) + \alpha\ \mathbf{Regularizer}(\mathcal{T}), \tag{10.1}$$

where V is the 3D structure, I the 2D image, $S_2(\cdot)$ a similarity measure between 2D images or image features, and $\mathbf{P}_F(\cdot)$ a forward projection operator. The forward projection is the most frequently employed approach, possibly because the above definition matches the defined goal of 3D–2D registration.

The second approach involves backprojection of information from one or more 2D image(s) into 3D space along the rays converging to the x-ray source (figure 10.2(b)). Hence, the similarity between the information in 3D and 2D images is maximized in 3D, which can be expressed by the following cost function:

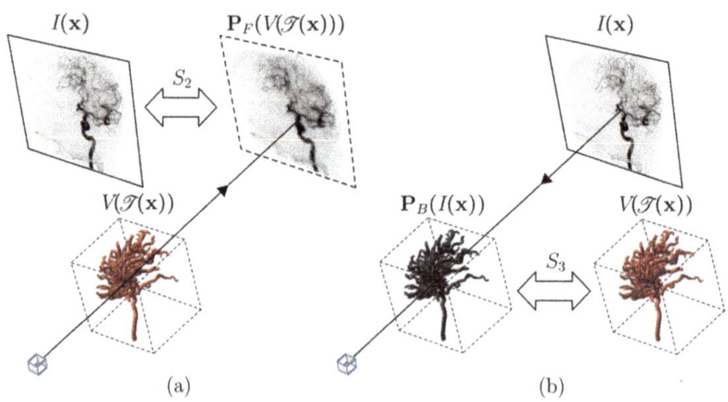

Figure 10.2. Registration of 3D and 2D images by (a) forward projection $\mathbf{P}_F$ and 2D–2D image information matching or (b) backward projection $\mathbf{P}_B$ and 3D–3D image information matching.

$$\underset{\mathcal{T}}{\operatorname{argmin}} C(\mathcal{T}) = -S_3(\mathbf{P}_B(I(\mathbf{x}), V(\mathcal{T}(\mathbf{x})) + \alpha\, \textbf{Regularizer}(\mathcal{T}), \tag{10.2}$$

where $\mathbf{P}_B(\cdot)$ is the backprojection operator and $S_3(\cdot)$ is a similarity measure between two 3D images or image features.

The regularization term in equations (10.1) and (10.2) is frequently used in deformable 3D–2D registration to ensure smoothness of the final transformation and to preserve the volume, area or length of the structures being aligned, and α is a non-negative weight that balances the influence of similarity and regularization terms. In 3D–2D registration of liver vasculature, for example, one might impose length preservation such that the resulting deformations do not change the length of vessels [2]. The image similarity term and the regularizer term can also be referred to as the external energy or data fidelity term and the internal energy term, respectively.

10.3 Classification of 3D–2D registration

There are five criteria that characterize a 3D–2D registration:

1. Image modality.
2. Spatial transformation.
3. Dimensional correspondence.
4. Number of views.
5. Registration basis.

Each of the criteria is described in the following corresponding subsections.

10.3.1 Image modality

3D–2D registration of vascular structures involves a 3D pre-interventional volume and 2D intra-interventional images, which can be of the same modality or of different modalities. Hence, 3D–2D registration can be monomodal or multimodal. Common pre-interventional volumes are CTA and MRA, while the intra-interventional images are usually fluoroscopy or x-rays, DSA and 3D-DSA acquired by a C-arm imaging system during endovascular IGIs. Registration between the DSA and 3D-DSA, for instance, can be considered monomodal. Registration of the CTA and the DSA can be considered multimodal, because the x-ray source used on the C-arm usually operates at different energies than those used in CTA.

A C-arm imaging system has a C-shaped body consisting of an aligned x-ray source and a detector attached to each end (figure 10.3). A patient undergoing treatment is placed on a moving table between the source and the detector. The x-rays emitted on one end of the C-arm travel through the patient and are captured and digitized by the detector on the other end. When an x-ray beam passes through the patient, some of the radiation is absorbed in a process known as attenuation. Anatomical structures that are denser have higher attenuation than those that are less dense. The remnant energy of the beam captured and quantized by the detector then determines the intensity value of the x-ray image [3].

The C-arm has two possible rotation axes of the gantry, i.e. cranial–caudal and left–right. The corresponding C-arm parameters that mainly define the viewpoint

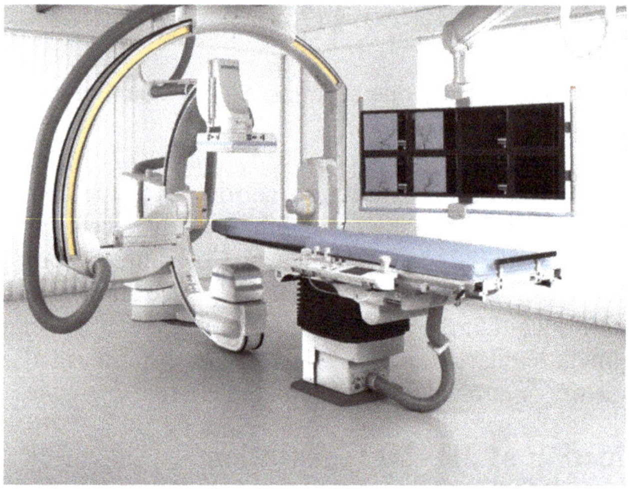

Figure 10.3. A modern C-arm imaging system for performing image-guided vascular interventions [5].

are the primary and secondary angle (PA and SA, respectively), while other parameters, such as source to object distance (SOD) and source to intensifier distance (SID) define the zoom factor and (u_0, v_0) the principal point [4]. The high rotational capability of the C-arm enables imaging of the patient from different viewpoints during IGI, thus it is widely used in minimally invasive cardio- and neuro-vascular IGIs. Furthermore, the C-arm can acquire a sequence of x-ray images. By injecting radio-opaque contrast agents into the blood flow, anytime during the IGI, the acquired sequence can highlight the dynamics of blood flow in the vascular structures.

10.3.2 Spatial transformation

The spatial transformation utilized in a 3D–2D registration can generally be categorized as rigid or non-rigid. Rigid registration is composed of rotations and translations of either the 3D vessel structures or the 2D detector (C-arm view). For vascular structures in pre-operative volumes, six rigid-body parameters need to be estimated: three translations and three rotations. Non-rigid registration introduces more complex deformations to the structure compared to rigid registration and, thus, has more degrees of freedom and generally a higher number of parameters. The most general linear spatial transformation is affine transformation, which adds anisotropic scaling and skewing along the cardinal axes on top of the rigid transformation (i.e. an additional six parameters). Further increasing the degrees of freedom may lead to unrestricted deformations of the images, thus constraints must be imposed through the regularization term to obtain realistic deformations. Constraints such as deformation smoothness and vessel length preservation are commonly used as internal energy terms in conjunction with the data fidelity term present in the cost functionals, see equations (10.1) and (10.2). The non-rigid transformation is often parameterized by B-splines and thin plate splines (TPS) since they ensure a smooth deformation.

In most applications of endovascular IGIs that involve the treatment of pathologies in cardiac [6] and cerebral vasculatures [7], and on vasculatures in the abdomen (liver [8]), and others, it is sufficient to use rigid transformation of the 3D image. The reason is that some vasculatures can be considered rigid, for instance, cerebral and even cardiac, if image acquisition is gated to electrocardiography signals. For vasculatures in the abdomen (e.g. liver and kidneys) a non-rigid transformation may need to be used, however, the rigid-body transformation is still required to initialize the posing of the 3D angiographic image.

10.3.3 Dimensional correspondence

The comparison of vessels and other vascular structures between the 3D volume and the 2D image can occur in 3D space or on the 2D imaging plane. If the comparison occurs on the 2D imaging plane, the intensities in the 3D volume, or other features, have to be rendered or transformed into the 2D imaging plane by forward projection. If the comparison occurs in the 3D space then intensities or other features of the structures in 2D images are backprojected along rays towards the x-ray source (figure 10.2). Backprojection is an important component of image reconstruction methods, which require multiple 2D views to extract high quality 3D image information. In IGIs two simultaneous 2D views acquired by biplane C-arm imaging systems are sometimes used, e.g. during embolization of arteriovenous malformations. The two mutually inclined 2D views can easily be used to reconstruct point features such as vessel centerlines in 3D to be matched to the vessel centerlines extracted from 3D volume to perform 3D–2D registration.

The intensity of 3D volumes can be projected to 2D by volume rendering methods for visualization and to achieve dimensional correspondence. Digitally reconstructed radiography (DRR) [9] is a simulation of volume projection by a ray casting operation. A DRR projection is formed by an integral function of voxel intensities encountered along each ray in a cone of rays, which all emanate from the x-ray source, pass through the volume and eventually hit the pixels on 2D image plane, as depicted in figure 10.4.

Different integral functions can determine the cast intensity values of pixels on the 2D DRR image. Composite DRRs process all the voxel intensities which the ray passes along its path. Each voxel is assigned an opacity and a color value based on the tissue type and those values are integrated along the ray to determine the final intensity value in the pixel. Different assignments for opacity and color maps are used in applications of DRR-based visualization [9]. Two simpler methods for volume visualization are minimum intensity projection (MinIP) and maximum intensity projection (MIP), which assign to the pixel either the minimum or maximum intensity value, respectively, as encountered along the ray path.

Generating the DRR or similar projections of the raw 3D volume is computationally demanding and may represent a bottleneck for a clinical application despite speed improvements in recent GPU implementations [10]. Two parameters mainly

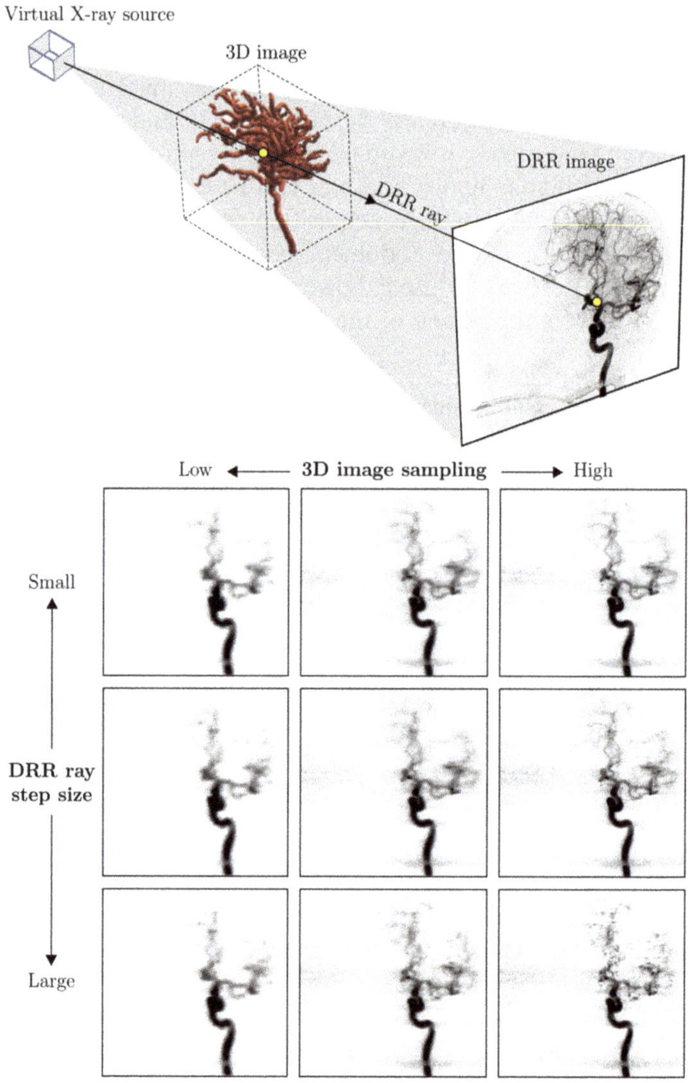

Figure 10.4. Digitally reconstructed radiograph (DRR) based on a 3D pre-interventional image, and the impact of 3D image sampling and DRR ray step length on the quality of the obtained DRR image.

affect the performance of a DRR projection: (i) 3D image sampling and (ii) ray step size. To reduce the computational demand the sampling of 3D volume can be reduced and the ray step length increased, however, this may have an adverse affect on the DRR quality (figure 10.4) and the 3D–2D registration. Namely, tuning these parameters for speed may drastically reduce the complexity of 3D vessel tree by poor visualization of smaller vessels and may therefore further ill-condition the process of matching 3D and 2D image information.

The second method for volume rendering is the projection of geometric primitives such as edges and vertices by 3D perspective projection. Geometric structures or a polygonal mesh formed from the surface or boundaries of structures of interest are rendered by wireframe methods. Texture mapping, shading and lighting operations can be applied on the surfaces of geometric structures. This type of projection is generally faster than ray casting methods, however, it requires accurate segmentation or feature detection and may result in the loss of important information encoded in the original intensity values.

10.3.4 Number of views

The number of simultaneous intra-interventional x-ray views is determined by the type of the C-arm employed during the intervention: one view is available on the monoplane, while two are available on the biplanar C-arm systems. Registration with two 2D views provides the advantage of better resolution of depth ambiguities and possible occlusions of the structures of interest and, in general, improves the convergence of 3D–2D registration to globally optimal solutions. Biplanar views are more commonly used in certain clinical applications such as embolization of arterial venous malformation (AVM), or in applications that require the use of deformable registration and/or employ backprojection and reconstruction-based approaches to achieve dimensional correspondence. However, most IGIs are carried out under a single C-arm view, while the C-arm is only rotated occasionally in order to disambiguate overlapping structures. The main reason for using a single x-ray view is to limit the potentially hazardous radiation dose delivered to the patient during IGI.

10.3.5 Registration basis

The registration basis determines the type of information extracted from both modalities and employed to quantitatively assess their similarity for the purpose of 3D–2D registration. When a 3D volume is acquired by the C-arm just before the intervention, the alignment of the 3D volume to intra-interventional 2D images may be established by C-arm calibration. Hence, the registration basis may be *calibration-based*. Another registration basis relies on stereotactic frames or external markers and is referred to as *extrinsic*. The anatomical information present in the 3D and 2D images is an *intrinsic* registration basis and may be further categorized as intensity-, feature- and gradient-based [11].

10.4 Review of registration bases

Methods for 3D–2D image registration in IGI were reviewed and categorized into extrinsic and intrinsic by Markelj *et al* [11]. The basis of registration can also be the coordinate frames of imaging devices obtained through the device calibration. The extrinsic methods employ artificial objects introduced manually into the imaged scene and generally require the acquisition of at least two mutually inclined x-ray projections [12, 13]. Conversely, the intrinsic methods base registration on the anatomical information contained in 3D and 2D images and seem readily applicable for registration of 3D to a single view 2D image. The intrinsic methods can be further categorized according to registration basis as intensity-, feature- and gradient-based [11]. These methods also enable a higher level of automation and seemingly easier integration into the clinical workflow of IGIs. General advantages and disadvantages of the registration bases are summarized in table 10.1.

10.4.1 Calibration-based methods

Calibration-based 3D–2D registration is possible if the C-arm is used to acquire both 3D and 2D images [14–16]. Such registration can be very accurate (0.2 mm)

Table 10.1. Summary of advantages and disadvantages of registration bases.

Registration basis	Advantages	Disadvantages
Calibration-based	• Simple usage • Very fast execution • Accurate registration	• Possible if 3D and 2D images acquired with the same imaging system (e.g. C-arm). • Patient movement invalidates registration, then a new 3D–2D image pair has to be acquired.
Extrinsic	• Fast execution • Accurate registration	• Artificial objects need to be affixed to the patient, which may be time-consuming, complex or even too invasive. • The artificial objects may occlude structures of interest.
Intensity-based	• Based on 3D and 2D anatomical information • No 3D or 2D image preprocessing needed	• Computationally expensive. • Close-to-optimal initial registration required. • Unreliable out-of-plane translation estimation.
Feature-based	• Based on 3D and 2D anatomical information • Fast execution	• Accurate and reliable extraction and matching of visual features are difficult. • Sensitive to image modality and variations in anatomy and image quality.
Gradient-based	• Based on 3D and 2D anatomical information • Fast execution • Robust against anatomy and image quality variation	• Close-to-optimal initial registration required. • Unreliable out-of-plane translation estimation.

and fast (a few seconds) [16], however, the main disadvantage is that even small patient movement during IGI may cause large registration errors. To recover the registration a new acquisition of the 3D image may be required, however, this increases the radiation dose and contrast agent usage and is time-consuming, therefore, it may be difficult to justify its use for the purpose of registration.

10.4.2 Extrinsic methods

The extrinsic methods base registration on matching artificial objects such as catheters, markers or other radio-opaque objects in the imaged scene. The advantage is that these objects are easy to detect in the images, however, the disadvantage is that they need to be firmly affixed to the patient. While some fixations may be too invasive, others may be too time-consuming or even overly complex to perform during IGI. Navab *et al* [17] used multi-modality markers visible on C-arm fluoroscopy with an optical tracking system to detect and correct for patient or C-arm motion, while Hamming *et al* [18] used similar markers for automatic initial image-to-world co-registration. Varnavas *et al* [12] used a radio-opaque ruler to determine in-plane translations of the 3D image by reconstructing and aligning a virtual fiducial marker. The marker was obtained based on manually selected corresponding locations on the radio-opaque ruler visible on two 2D projections. Truong *et al* [13] extracted a catheter visible in a 3D image and performed a global rigid-body fit to minimize the distance between the medial lines of the catheter and of the corresponding vessel, reconstructed in 3D through manual selection of medial points on two (biplane) x-rays. Otake *et al* [19] estimate the relative pose between x-ray images and the 3D anatomical structure using an in-image robust tracking fiducial and then register CTA with multiple x-rays by intensity-based mutual information and gradient information 3D–2D image similarity measures, which are among the intrinsic methods reviewed next.

10.4.3 Intensity-based methods

The intensity-based methods establish the dimensional correspondence between 3D and 2D images by using DRR, MIP or a similar 3D image visualization technique that best models the actual projection of pre-operative 3D image into 2D detector plane. Registration is then based on matching the projected 3D image to the intra-operative x-ray image(s) by a similarity measure such as mutual information [20], gradient information [19], gradient difference [21], pattern intensity [22], gradient correlation [23] or sum of squared differences [24]. Dong *et al* [25] introduced a similarity measure based on the distance between coefficients of orthogonal Zernike moment decompositions of the DRR and the 2D image. Flach *et al* [26] perform deformable registration of CT to low dose flouroscopic raw data by optimizing, in an alternating manner, the sum of squared distances as data fidelity term and a fluid-based diffusion as regularizer to obtain smooth deformation. They compare the 3D–2D registration results to 3D–3D registration between CT and low dose tomographic flouroscopy. Unfortunately, most of the intensity-based image similarity measures have poor sensitivity with respect to translation of 3D images along the direction of projection (i.e. out-of-plane translation) and require close initialization due to the presence of local minima in the similarity measure. Furthermore, generating the projections of the raw 3D image is computationally demanding and may represent a bottleneck for a clinical application despite speed improvements in recent GPU implementations [10].

10.4.4 Feature-based methods

In the intrinsic feature-based category of 3D–2D registration, image features such as vessel centerlines, binary vessel masks, points or certain geometric primitives are extracted from the images and utilized for registration. Therefore, methods such as vessel segmentation and centerline extraction need to be performed on 3D or 2D images in order to compute the similarity between the images.

Metz *et al* [27] aligned coronary centerlines of CTA and x-ray images using a similarity measure composed of the distance transform of a projected vessel tree model and a fuzzy segmentation of x-rays. Their method also accounts for heart beat and respiratory motion by synchronizing heart phases. Rivest-Henault *et al* [28] minimized the distances between the centerlines of the projected CTA and x-ray images using different optimization algorithms for translation, rigid and affine transformations. At the second stage they perform non-rigid alignment on biplane x-rays using distances between centerlines with epipolar constraint as the image term and displacement, smoothness and myocardium constraints as the internal energy terms. Turgeon *et al* [29] registered binarized projections of segmented 3D coronary arteries with segmented x-ray angiography images using entropy correlation coefficient similarity on both single and biplane angiograms. Ruijters *et al* [30] devised a similarity measure based on the distance transform of segmented CTA projections and enhanced x-ray images in the form of a vesselness map. Groher *et al* [31] employed a graph-based similarity specifically developed for registration of liver vasculatures, which matches a segmented 3D vessel tree model to the enhanced intra-operative image and simultaneously derives a segmentation of the 2D image. This approach has been advanced to perform non-rigid alignment [8]. In a later work, Groher *et al* [2] performed a deformable registration of the 3D segmented model to the enhanced x-ray image by a cost function consisting of an external term that minimizes the distance between the projected centerlines and locations with high values in the enhanced image, and the internal term enforcing vessel length preservation.

More recently, Baka *et al* [32] employed training of a population of CTA coronary models by measuring landmark coordinates on cardiac surfaces and estimating the motion. The obtained statistical motion model of CTA was registered to the x-ray sequence by minimizing distances and orientation differences between projected 3D vessel points and extracted 2D centerlines across all frames. Temporal alignment between the CTA and x-ray was modeled by a piecewise linear function and respiratory motion was constructed by quadratic interpolation of poses in the first, central and last frames of the sequence. Metz *et al* [6] proposed a 3D+t/2D+t (t: time) registration method that uses a patient specific dynamic coronary model derived from the CTA scan obtained by a vessel centerline extraction and subsequent motion estimation. The model is aligned to the 2D+t x-ray sequence by time varying rigid transformations, which takes breathing motion (which is also rigid) and the temporal relation between CTA and x-ray time points into account. The cost function at any time point is measured as average vessel centerline distance between the CTA and the most probable x-ray centerlines. Baka *et al* [33] construct probability distributions of moving and scene point sets of vessel centerlines in the form of Gaussian mixture models (GMM) and use a similarity metric that minimizes the difference between Gaussian mixtures of both point sets for a 3D–2D registration. The Jacobian matrix of the cost function was analytically computed to perform gradient descent optimization. Later, orientations were added to the point sets to create 4D GMM distributions. Kim *et al* [34] extract vessel centerlines of 3D and 2D vasculature and perform deformable registration by using a thin plate spline based robust point matching algorithm, which alternates between the estimation of the correspondence and the transformation of the two point sets. They report that outliers in both point sets are well handled by the method. Aksoy *et al* [35] decouple the estimation of rotation and translation before matching segmented CTA to segmented x-ray vessels. Rotation is recovered by matching a set of rotated DRR templates of CTA to the binary x-ray vessels using scale and shift invariant similarity measures computed from magnitudes of the Fourier transformation of the images. In the second step, the 3D translation is recovered in the spatial domain by minimizing the distance and maximizing the overlap ratio between the 3D vessel model and the 2D vessels.

Some authors [36, 37] used reconstruction of 3D images from several x-ray images acquired from different viewpoints in order to perform registration to the pre-operative volume with 3D–3D registration methods. However, the 2D x-ray images need to be acquired simultaneously to obtain a reconstruction without motion induced artifacts. Furthermore, the quality of the reconstructed model depends on the number of views. Serradel *et al* [38] used a generative model for CTA from synthetic samples and simultaneously reconstructed the 3D structure of a non-rigid coronary tree by estimating point correspondences between a single view x-ray image and a reference 3D shape. Features are nodes generated in 3D and points of interest that are extracted by the vesselness filter in the x-ray [39]. The cost function minimizes the reprojection error by alternating matches of corresponding features and perturbing non-rigid parameters stored as a principal component analysis (PCA) model. Nodes are matched as an optimal assignment problem via minimization of Mahalanobis distance between the two points and the distance between their orientations.

Because the raw 3D, 2D, or both 3D and 2D intensity information is reduced to a small set of features, the feature-based methods are usually fast. However, the accuracy and robustness of these methods are heavily dependent on the quality of segmentations and extracted features, which must be devised for each image modality and target anatomy of interest. As varying conditions are usually encountered during IGI, these methods may be unreliable, or may require case-by-case tuning, and thus seem less suitable for practical use.

10.4.5 Gradient-based methods

In gradient-based methods [40–42] a small subset of high-magnitude gradients (the edges of structures of interest) can be corresponded between 3D and 2D images through projection [40], backprojection [41, 43] or reconstruction [42]. The advantage of these methods is that the process of corresponding subsets of 3D and 2D gradients, or gradient distributions encoded in gradient covariance matrices [43], is more efficient than generating projection images such as DRRs or MIPs. Furthermore, segmentation or feature extraction that may otherwise be modality- or anatomy-dependent is generally not required to extract the gradient features. Hybrid feature- and gradient-based methods have also emerged, for example, to register 3D and 2D cerebral angiograms. Mitrović *et al* [44] performed a model-to-image 3D–2D registration by matching geometric primitives of the 3D vessels such as centerlines, radii and their principal local orientations to high-magnitude intensity gradients of biplane x-rays. The aforementioned methods, however, were mainly used in registration of 3D to biplane [44] or even multiplane x-ray images [41, 42]. When used for 3D to monoplane x-ray registration, the similarity measures employed in these methods exhibit poor sensitivity to out-of-plane translations, similarly to those used in the intensity-based methods.

10.5 Review of transformation estimation approaches

The registration basis, consisting of the image similarity measure and, possibly, regularizer, defines a cost function, which needs to be optimized, i.e. minimized or maximized, to estimate the transformation of either the 3D volume or the 2D detector. A standard approach is to use iterative optimization techniques. Another approach is by stratified optimization, which divides the transformation parameters into subsets and estimates the parameters in each subset in a sequential order. There are also regression-based approaches that employ multiple training datasets with known optimal registration parameters to train a regression model, which is then used to estimate the registration parameters for a new pair of 3D and 2D images. General advantages and disadvantages of the three transformation estimation approaches are summarized in table 10.2.

10.5.1 Iterative methods

Iterative optimization methods search for the optimal solution by minimizing or maximizing a cost function consisting of the similarity measure between both modalities and, in particular, deformable registration with an additional regularizer of the transformation. Typically, the choice of the cost function affects the choice of optimization methods.

In gradient-based optimizers, the gradients and/or Hessian of the cost function are computed to determine the step or trust region size and step direction. If the cost function is linear or quadratic in the vicinity of the initial alignment conditions then gradient-based optimizers such as Newton, quasi-Newton and conjugate gradients will exhibit fast convergence to the global solution. Commonly used gradient-based

Table 10.2. Summary of advantages and disadvantages of transformation estimation approaches.

Estimation approach	Advantages	Disadvantages
Iterative	• Accurate • Easy to implement	• Variable convergence times • Possible convergence to local optima • Affected by initial alignment
Stratified	• Accurate • Faster than iterative • Less affected by initial alignment	• Requires complex optimization strategy for each subset • Applicable for simple transformations (e.g. rigid)
Regression-based	• Fast and fixed time • Not affected by local optima • Not affected by initial alignment	• Less accurate • Success depends on trained data • Depends on accurate extraction of features

optimizers in the literature are Broyden–Fletcher–Goldfarb–Shanno (BFGS), Polak Ribiere and steepest gradient descent [2, 26, 27, 33]. If the cost function cannot be negative as in distance-based similarities, it can be formulated as a regression equation, then iterative nonlinear least squares methods such as Gauss–Newton and Levenberg–Marquart are used to find the local solution [33]. Point cloud registration methods such as iterative closest point can be solved by a least squares method, which minimizes the squared distances between two points sets. If the energy function is a well formulated Euler–Lagrange equation, consisting of internal and external energy terms as in the case of deformable registration, gradient descent and nonlinear conjugate gradient methods are frequently preferred [2, 26, 28].

In cases where analytical derivative computations are infeasible or computations of finite differences is expensive or cannot approximate gradients accurately, derivative-free optimization methods are employed. Some prominent examples are best neighbor, Powell, Nelder–Mead (Down Hill Simplex) and BOBYQA. Powell [6, 30] and best neighbor are the simplest algorithms, inspecting the cost function with a step in all predetermined search directions and then taking the best one. They are, however, prone to local extrema. Nelder–Mead [28, 29, 31, 45] evaluates the function value at each vertex of a polytope and the one with the worst value is replaced by another one using expansion, reflection or contraction operation. BOBYQA uses a quadratic approximation of the cost function by interpolation in a trust region and replaces an interpolation point in each iteration. Nelder–Mead and BOBYQA are popular choices for non-convex functions since they are less sensitive to local extrema than gradient-based optimizers. Henault *et al* [28] report that the Nelder–Mead algorithm performs best in global alignment of vessel centerlines for rigid and affine transformations. Nelder–Mead is the most frequently used derivative-free deterministic optimizer in 3D–2D angiography registration literature.

The greatest difficulty that the gradient-based optimizers have is convergence to local extrema. If the cost function is not convex around the initial alignment conditions then they will converge to a local extrema. Several authors have tried global optimization strategies to avoid the local extrema in cases of high or arbitrary initial alignment offsets. Multi-resolution approaches start with low resolution images and progressively proceed to higher resolutions after convergence in each resolution [19]. Stochastic techniques generate random samples of search space and a local optimizer is started at those positions. Stochastic methods are more suitable for highly nonlinear functions with abundant local extrema. Some examples used are random search, simulated annealing, evolutionary algorithms and sequential Monte Carlo random sampling [28, 30, 46, 47]. Random search is the simplest stochastic method that samples new positions in a given radius of the current position. Simulated annealing algorithm generates a new point randomly by a probability distribution with a scale proportional to the current temperature, which determines the distance of the new point from the current one. The algorithm accepts all new points that lower the value of the cost function, but also, with a certain probability, points that raise the value of the cost function. The algorithm systematically lowers the temperature, storing the best point found so far. By accepting points that raise the value of the cost function, the algorithm avoids being trapped in local minima, and is able to explore globally for more possible solutions. The covariance matrix adaptation evolution strategy (CMA-ES) [19] is an evolutionary algorithm where new candidate solutions are sampled from a multivariate normal distribution. The mean of the distribution is updated such that the likelihood of previously successful candidate solutions is maximized. Mutation is performed by adding a random vector, a perturbation with zero mean. Pairwise dependences between the variables in the distribution are represented by a covariance matrix. The covariance matrix is updated by the covariance matrix adaptation (CMA) method that maximizes the likelihood of previously successful search steps. CMA-ES has very high probability of convergence to a global solution for a large class of functions regardless of initial conditions. Florin *et al* [47] report that a sequential Monte Carlo sampling and condensation technique performs better than random search and gradient-based methods for global optimization. Sequential Monte Carlo sampling draws samples from a posterior probability distribution function whose weights are updated according to the principle of importance density [48]. Otake *et al* [10] use a multi-start strategy for searching the global optimum. In a global multi-start method, the search space is partitioned to multiple subspaces and separate CMA-ES optimizers are run in a parallel fashion.

Discrete optimization techniques discretize the parameter space into subintervals. Recent Markov random field (MRF) formulations of a registration energy functional usually include a unary potential that represents the data term, and a pairwise potential between labels of discretized parameter space that represents the regularization term. An MRF-based energy function is formulated as the sum of all potentials. Any similarity measure can be approximated by MRF models [49]. The main advantage of this model is that the MRF energy function can be optimized by linear programming. Zikic *et al* [50] propose an MRF model using only second order terms for more efficient optimization. The approximation at a certain point in the parameter space is the normalized sum of evaluations of the original energy at projections of that point to two-dimensional subspaces. Also, a strategy for refinement of the search space is employed over iterations so as to increase registration accuracy and keep the number of labels small for efficiency.

An alternative approach for searching the global optimum for non-convex cost functions is template-based optimization. In this approach, all possible spatial transformations of a certain degree of freedom within a range are sampled and their DRRs are compared to the 2D image by a robust similarity measure [35]. Local extrema are surely avoided by exhaustive searches in a limited computation time, however, discretized parameter values have to be interpolated by either a function or a local optimizer.

10.5.2 Stratified methods

Optimization strategies that stratify the transformation parameters into separate subsets and then perform a sequential estimation of the subsets of parameters may be employed. This is particularly useful for estimation of 3D rigid-body transformation in order to increase the sensitivity of any similarity measure to the out-of-plane translation of the 3D image. Namely, the sensitivity is generally highest when all other rigid-body parameters are close to their optimal values. Because the dimension of the search space is reduced in the individual sequential steps, the registration process is usually faster than with iterative optimization and an exhaustive search can be used in low-dimensional parameters space to overcome large initial alignment errors.

Using the stratified parameter estimation, several researchers first determined the in-plane translation parameters by exhaustive grid search [51, 52] or frequency domain methods [53]. Kerrien *et al* [51] found the in-plane translations by optimizing normalized cross correlation (NCC) over a fixed grid, followed by optimization of all rigid-body parameters. In a two-stage method, Kita *et al* [53] first determined the in-plane translations by optimizing NCC in the frequency domain. By optimizing NCC over fixed grids in a three-stage approach, Hentschke and Tönnies [52] first determined the in-plane translations, then the out-of-plane translation and in-plane rotation and, finally, the two remaining rotations. Kubias *et al* [54] determined the in-plane prior to the out-of-plane parameters in a multi-resolution and multi-stage optimization strategy using low- and high-resolution images in consecutively applied global and local optimizers, respectively. To recover the rotations and scale, Van der Bom *et al* [55] used projection-slice theorem, followed by phase correlation to recover the in-plane translations, however, the method resulted in high alignment errors around 20 mm. Aksoy *et al* [35] matched rotation templates (a set of DRRs of segmented 3D images in a discrete set of rotations) to a segmented x-ray image by a scale and translation invariant measure computed in the frequency domain. After selecting the optimal rotations, all rigid-body parameters were iteratively optimized through minimization of the overlap between the best matching pair of segmented DRR and the x-ray image. Despite promising results, the estimation of the out-of-plane translation in monoplane 3D–2D registration was not addressed adequately in any of the above methods.

10.5.3 Regression-based methods

Regression-based approaches directly relate features of images to the spatial transformation parameters by a linear or a nonlinear function, hence, iterative optimization procedures are not employed during the registration process. The function is trained usually with simulated 2D images before being applied to real intra-interventional images. Gouveia *et al* [56] have evaluated seven regression methods for 3D–2D registration. Input features consisted of first and second order moments and PCA of the 2D image intensities, while the outputs are the registration parameters. Multivariate regression estimates the regression coefficients of a linear and polynomial equation of input features with a least squares method. The K nearest neighbor generates predictions by averaging output responses of k nearest input points in the training set. Multilayer perceptrons (MLP) are a popular choice for nonlinear regression due to their capability of approximating arbitrary functions. In the training phase, synaptic weights are optimized such that the difference between true and actual outputs is minimized by conjugate gradients and Levenberg—Marquart optimization algorithms. Their activation function is typically a hyperbolic tangent function. The radial basis function (RBF) network has a similar structure to the MLP except that a Gaussian function was used as the activation function. Support vector machine regression (SVR) maps input data to a higher dimensional space by the RBF kernel function and compute the output by a weighted linear combination of the kernels. The results of Gouveia *et al* [56] show that MLP with Levenberg Marquart optimization and RBF are robust to large initial alignment offsets and yield the most accurate results with lower variance, but are slightly less accurate than traditional iterative registration approaches.

10.6 Validation procedures

Before a 3D–2D image registration can be incorporated into a clinical image-guidance system it must undergo extensive and objective validation. Although several 3D–2D image registration methods [11] were developed for image-guidance systems, i.e. for 3D roadmapping [16, 57], their translation into clinical use is limited because these methods generally lack an extensive and objective validation.

Performing such a validation is difficult due to the wide range of materials, methods and definitions that are required, namely: (i) a large number of patient image datasets needs to be acquired in the clinical context of image-guided intervention; (ii) a corresponding reference or gold standard registration, which has to be accurate and reliable, needs to be established on these datasets; (iii) a procedure for validating 3D–2D image registration along with the definition of performance metrics needs to be specified. Standard procedures and performance metrics for validation of 3D–2D registration in general were introduced by Van der Kraats *et al* [58] and later revised by Markelj *et al* [59].

Unfortunately, the creation of validation datasets has received little attention in the literature. There are currently four publicly available validation datasets of 3D–2D registration, one of a cadaveric spine segment [60], one of a cadaveric swine head [61], one of a spine and a pelvis generated from a visible human dataset [59] and one of cerebral angiograms [7]. There was another dataset of a cadaveric spine segment created by Van der Kraats *et al* [58], but it seems to be no longer publicly available. The clinical context associated with the aforementioned image datasets is spine surgery [58–60], radiotherapy of the head [61] and endovascular image-guided neurosurgery [7]. Hence, the dataset of cerebral angiograms [7], to the best of our knowledge, is the only dataset available to objectively validate and compare the performance of methods for 3D–2D registration of vascular structures.

In the following subsections, the approaches toward gold standard creation, measures of registration error and procedures for evaluating the performance of 3D–2D registration methods are reviewed and discussed.

10.6.1 Gold standard creation

The main challenge of using the 3D and 2D patient images for objective and quantitative validation of 3D–2D registration method(s) is how to obtain an accurate and reliable gold standard. Two tasks need to be carried out: (i) calibrate projection geometry of the 2D image acquisition device and (ii) devise materials and methods to find the optimal spatial transformation of the 3D image.

Most existing C-arm systems do not provide accurate parameters of the projection view (PA, SA, SOD, SID and (u_0, v_0)), therefore, these parameters have to be calibrated for each C-arm pose. A common parameterization of the 2D imaging system on C-arm is given in [4]. For some C-arm systems the deviations from ideal geometry and pose are reproducible and may be compensated by prior calibration of the C-arm [16, 62, 63]. Depending on the mechanical design of the C-arm system, however, the deviations from ideal geometry and pose might not be reproducible and such a C-arm has to be calibrated on-line during image-guided intervention. For such situations, Otake *et al* [19] used a robust tracking fiducial made of ball bearings and steel wire shaped as an ellipse and lines that provided C-arm calibration directly from a single 2D fluoroscopy image.

The optimal spatial transformation of a 3D image can be established in several ways that mainly differ in the complexity of materials and methods used and, possibly, require a different protocol of image acquisition that may be more or less compatible with the workflow during image-guided interventions. Van de Kraats *et al* [58] used a calibrated C-arm to acquire 2D x-rays from several projection views and performed reconstruction of a 3DRX image. The gold standard registration of CT and MR volumes was obtained through alignment to the 3DRX by intensity-based 3D–3D image registration [58]. In most clinical contexts, however, using more than one or two 2D x-rays for establishing the gold standard may raise ethical concerns due to excessive irradiation of the patient. Markelj *et al* [59] defined the 2D image projection geometry so as to create synthetic 2D projection images from the 3D images, hence, the gold standard is inherently given. However, such a simple approach to gold standard creation does not capture the conditions, e.g. image noise, occlusions, geometric deformations, etc, encountered on real 2D images acquired during the intervention and is therefore not appropriate for objective validation.

For patient images acquired during an image-guided intervention the gold standard may be obtained by manual alignment, i.e. by perturbing the transformation of the 3D image until its projection overlaps with the 2D image [64] or by a reference registration method based on manually co-locating prominent anatomical landmarks such as bifurcations and vessel curves on 2D and 3D images or based on manual or semi-automated segmentation of vessels in 3D and 2D [8, 35]. Currently these are the approaches used to establish the gold standard in deformable 3D–2D registration, e.g. for the liver [8] and acquisitions of cardiac vasculatures not gated to electrocardiography signal [6]. However, it is difficult to establish such a gold standard in a consistent manner across a large patient image dataset due to subjective and unreliable manual input and, in cases such as the the liver vasculature, also due to insufficient complexity of the vessel network. Hence, the accuracy of the gold standard may vary substantially between different patient image datasets and, therefore, such a gold standard cannot be used to objectively and reliably validate the 3D–2D registration methods.

By attaching fiducial markers to the patient one can recover both the 2D image acquisition geometry and the optimal spatial transformation of the 3D image [7, 60, 61]. Therefore, this approach seems most promising for the creation of a gold standard on patient image datasets. Tomaževič *et al* [60] and Pawiro *et al* [61] used cadaver-implanted fiducial markers, which is clearly too invasive to perform on (live) patients. Mitrović *et al* [7] used an elastic headband with integrated steel balls as fiducial markers. The elastic headband can be easily attached to a patient's head during the image-guided endovascular neurosurgery, during which both 3D and 2D images are usually acquired by the C-arm. To acquire the gold standard on vasculature other than the cerebral vasculature, the fiducial marker carrier device needs to be redesigned. The gold standard is based on the registration of the position of fiducial markers extracted from 3D and 2D images, whereas two 2D projection images need to be acquired to calibrate the C-arm in the two corresponding projection views (figure 10.5). The advantage of such an approach is the possibility of automating all the steps to obtain the gold standard, i.e. extraction and correspondence of fiducial markers in 3D and 2D, retrospective C-arm calibration and marker co-registration [65]. Furthermore, for rigid-body 3D–2D registration, the accuracy of a gold standard based on fiducial marker co-registration can be assessed with the methodology presented by Fitzpatrick *et al* [66]. For instance, on ten patient image datasets of cerebral angiograms Madan *et al* [65] reported the accuracy of the fiducial-based gold standard from 0.1 to 0.2 mm, which is at least twice better than the level of accuracy expected from 3D–2D registration methods and, therefore, seems suitable for objective validation of the methods.

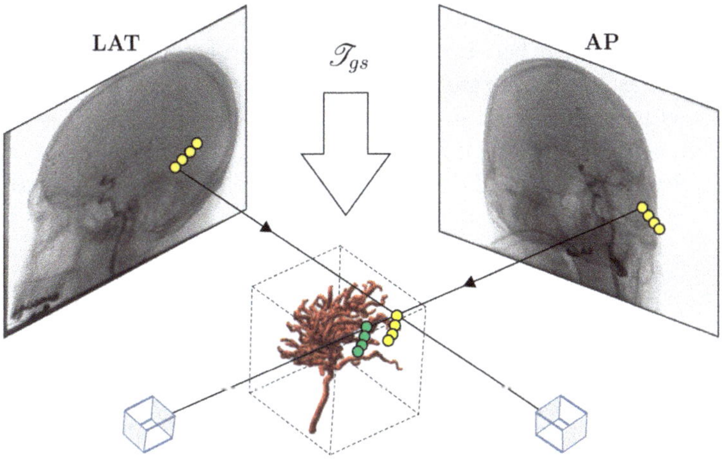

Figure 10.5. Gold standard 3D–2D registration $\mathcal{T}_{gs}$ established by aligning the positions of fiducial markers extracted from 3D and 2D images [7].

10.6.2 Registration error

Various measures of registration error are used depending on the task of 3D–2D registration [58]. For instance, 3D roadmapping [57], in which the 3D image is projected and overlayed onto the 2D angiogram, requires a good overlap between vessels in the 2D projection, therefore, the registration error should be measured in 2D. On the other hand, during image-guided biopsy or delivery of treatment devices their exact placement in 3D patient space is important, hence, to guide or position these tools and devices the registration error should be measured in 3D.

Registration errors can be measured by the distance between positions of 3D or 2D image features (e.g. fiducials, anatomical landmarks, object contours or surfaces) after the 3D–2D registration and their positions in the gold standard registration. Common image features are (target) points $\mathbf{t}_i$ that lie on the structures of interest, i.e. on angiograms $\mathbf{t}_i$ are usually the centerline points of a 3D vessel tree [7], which can be extracted from a segmentation of the vessels. A possible approach to extract the vessel centerlines is to perform interactive thresholding of the 3D angiogram and obtain centerlines by Lee's thinning algorithm [67], followed by removal of short, spurious and possibly incorrect centerlines and vessel branches whose length is less than twice the corresponding vessel diameter [68].

A widely used performance measure in 3D is the target registration error (TRE), while the mean over all target points K is used to compute the registration error:

$$\mathrm{mTRE} = \frac{1}{K}\sum_{i=1}^{K} ||\mathcal{T}_{\mathrm{reg}}(\mathbf{t}_i) - \mathcal{T}_{\mathrm{gs}}(\mathbf{t}_i)||, \qquad (10.3)$$

where $\mathcal{T}_{\mathrm{reg}}$ and $\mathcal{T}_{\mathrm{gs}}$ denote the transformation obtained by 3D–2D registration and the gold standard, respectively.

A straightforward performance measure in 2D is the projection distance (PD) computed as the distance between the registered and gold standard locations of target points in the 2D image space. Since target points $\mathbf{t}_i$ are defined in 3D image space they need to be projected into 2D using the forward projection operator $\mathbf{P}_F$, which translates the points $\mathbf{t}_i$ from 3D to the 2D imaging plane along rays emanating from the x-ray source $\mathbf{r}_s$. The 2D registration error is computed as mean PD:

$$\text{mPD} = \frac{1}{K}\sum_{i=1}^{K}\|\mathbf{P}_F\mathcal{T}_{\text{reg}}(\mathbf{t}_i) - \mathbf{P}_F\mathcal{T}_{\text{gs}}(\mathbf{t}_i)\|. \tag{10.4}$$

The value of mPD depends on the distance of target points to the 2D image plane. Instead, several researchers use the reprojection distance (RPD) defined as the minimum distance between the line $\mathcal{L}_i$, which passes through the x-ray source $\mathbf{r}_s$ and the 3D target point in the registered position $\mathcal{T}_{\text{reg}}(\mathbf{t}_i)$, and the corresponding 3D target point in the gold standard position $\mathcal{T}_{\text{gs}}(\mathbf{t}_i)$. Hence, the 2D registration error that is independent of the distance to the 2D image plane is computed as mean RPD:

$$\text{mRPD} = \frac{1}{K}\sum_{i=1}^{K} d_{\min}\left[\mathcal{L}_i(\mathbf{r}_s, \mathcal{T}_{\text{reg}}(\mathbf{t}_i)), \mathcal{T}_{\text{gs}}(\mathbf{t}_i)\right], \tag{10.5}$$

where $d_{\min}[\cdot]$ denotes the minimum distance between a line and point. A geometric representation of the TRE, RPD and PD registration errors is shown in figure 10.6.

10.6.3 Performance evaluation

The evaluation methodology of van de Kraats *et al* [58] and Markelj *et al* [59] involves creation of synthetic transformations or deformations of the 3D image with respect to gold standard registration, which represent the starting positions for 3D–2D registration. The starting positions are generated according to initial misregistrations of the 3D image from the gold standard in some range of mTRE (e.g. 0–20 mm). The mTRE is usually uniformly distributed in the specified range

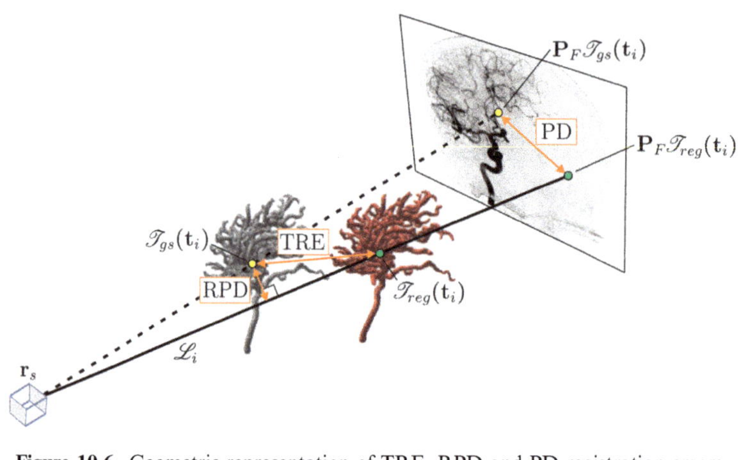

Figure 10.6. Geometric representation of TRE, RPD and PD registration errors.

and the number of starting positions per 1 mm mTRE subinterval is also determined. Typically there are 20 starting positions per interval and thus a total of 400 starting positions per dataset.

For 3D and 2D images both acquired on a C-arm system, one could also use the machine-based registration obtained from DICOM-accessible C-arm parameters as more realistic starting positions [64]. However, the number of such starting positions is proportional to the number of datasets, which is usually low, while such an approach is also limited to certain clinical contexts.

Common metrics of registration performance involve registration accuracy, failure criteria, success rate, capture range and execution time. The standardized evaluation methodology proposed by van de Kraats *et al* [58], and later revised by Markelj *et al* [59], employs the mTRE, mRPD and mPD as measures of registration accuracy. The most general measure is the mTRE, however, as noted previously, the mPD and mRPD may suffice in certain clinical applications [16, 57] and are typically reported if the registration is performed between a 3D and a single 2D image.

In the methodology by van de Kraats *et al* [58], a registration failure criterion is specified by the minimum acceptable level of registration error and depends on the clinical application. On cerebral angiograms, Mitrović *et al* [7] established that mTRE or mRPD below 2 mm is sufficient for the purpose of 3D roadmapping and 3D–2D image fusion. Other metrics are then based on the failure criterion, i.e. the success rate measures the percentage of successful registration trials and the capture range is defined as the initial misregistration, at which some high-enough success rate, e.g. 95% [58], is achieved.

The selection of failure criteria may bias the performance evaluation, since trimming the distribution of registration errors through rejection of failed registration trials directly impacts the assessment of registration accuracy, success rate and capture range. To avoid the use of failure criteria, Markelj *et al* [59] employ accumulative subintervals of initial misregistration, e.g. 0–4, 0–8, 0–12, 0–16, and 0–20 mm, in which the initial mTREs are uniformly distributed. In each of the subintervals they capture the distribution of registration error and then determine the accuracy as a percentile (50% and 95%) of the estimated distribution.

10.7 Validation of 3D–2D registration on cerebral angiograms

The current state-of-the-art and challenges in 3D–2D image registration are best observed by rigorous and extensive validation on datasets with established gold standard registration. The following experiments involved ten patient image datasets, which are publicly available[1] and contain 3D and 2D cerebral angiograms [7], namely 3D and 2D digitally subtracted angiograms or 3D- and 2D-DSAs, respectively. The 2D-DSAs were acquired in the anterior–posterior (AP) and lateral (LAT) projection views, thus forming 20 pairs of 3D and 2D

[1] URL: http://lit.fe.uni-lj.si/tools.php?lang=eng.

images. The gold standard 3D–2D registrations were established by co-registration of fiducial markers [7].

The experiments involved 3D and 2D image registration trials using two recent methods, the first based on stratified 3D rigid-body parameter optimization for matching rotation templates and vessel tree features [35] and the second based on iterative BOBYQA optimization and image similarity computed by comparing 3D and 2D gradient covariances [43]. We refer to the two methods as *stratified* and *iterative*, respectively. While the first is expected to be robust to high initial registration errors, the second is expected to yield accurate 3D–2D registration if initialized close to the optimal registration. Running these two methods sequentially should, therefore, result in a registration that is robust to initial error and a registration that is highly accurate. To verify this hypothesis, the third method consists of a sequential execution of the stratified and iterative method and was referred to as *combined.*

In the following subsection we first describe the experimental set-up and then present validation results according to two validation methodologies [58, 59], one with and one without the use of failure a criterion.

10.7.1 Experimental set-up

Registration errors were measured by mTRE and mRPD based on the initial and final alignment of 3D targets with respect to their gold standard position. The 3D targets were the vessels' centerlines, extracted from 3D-DSA in each of the ten datasets [7]. The initial starting positions of 3D images were defined in terms of mTRE, generated in the range 0–100 mm with respect to the gold standard position by randomly sampling rigid-body transformations.

Translations were randomly sampled in the range [−100, 100] mm, while rotations were sampled in the range [−5, 5] degrees, such that the desired initial mTRE was achieved. The following ranges of translations and rotations correspond to the initial misalignment of the pre-operative 3D and intra-operative 2D images that is expected in a typical interventional C-arm suite [62, 63] and may be due to the use of uncalibrated C-arm pose or patient movement. For each 3D–2D image pair, one set of rigid-body parameters was randomly generated in each 1 mm subinterval of mTRE, hence, in total 100 per pair. Since there were 20 pairs of 3D- and 2D-DSAs and 100 initial rigid-body parameters per each image pair and three registration methods were tested, we altogether performed 6000 3D–2D registrations.

10.7.2 Evaluation based on failure criteria

The methodology of van de Kraats *et al* [58] requires setting a threshold on registration error, which delineates between a successful and failed registration trial. As proposed by Mitrović *et al* [7] for cerebral angiograms, the registration failure criterion was set to 2 mm for both mTRE and mRPD registration error metrics. Hence, a 3D–2D registration was considered successful if mTRE or mRPD was less than 2 mm. The overall registration accuracy was defined as MEAN ± STD of mRPD of all successful registrations and the overall success rate (SR) was defined as the percentage of successful registrations. Capture range (CR) was defined as the first mTRE or mRPD subinterval of length 1 mm, in which more than one registration out of 20 failed. This setting corresponded to a 95% confidence level for the CR estimate.

Evaluation results for the three methods are shown in tables 10.3 and 10.4 for the mTRE and mRPD metric, respectively. The stratified method achieved a higher SR than the iterative method, but was generally less accurate. The sequentially combined methods were the most accurate and had the highest SR and CR. According to the mRPD metric (table 10.4) the obtained results are generally satisfactory for the clinical application of 3D roadmapping [16, 57], while the results for the mTRE metric fall below expectations, since the best SR is 48% and the best CR is 1 mm. Examples of final registrations according to mTRE and mRPD metrics are shown in figure 10.7.

For additional insight into registration performance, figure 10.8 shows a cumulative success rate (cSR) computed with respect to the initial mTRE such that the cumulative number of successful registration trials was divided by the

Table 10.3. Results of 3D–2D registrations on ten pairs of cerebral angiograms [44]. Registration accuracy is reported as MEAN ± STD of mTRE of successful registrations (mTRE < 2 mm), success rate (SR) and capture range (CR) across 1000 registrations of 3D- and 2D-DSA image pairs.

View	Method	MEAN ± STD [mm]	SR [%]	CR [mm]
AP	Stratified	1.34 ± 0.41	28.0	1.0
	Iterative	0.95 ± 0.54	7.4	3.0
	Combined	1.12 ± 0.51	45.6	1.0
LAT	Stratified	1.34 ± 0.42	17.1	1.0
	Iterative	—	0.0	1.0
	Combined	0.95 ± 0.48	48.1	1.0

Table 10.4. Results of 3D–2D registrations on ten pairs of cerebral angiograms [44]. Registration accuracy is reported as MEAN ± STD of mRPD of successful registrations (mRPD < 2 mm), success rate (SR) and capture range (CR) across 1000 registrations of 3D- and 2D-DSA image pairs.

View	Method	MEAN ± STD [mm]	SR [%]	CR [mm]
AP	Stratified	0.99 ± 0.48	64.8	3.0
	Iterative	0.62 ± 0.41	33.1	11.0
	Combined	0.39 ± 0.23	95.8	49.0
LAT	Stratified	1.03 ± 0.47	75.2	3.0
	Iterative	0.74 ± 0.44	34.0	9.0
	Combined	0.40 ± 0.20	98.9	91.0

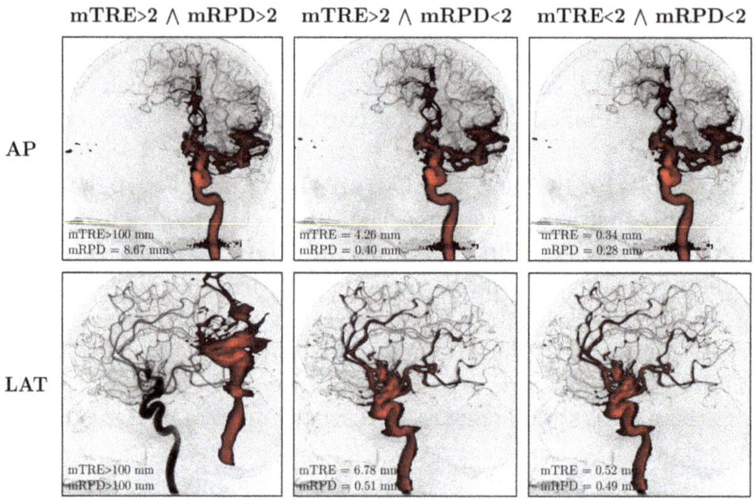

Figure 10.7. Final alignment of cerebral angiograms in AP and LAT views with respect to mTRE and mRPD shown as a superposition of 2D-DSA (grayscale) and a DRR (red) of 3D-DSA after 3D–2D registration.

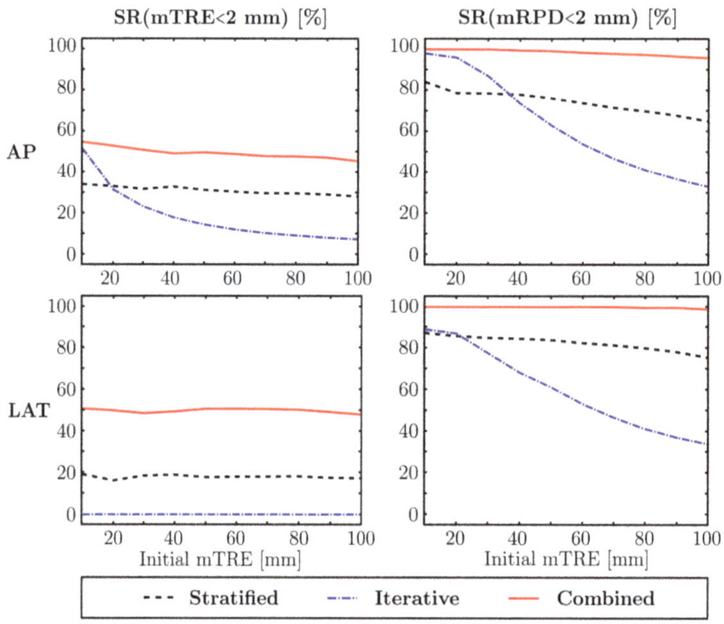

Figure 10.8. Cumulative SRs for a failure criterion of 2 mm (final mTRE, mRPD) shown with respect to initial mTRE across ten AP and LAT datasets of cerebral angiograms [7].

number of all registration trials up to some initial mTRE. When the initial mTRE was less than 20 mm, the iterative method achieved a higher SR than the stratified method, however, the SR then decreased drastically. Clearly, the iterative method requires a good initial starting position for the registration to succeed. On the other hand, the SR of the stratified method is nearly constant (with respect to mTRE and mRPD) regardless of initial mTRE. The combined method absorbs the advantages of both stratified and iterative methods, such that the stratified method provides a good and robust initial starting position for the iterative method which then delivers highly accurate registration with ~0.4 mm mean mRPD error with nearly constant and high SR of up to 99% and high CR up to 91 mm for mRPD metric.

Achieving a high SR for the mTRE metrics, however, remains an open challenge. One of the main reasons for lower registration performance is poor sensitivity of the employed 3D–2D image similarity measures, and the state-of-the-art image similarity measures in general, to out-of-plane translation of the structures being registered. Since even a large out-of-plane translation reflects in small changes of the scale of structures, improved similarity measures that are highly sensitive to small step in out-of-plane translation are needed.

10.7.3 Evaluation without a failure criterion

To verify the conclusions made in the previous subsection, but without a predefined threshold on the final registration accuracy, we performed validation using the methodology by Markelj *et al* [59]. For this purpose, the distribution of registration errors (mTRE and mRPD) was probed at the 50th and 95th percentile in progressively increasing accumulative intervals of initial mTRE, i.e. 0–20, 0–40, 0–60, 0–80 and 0–100mm. Note that the initial mTREs were uniformly distributed in each of these intervals.

Tables 10.5 and 10.6 show the results for the mTRE and mRPD metrics, respectively. The stratified method is able to constrain the mTRE to within ~16 mm (P_{95}), regardless of the initial mTRE, while the iterative method clearly fails to bound the mTRE. Nevertheless, the combined method was able to further constrain the final mTRE to below ~8 mm in the range of 0–80 mm of initial mTRE. The median of final mTRE also improved compared to the stratified method and was around 2 mm (table 10.5). This aspect of the methods' performance was previously not revealed by the evaluation based on a 2 mm mTRE failure threshold.

For the mRPD metric, table 10.6 shows that the iterative method has excellent performance in the range of 0–20 mm of initial mTRE, but the performance degrades substantially for large ranges of initial mTRE. Hence, good initialization is very important for the iterative method. The combined method results show that the stratified method is able to deliver a good initialization for the iterative method, since the obtained final mRPD is constrained to within ~0.8 mm for 0–80 mm and even 0–100 mm of initial mTRE on the AP and LAT views, respectively.

The distributions of final mTRE and mRPD in the corresponding accumulative intervals are demonstrated by box–whisker plots in figure 10.9.

10.8 Challenges in translation to clinical application

The major areas in 3D–2D registration for image-guided angiography interventions (IGIs) that need improvement are the ability to function under changing conditions and robust performance under large initial alignment errors. Ideally a robust 3D–2D

Table 10.5. Results of 3D–2D registrations on ten pairs of cerebral angiograms [44]. Registration accuracy is reported as the 50th (P_{50}) and 95th (P_{95}) percentile of mTRE in a corresponding accumulative interval of the initial mTRE.

View	Accumulative interval of initial mTRE	Stratified		Iterative		Combined	
	[mm]	P_{50} [mm]	P_{95} [mm]	P_{50} [mm]	P_{95} [mm]	P_{50} [mm]	P_{95} [mm]
AP	0–20	2.71	8.84	4.44	15.30	1.88	5.69
	0–40	2.84	9.51	10.30	37.66	2.02	5.60
	0–60	3.05	10.45	20.26	57.90	2.02	6.90
	0–80	3.24	13.01	31.29	76.80	2.04	8.24
	0–100	3.39	16.47	43.27	96.15	2.22	14.90
LAT	0–20	4.30	12.42	12.80	>100.00	2.00	5.92
	0–40	4.03	12.89	17.57	>100.00	2.01	6.03
	0–60	4.13	12.75	34.22	>100.00	1.96	6.03
	0–80	4.22	13.36	91.14	>100.00	1.98	6.65
	0–100	4.34	14.52	>100.00	>100.00	2.09	7.37

Table 10.6. Results of 3D–2D registrations on ten pairs of cerebral angiograms [44]. Registration accuracy is reported as the 50th (P_{50}) and 95th (P_{95}) percentile of mRPD in corresponding accumulative interval of the initial mTRE.

View	Accumulative interval of initial mTRE	Stratified		Iterative		Combined	
	[mm]	P_{50} [mm]	P_{95} [mm]	P_{50} [mm]	P_{95} [mm]	P_{50} [mm]	P_{95} [mm]
AP	0–20	1.20	4.92	0.40	1.81	0.32	0.71
	0–40	1.17	5.45	0.62	28.25	0.32	0.69
	0–60	1.24	6.40	1.37	46.28	0.33	0.73
	0–80	1.30	8.80	10.32	59.91	0.33	0.78
	0–100	1.39	12.41	19.10	74.88	0.34	1.81
LAT	0–20	1.18	4.36	0.56	3.12	0.34	0.76
	0–40	1.14	4.13	0.85	13.32	0.34	0.74
	0–60	1.14	3.94	1.68	23.70	0.34	0.75
	0–80	1.18	4.34	6.34	39.78	0.34	0.76
	0–100	1.26	6.26	9.59	58.41	0.35	0.78

registration algorithm should not be sensitive to image noise and artifacts. In order for the method to perform reliably under variable circumstances, the errors must be low and predictable.

The development of 3D–2D registration methods that are not affected by initial alignment errors and have high final success rates as measured by registration errors

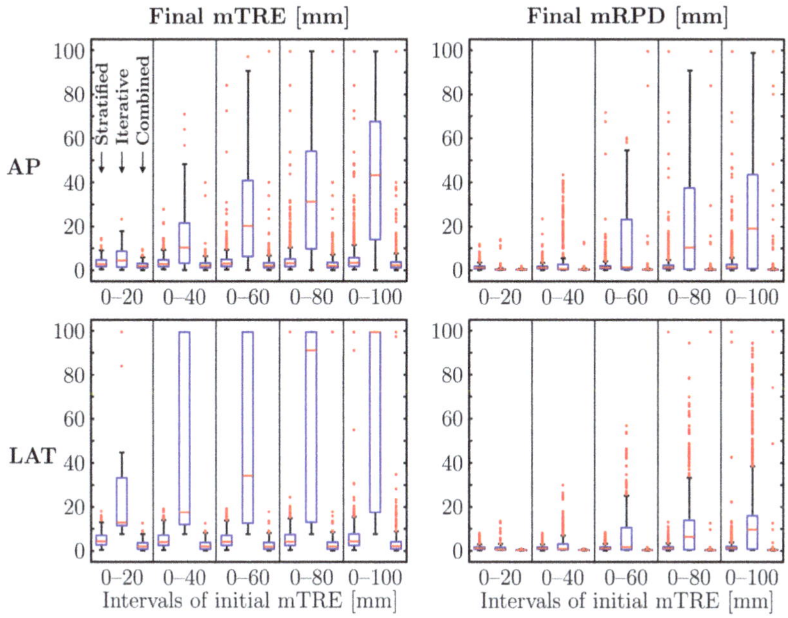

Figure 10.9. Box–whisker plots of mTRE and mRPD registration errors in accumulative intervals of initial mTRE for the three tested 3D–2D registration methods.

in 3D (mTRE) are still open research targets. Some of the intrinsic methods based on iterative optimization report high success rates and low alignment errors, but require close initialization due to an abundance of local optima. While derivative-free optimizers such as Nelder–Mead and simulated annealing can avoid being trapped in local optima, it is not possible to ensure that they will converge to the global solution. To address these problems, a combination of stratified and iterative optimization seems promising.

Another deficiency of 3D–2D registration methods is high specialization for particular applications, hence, generalization of the methods and results to other applications is often not possible. Intensity-based registration methods are dependent on the reproducibility of intensity patterns, which may vary between different vascular imaging techniques, but also due to varying levels of injected contrast or due to blood flow induced variations. Feature-based registration methods rely on accurate extraction and matching of features, which is a difficult task on complex vascular networks and for different imaging techniques [69]. Furthermore, these methods may not be reliable when image quality and anatomical conditions change significantly. A single 3D–2D registration algorithm reliable enough to be employed in all IGI scenarios concerning an anatomy may not be still available. Moreover, some of the proposed methods require manual interactions from the surgeon during the intervention, which may not be desirable under real-time constraints.

Another bottleneck for IGI applications is time complexity. The real-time constraints require the algorithm complexities to be tractable and to converge to optimal solution in a few number of steps. Efficiency of iterative optimization methods may suffer from uncertainty in the number of steps required. The worst case time complexity of the searching method must have a reasonable bound for IGI applications.

The creation of validation datasets consisting of patient images acquired during IGI has received little attention in the literature. Only one dataset of cerebral angiograms with an accurate gold standard is currently publicly available for the purposes of objective validation and comparison of the performance of 3D–2D registration methods developed for vascular structures. To perform validation of methods for vascular structures in other anatomical regions, corresponding patient image datasets need to be acquired and a gold standard needs to be established. While the tools for the creation of accurate gold standards for rigid-body 3D–2D registration are well known, the development of methods and tools for creating such an accurate gold standard for deformable 3D–2D registration remains an open challenge.

References

[1] Redwood S, Curzen N and Thomas M 2010 *Oxford Textbook of Interventional Cardiology* (Oxford: Oxford University Press)

[2] Groher M, Baust M, Zikic D and Navab N 2010 Monocular deformable model-to-image registration of vascular structures *Biomedical Image Registration* (*Lecture Notes in Computer Science* vol 6204) (Berlin: Springer) pp 37–47

[3] Prince J and Links J 2014 *Medical Imaging Signals and Systems* (London: Pearson)

[4] Shechter G, Shechter B, Resar J and Beyar R 2005 Prospective motion correction of x-ray images for coronary interventions *IEEE Trans. Med. Imaging* **24** 441–50

[5] Siemens 2015 https://www.siemens-healthineers.com/refurbished-systems-medical-imaging-and-therapy/ecoline-refurbished-systems/angiography-ecoline/artis-zee-biplane-eco

[6] Metz C, Schaap M, Klein S, Baka N, Neefjes L, Schultz J, Niessen W and van Walsum T 2013 Registration of 3D+t coronary CTA and monoplane 2D+t x-ray angiography *IEEE Trans. Med. Imaging* **32** 919–31

[7] Mitrović U, Špiclin Z, Likar B and Pernuš F 2013 3D–2D registration of cerebral angiograms: a method and evaluation on clinical images *IEEE Trans. Med. Imaging* **32** 1550–63

[8] Groher M, Zikic D and Navab N 2009 Deformable 2D–3D registration of vascular structures in a one view scenario *IEEE Trans. Med. Imaging* **28** 847–60

[9] Bankman I N (ed) 2008 *Handbook of Medical Image Processing and Analysis* 2nd edn (New York: Academic)

[10] Otake Y, Wang A S, Stayman J W, Uneri A, Kleinszig G, Vogt S, Khanna A J, Gokaslan Z L and Siewerdsen J H 2013 Robust 3D–2D image registration: application to spine interventions and vertebral labeling in the presence of anatomical deformation *Phys. Med. Biol.* **58** 8535

[11] Markelj P, Tomazevič D, Likar B and Pernuš F 2012 A review of 3D–2D registration methods for image-guided interventions *Med. Image Anal.* **16** 642–61

[12] Varnavas A, Carrell T and Penney G 2013 Increasing the automation of a 2D–3D registration system *IEEE Trans. Med. Imaging* **32** 387–99

[13] Truong M, Aslam A, Ginks M, Rinaldi C, Rezavi R, Penney G and Rhode K 2009 2D–3D registration of cardiac images using catheter constraints *Comput. Cardiol.* **2009** 605–8

[14] Rhode K S *et al* 2005 A system for real-time XMR guided cardiovascular intervention *IEEE Trans. Med. Imaging* **24** 1428–40

[15] Gorges S, Kerrien E, Berger M O, Trousset Y, Pescatore J, Anxionnat R, Picard L and Bracard S 2006 3D augmented fluoroscopy in interventional neuroradiology: precision assessment and first evaluation on clinical cases *Workshop on Augmented Environments for Medical Imaging and Computeraided Surgery, AMIARCS* **vol 2006** pp 1–10

[16] Ruijters D, Homan R, Mielekamp P, van de Haar P and Babič D 2011 Validation of 3D multimodality roadmapping in interventional neuroradiology *Phys. Med. Biol.* **56** 5335–54

[17] Navab N, Heining S-M and Traub J 2010 Camera augmented mobile C-arm (CAMC): calibration, accuracy study, and clinical applications *IEEE Trans. Med. Imaging* **29** 1412–23

[18] Hamming N M, Daly M J, Irish J C and Siewerdsen J H 2009 Automatic image-to-world registration based on x-ray projections in cone-beam CT-guided interventions *Med. Phys.* **36** 1800–12

[19] Otake Y, Armand M, Armiger R S, Kutzer M, Basafa E, Kazanzides P and Taylor R 2012 Intraoperative image-based multiview 2D/3D registration for image-guided orthopaedic surgery: incorporation of fiducial-based C-arm tracking and GPU-acceleration *IEEE Trans. Med. Imaging* **31** 948–62

[20] Zollei L, Grimson E, Norbash A and Wells W 2001 2D–3D rigid registration of x-ray fluoroscopy and CT images using mutual information and sparsely sampled histogram estimators *Proc. IEEE Conf. on Computer Vision and Pattern Recognition* (Washington, DC: IEEE Computer Society) doi:https://doi.org/10.1109/CVPR.2001.991032

[21] Penney G P, Weese J, Little J A, Desmedt P, Hill D L G and Hawkes D J 1998 A comparison of similarity measures for use in 2D–3D medical image registration *IEEE Trans. Med. Imaging* **17** 586–95

[22] Brown L M G and Boult T E 1996 Registration of planar film radiographs with computed tomography *Workshop on Mathematical Methods in Biomedical Image Analysis* (Washington, DC: IEEE Computer Society) pp 42–51

[23] Demirci S, Baust M, Kutter O, Manstad-Hulaas F, Eckstein H-H and Navab N 2013 Disocclusion-based 2D–3D registration for angiographic interventions *Comput. Biol. Med.* **43** 312–22

[24] Maintz J B A and Viergever M A 1998 A survey of medical image registration *Med. Image Anal.* **2** 1–36

[25] Dong S, Kettenbach J, Hinterleitner I, Bergmann H and Birkfellner W 2008 The Zernike expansion—an example of a merit function for 2D–3D registration based on orthogonal functions *Proc. Medical Image Computing and Computer Assisted Interventions* pp 964–71

[26] Flach B, Brehm M, Sawall S and Kachelrie M 2014 Deformable 3D–2D registration for CT and its application to low dose tomographic fluoroscopy *Phys. Med. Biol.* **59** 7865

[27] Metz C, Schaap M, Klein S, Rijnbeek P, Neefjes L, Mollet N, Schultz C, Serruys P, Niessen W and van Walsum T 2011 Alignment of 4D coronary CTA with monoplane x-ray angiography *6th Inter. Workshop, AE-CAI 2011, Held in Conjunction with MICCAI 2011* **2011** pp 106–16

[28] Rivest-Henault D, Sundar H and Cheriet M 2012 Nonrigid 2D/3D registration of coronary artery models with live fluoroscopy for guidance of cardiac interventions *IEEE Trans. Med. Imaging* **31** 1557–72

[29] Turgeon G A, Glen Lehmann G G, Drangova M, Holdsworth D and Peters T 2005 2D–3D registration of coronary angiograms for cardiac procedure planning and guidance *Med. Phys.* **32** 3737–49

[30] Ruijters D, ter Haar Romeny B M and Suetens P 2009 Vesselness-based 2D–3D registration of the coronary arteries *Int. J. Comput. Assist. Radiol. Surg.* **4** 391–7

[31] Groher M, Padoy N, Jakobs T F and Navab N 2006 New CTA protocol and 2D–3D registration method for liver catheterization *Proc. Medical Image Computing and Computer Assisted Interventions* pp 873–81

[32] Baka N, Metz C, Schultz C, Neefjes L, van Geuns R, Lelieveldt B, Niessen W, van Walsum T and de Bruijne M 2013 Statistical coronary motion models for 2D+t/3D registration of x-ray coronary angiography and CTA *Med. Image Anal.* **17** 698–709

[33] Baka N, Metz C, Schultz C, van Geuns R-J, Niessen W and van Walsum T 2014 Oriented Gaussian mixture models for nonrigid 2D/3D coronary artery registration *IEEE Trans. Med. Imaging* **33** 1023–34

[34] Kim H-R, Kang M-S and Kim M-H 2014 Non-rigid registration of vascular structures for aligning 2D x-ray angiography with 3D CT angiography *Advances in Visual Computing* (*Lecture Notes in Computer Science* vol 8887) ed G Bebis *et al* (Berlin: Springer) pp 531–9

[35] Aksoy T, Unal G, Demirci S, Navab N and Degertekin M 2013 Template-based CTA to x-ray angio rigid registration of coronary arteries in frequency domain with automatic x-ray segmentation *Med. Phys.* **40** 101903

[36] Tomazevič D, Likar B and Pernuš F 2007 3D–2D image registration: the impact of x-ray views and their number *Proc. Med. Image Comput. Comput. Assist. Interv.* **4791** 450–7

[37] Prummer M, Hornegger J, Pfister M and Dorfler A 2006 Multi-modal 2D–3D nonrigid registration *Proc. of SPIE* **vol 6144** 61440X

[38] Serradell E, Romero A, Leta R, Gatta C and Moreno-Noguer F 2011 Simultaneous correspondence and non-rigid 3D reconstruction of the coronary tree from single x-ray images *IEEE Int. Conf. on Computer Vision* (Piscataway, NJ: IEEE) 850–7

[39] Frangi A F, Niessen W J, Vincken K L and Viergever M A 1998 Multiscale vessel enhancement filtering *Proc. Med. Image Computing and Computer Assisted Interventions* pp 130–7

[40] Livyatan H, Yaniv Z and Joskowicz L 2003 Gradient-based 2-D/3-D rigid registration of fluoroscopic x-ray to CT *IEEE Trans. Med. Imaging* **22** 1395–406

[41] Tomaževič D, Likar B, Slivnik T and Pernuš F 2003 3-D/2-D registration of CT and MR to x-ray images *IEEE Trans. Med. Imaging* **22** 1407–16

[42] Markelj P, Tomaževič D, Pernuš F and Likar B 2008 Robust gradient-based 3-D/2-D registration of CT and MR to x-ray images *IEEE Trans. Med. Imaging* **27** 1704–14

[43] Špiclin Z, Likar B and Pernuš F 2014 Fast and robust 3D to 2D image registration by backprojection of gradient covariances *Biomedical Image Registration* (*Lecture Notes in Computer Science* vol 8545) ed S Ourselin and M Modat (Berlin: Springer) pp 124–33

[44] Mitrović U, Špiclin Z, Likar B and Pernuš F 2013 Method for 3D-2D registration of vascular images: application to 3D contrast agent flow visualization *Clinical Image-Based Procedures. From Planning to Intervention* (*Lecture Notes in Computer Science* vol 7761) ed K Drechsler, M Erdt, M Linguraru, C Oyarzun Laura, K Sharma, R Shekhar and S Wesarg (Berlin: Springer) pp 50–8

[45] Groher M, Bender F, Hoffmann R-T and Navab N 2007 Segmentation-driven 2D-3D registration for abdominal catheter interventions *Medical Image Computing and Computer-Assisted Intervention - MICCAI 2007, Part II* vol 4792 ed N Ayache, S Ourselin and A Maeder (Berlin: Springer) pp 527–35
[46] Vermandel M, Betrouni N, Palos G, Gauvrit J Y, Vasseur C and Rousseau J 2003 Registration, matching, and data fusion in 2D/3D medical imaging: application to DSA and MRA *Medical Image Computing and Computer-Assisted Intervention* (Berlin: Springer) pp 778–85
[47] Florin C, Williams J, Khamene A and Paragios N 2005 Registration of 3D angiographic and X-ray images using sequential Monte Carlo sampling *Computer Vision for Biomedical Image Applications* (*Lecture Notes in Computer Science* vol 3765) ed Y Liu, T Jiang and C Zhang (Berlin: Springer) pp 427–36
[48] Doucet A, Godsill S and Andrieu C 2000 On sequential Monte Carlo sampling methods for Bayesian filtering *Stat. Comput.* **10** 197–208
[49] Glocker B, Komodakis N, Tziritas G, Navab N and Paragios N 2008 Dense image registration through MRFs and efficient linear programming *Med. Image Anal.* **12** 731–41
[50] Zikic D, Glocker B, Kutter O, Groher M, Komodakis N, Kamen A, Paragios N and Navab N 2010 Linear intensity-based image registration by Markov random fields and discrete optimization *Med. Image Anal.* **14** 550–62
[51] Kerrien E, Berger M, Maurincomme E, Launay L, Vaillant R and Picard L 1999 Fully automatic 3D–2D subtracted angiography registration *Proc. Second Int. Conf. on Medical Image Computing and Computer-Assisted Intervention* **vol 1679** pp 664–71
[52] Hentschke C M and Tönnies K D 2010 *Automatic 2D/3D-Registration of Cerebral DSA Data Sets Bildverarbeitung für die Medizin, BVM* (Aachen: Springer) pp 162–6
[53] Kita Y, Wilson D L and Noble A 1998 Real-time registration of 3D cerebral vessels to x-ray angiograms *Medical Image Computing and Computer-Assisted Intervention* vol 1496 (Berlin: Springer) pp 1125–33
[54] Kubias A, Deinzer F, Feldmann T and Paulus D 2007 Extended global optimization strategy for rigid 2D/3D image registration *Computer Analysis of Images and Patterns* (*Lecture Notes in Computer Science* vol 4673) ed W Kropatsch, M Kampel and A Hanbury (Berlin: Springer) pp 759–67
[55] van der Bom M J, Bartels L W, Gounis M J, Homan R, Timmer J, Viergever M A and Pluim J P W 2010 Robust initialization of 2D–3D image registration using the projection-slice theorem and phase correlation *Med. Phys.* **37** 1884–92
[56] Gouveia A, Metz C, Freire L and Klein S 2012 Comparative evaluation of regression methods for 3D–2D image registration *Artificial Neural Networks and Machine Learning* (*Lecture Notes in Computer Science* vol 7553) ed A Villa, W Duch, P Érdi, F Masulli and G Palm (Berlin: Springer) pp 238–45
[57] Rossitti S and Pfister M 2009 3D road-mapping in the endovascular treatment of cerebral aneurysms and arteriovenous malformations *Interv. Neuroradiol.* **15** 283–90
[58] van de Kraats E B, Penney G P, Tomaževič D, van Walsum T and Niessen W J 2005 Standardized evaluation methodology for 2-D–3-D registration *IEEE Trans. Med. Imaging* **24** 1177–89
[59] Markelj P, Likar B and Pernuš F 2010 Standardized evaluation methodology for 3D/2D registration based on the Visible Human data set *Med. Phys.* **37** 4643–7

[60] Tomaževič D, Likar B and Pernuš F 2004 'Gold standard' data for evaluation and comparison of 3D/2D registration methods *Comput. Aided Surg.* **9** 137–44

[61] Pawiro S A *et al* 2011 Validation for 2D/3D registration I: a new gold standard data set *Med. Phys.* **38** 1481–90

[62] Siewerdsen J H, Moseley D J, Burch S, Bisland S K, Bogaards A, Wilson B C and Jaffray D A 2005 Volume CT with a flat-panel detector on a mobile, isocentric C-arm: pre-clinical investigation in guidance of minimally invasive surgery *Med. Phys.* **32** 241–54

[63] Daly M J, Siewerdsen J H, Cho Y B, Jaffray D A and Irish J C 2008 Geometric calibration of a mobile C-arm for intraoperative cone-beam CT *Med. Phys.* **35** 2124–36

[64] Mitrović U, Špiclin Z, Likar B and Pernuš F 2013 Evaluation of 3D–2D registration methods for registration of 3D-DSA and 2D-DSA cerebral images *Proc. SPIE* **8669** 866931

[65] Madan H, Likar B, Pernuš F and Špiclin Z 2015 Device and methods for 'gold standard' registration of clinical 3D and 2D cerebral angiograms *Proc. SPIE* **9415** 94151G

[66] Fitzpatrick J, West J and Maurer C R Jr 1998 Predicting error in rigid-body point-based registration *IEEE Trans. Med. Imaging* **17** 694–702

[67] Lee T C, Kashyap R L and Chu C N 1994 Building skeleton models via 3-D medial surface axis thinning algorithms *CVGIP: Graph. Models Image Process.* **56** 462–78

[68] Groher M, Jakobs T F, Padoy N and Navab N 2007 Planning and intraoperative visualization of liver catheterizations: new CTA protocol and 2D–3D registration method *Acad. Radiol.* **14** 1325–40

[69] Lesage D, Angelini E D, Bloch I and Funka-Lea G 2009 A review of 3D vessel lumen segmentation techniques: models, features and extraction schemes *Med. Image Anal.* **13** 819–45

IOP Publishing

Vascular and Intravascular Imaging Trends, Analysis, and Challenges, Volume 1
Stent applications
Petia Radeva and Jasjit S Suri

Chapter 11

Endovascular navigation with intravascular imaging

Su-Lin Lee, Angelos Karlas and Alessio Dore

While the current clinical usage of x-ray fluoroscopy for the navigation of endovascular catheters is widespread, the negative effects of radiation and the toxicity of imaging contrast agents has driven researchers to find a safer way to localise devices during these procedures. Fluoroscopic image overlay of angiography to provide a map of the vasculature is already in clinical use but this does not adapt to changes in vessel shape and motion. Current research into the tracking of devices in fluoroscopic sequences and the integration of sensing devices such as electro-magnetic tracking have made some progress into the reduction of x-ray use and procedural time but are difficult to use in some endovascular applications. While intravascular imaging has seen application for tissue characterisation, investigations into its use for other applications has been limited. In this chapter, we first review the current research into endovascular navigation using intravascular imaging and sensing before introducing two potential navigation systems, both incorporating the use of IVUS imaging. We conclude with the identification of the current limitations and emerging research opportunities in this new area, with an aim to bringing intravascular imaging for navigation to clinical use.

11.1 Introduction

The current clinical practice for the use of intravascular imaging modalities is in conjunction with x-ray fluoroscopy to guide the placement of the imaging catheter. Whilst x-ray fluoroscopy provides a general overview of the region of interest, contrast agent enhancement is required for detailed visualisation of the vessels; 3D visualisation of the vessels requires even more contrast agent whilst a rotational angiography is performed. The need for an intra-operative navigation system for endovascular procedures is then clear: a reduction in the use of iodine-based contrast

doi:10.1088/2053-2563/ab01fach11

agent as well as x-ray fluoroscopy would result in a safer procedure for both patients and clinicians alike. While the current clinical availability of the use of angiographic roadmaps, obtained either preoperatively or intraoperatively, integrated with x-ray fluoroscopy allows the clinician to locate devices within the vasculature without the extra use of a contrast agent, this still requires the use of the radiative imaging modality.

In this chapter, we first review the state-of-the-art in the use of intravascular imaging for intra-operative navigational use before describing our recent research into the use of intravascular ultrasound (IVUS) imaging for guidance in arterial procedures. We then identify the research priority areas in the near future for endovascular navigation using intravascular imaging to reach clinical use.

11.2 Existing research into intravascular imaging for navigation

The current commercially available navigation systems for intravascular procedures focus on instrument localisation based on external imaging. X-ray fluoroscopy is the current state-of-the-art imaging in theatres and, while it is able to provide a live view of endovascular devices within the body, it brings a host of unfortunate side effects caused by the radiation and the need for nephrotoxic contrast agents for vessel delineation.

For improved endovascular navigation, one may look towards interventional cardiac procedures, where the use of navigation is in a more mature state. Intracardiac catheters for electrophysiological mapping and cardiac ablation can be tracked using commercially available systems such as the Biosense-Webster CARTO® and St Judes EnSite™ NavX™. The insertion of these catheters is still performed with x-ray fluoroscopy but its use is limited, after which the clinician is usually dependent on the tracking system and/or a registered preoperative scan. This is due to a number of factors, the main one being the different motion exhibited by the heart—while the heart does beat and is affected by respiration, the motion is consistent and generally known. Also, the coverage of vasculature, especially the aorta, is much greater than that of the heart, making tracking via electric or electromagnetic fields difficult.

The use of intravascular imaging, introduced via a catheter, can add an additional level of information to the clinician, but the interpretation of this information together with localisation of the catheter within the anatomy is not straightforward. For example, the 2D projection of the x-ray images does not indicate the through-plane shape of the vasculature, making the retargeting of sites identified via intravascular imaging difficult. An advanced navigation system is required to provide clinicians with both the local data from the intravascular imaging and the global view of the vasculature. We review here the current use of various intra-vascular imaging methods for navigational purposes.

11.2.1 IVUS

IVUS is the most widely used intravascular imaging techniques and employs a tiny ultrasound transducer mounted on the tip of a catheter to image the interior of blood vessels. A series (typically 256) of ultrasound pulses are emitted and the consequent echoes are detected at different angular directions. Common IVUS systems employ 1D piezoelectric transducer arrays and generate 360° images on planes perpendicular to the blood flow. Conventional IVUS catheters used in the coronary arteries have a theoretical resolution of 19–39 μm (20–45 MHz) with >5 mm penetration.

While IVUS imaging is relatively affordable, based on disposable equipment alone, it is more expensive than the use of x-ray fluoroscopy and is an invasive imaging procedure requiring the insertion and withdrawal of a catheter. However, the imaging modality itself is much safer, with no ionising radiation and no requirement for toxic contrast agents. Processing of the ultrasound images can be challenging but as automatic segmentation and characterisation of images are already available and implemented in commercial systems, this lends well to the use of this modality for intra-operative navigational purposes.

11.2.1.1 Registration to fluoroscopy

A common approach to the use of IVUS imaging for navigational purposes is through the registration of angiography to the series of collected IVUS images. A better understanding of the entire vascular network is obtained through the 3D angiography whilst the IVUS images provide the cross-sectional characterisation of the artery under consideration.

Accurate registration of IVUS images to angiography does require tracking of the catheter in the fluoroscopic images. It is not the aim of this chapter to review this body of work, but many methods for the extraction of the catheter configuration have already been proposed. Fluoroscopy-based computer vision techniques have used optimal B-spline curve fitting [3], adaptive spatio-temporal filtering [34], learning classification approaches [6] and dynamic optimisation [46], amongst others.

Wahle *et al* [43] presented an initial system for the fusion of biplane angiography with IVUS imaging. A 3D model of the vessel was first obtained from the angiography data. While the IVUS images were collected, the biplane C-arm images were also recorded and a dynamic programming approach was used to detect the full catheter trajectory. A catheter model encapsulating bending, torsion, position, orientation and twisting was also incorporated to ensure that the IVUS images were oriented correctly on the catheter path. The authors also proposed an automatic statistics-based algorithm for the identification of correct 3D orientation of IVUS images during registration to the angiographic data [44]. Evans *et al* [12] took a similar approach, also using ECG-gated biplane fluoroscopy to track the IVUS catheter and then using affine transformation matrices to fuse the IVUS images to the catheter positions. The benefits of biplane fluoroscopy are clear—the 3D positions of the catheters can be tracked from the images; however, biplane imaging systems are more expensive and their limited movement can affect the surgical workflow and thus they are still relatively uncommon in hospitals.

Tu *et al* [40] approach the registration process for coronary procedures with distance mapping to a known, manually labelled position. They also skip the 3D reconstruction of the catheter trajectory, using only the centreline of the 3D vasculature. Distance mapping may not be suitable for more tortuous vasculature but is effective in more straightforward vessels. Manual point selection may be error prone but does facilitate the registration process. Wang *et al* [45] simplifies the manual requirement of their approach by only having the operator defining a segment of clinical significance. Any endovascular devices in this fluoroscopic 'field-of-view' were then detected and tracked using a Haar-based probabilistic boosting tree classifier and a Bayesian model, respectively.

11.2.1.2 Feature detection

Navigation using IVUS requires the identification of landmarks in the IVUS image sequence, both for registration purposes as well as localisation within the vasculature. Alberti *et al* [2] have developed a method based on classification of textural features and a multiscale stacked sequential learning scheme to automatically detect and measure bifurcations in coronary IVUS sequences. In addition to the bifurcations, the corresponding image frames, the angular orientation of the bifurcation and the extension are all identified.

Features can also include those from implanted devices, although this requires the IVUS imaging to be performed after the procedure. The fully automatic detection of stent struts in IVUS images was performed using a cascade of GentleBoost classifiers in work by Rotger *et al* [30]; here, structural features of the stent were used to code the information of the different subregions of the struts. More recently from the same group, automatic strut detection is first preceded by a stent shape estimation from the IVUS images using a supervised context-aware multi-class classification scheme [8]. The stent strut identification exploits both the estimated stent shape and the local appearance of the strut features.

11.2.1.3 Forward facing probes

Forward-looking IVUS image probes have been suggested and prototypes developed but to this date, these have not been made commercially available. In a navigational context, a forward facing IVUS catheter would be able to assist clinicians with the detection of vessel branches and vessel obstructions for guidewire advancement, without requiring the use of contrast agent enhanced x-ray fluoroscopy.

Stephens *et al* [38] developed two forward-looking array designs for intracardiac use; these catheters were used within the heart simultaneously with an ablation catheter. While the initial designs were promising, the quality of the ultrasound images was less than that of commercially available catheters. In 2008, Volcano (San Diego, USA) acquired Novelis and their proprietary forward-looking IVUS (FLIVUS) technology with a view to integrating this into their existing platform. It has been suggested that they have been developing the technology and are looking to bring the product to market in the very near future but with the recent acquisition of Volcano by Philips (2014), it is now not clear if the product will appear.

11.2.2 OCT

Intravascular optical coherence tomography (OCT) imaging also requires the use of a contrast agent, which while safe for most of the population, may cause adverse reactions. Iodinated contrast agents, as also used in computed tomography angiography (CTA), can accumulate in the kidneys and lead to contrast-induced nephropathy [16]. The use of OCT has been compared to IVUS and studies have shown that the increased resolution of OCT can be used to better detect stent malposition. However, while there are many benefits to OCT, the fact remains that it is less common in theatres than IVUS.

Unal *et al* [41] detected stent struts in OCT images for assessing the amount of in-stent restenosis post percutaneous coronary intervention. Their results show great promise for the detection of features (albeit features of already implanted stents) using OCT, with possible application to navigation.

11.2.3 Intravascular magnetic resonance imaging

Magnetic resonance (MR) imaging is a safe imaging modality without any ionising radiation and there has been an increasing amount of research into its use for endovascular procedural guidance via MR fluoroscopy [31]. This is not strictly speaking an endovascular imaging modality, but MR is capable of real-time 3D localisation of the tip of the endovascular catheter and tissue characterisation. However, MR imaging for guidance of endovascular procedures is not currently in clinical use as there remain many research issues in the development of MR compatible endovascular devices and limitations to real-time MR imaging such as image resolution [18]. Also, the cost of MR is significantly higher than that of other interventional imaging modalities.

11.2.4 Other sensing

Apart from imaging, a number of other sensing devices are also available for endovascular use. Investigations into their use for *in vivo* navigation have been performed, with initial results presented.

11.2.4.1 Electromagnetic sensing

The use of electromagnetic (EM) tracking with catheters has been explored extensively and is already in use in commercial systems for tracking cardiac catheters (e.g. Biosense-Webster CARTO). These can be used in conjunction with a preoperative scan of the vasculature, in which case registration is required. Fiducial markers on the skin may be used or natural features such as bifurcations or existing calcifications in the vasculature.

Liu *et al* [23] have employed EM tracking to determine real-time catheter pose with respect to the surrounding vascular wall. The geometric information about the vascular walls was preoperatively obtained using MRI and registration between the preoperative image data and intra-operative vascular phantom were performed using a two stage registration scheme consisting of the iterative closest point (ICP) algorithm.

Wood *et al* [47] have investigated the use of EM sensors on many devices, including endovascular guidewires. Here, rather than simply attaching the EM sensors to the catheter, and thus affecting manipulation of the devices, they have created guidewires from the sensors, embedding them within the device itself. This leads to more natural manipulation of the device without added bulk. Validation was performed on phantoms. Also validated on silicone phantoms was work performed by Cochennec *et al* [9] using the Stealthstation® (Medtronic, USA), a commercially available clinical EM-based surgical navigation system, to guide catheter cannulation. They found that its use, though increasing the time for cannulations, reduced the use of x-ray fluoroscopy and improved cannulation performance scores.

One of the most recent and advanced navigation systems available is the CustusX (SINTEF, Dept Medical Technology, Trondheim, Norway), originally developed for minimally invasive procedures. Again, guidewires were created with sensors embedded within. This still requires the connection of trailing wires to the EM control system and there are limitations as to the size of the field created by the EM field generator. The NDI Aurora (NDI, Waterloo, ON, Canada), used in this system, has a field size of 0.125 square metres, smaller than that required to cover the length of the descending aorta in the average person. Some of this may be circumvented through the use of extra sensors used to roughly track the position of the anatomy, but any ferromagnetic device within or near to the electromagnetic field will affect the field and hence results. The authors have also reviewed the use of EM sensing for navigation, along with possible methods for error compensation, in endovascular aortic repair [39].

There have been clinical and pre-clinical investigations into the use of EM sensing in endovascular interventions. Abi-Jaoudeh *et al* [1] demonstrated the feasibility of inserting a thoracic stent graft with a navigation system incorporating both 3D images and EM sensing. Using the CustusX system, Manstad-Hulaas *et al* [24] has also shown successful catheterisations with fewer attempts required to insert the guidewire correctly than without the navigation system.

As is common with any system dependent on a static preoperative volumetric scan of the anatomy, however, motion and deformation affects the results. The aorta is not fixed within the body and may deform as the patient moves. Likewise, the introduction of more rigid devices into the vasculature may cause deformation; a stiff guidewire may affect a 'straightening' of the vessel. This may affect registration results to the intra-operative EM coordinate system. Motion, in the form of cardiac pulsation or respiration, can also affect navigation results.

11.2.4.2 Shape sensing

Of recent interest is research into the use of fibre-Bragg grating (FBG) for shape sensing. This is an optical sensor made of a multi-core fibre, with changes in the optical length detected in each of the single cores. They are particularly sensitive to strain and temperature and thus have been used to sense changes in these in aerospace industries and industrial engineering, among others. 'Fibre optic shape sensing', an emerging technology based on fibre-Bragg grating, has been demonstrated and patented by Luna Technologies [14], with results showing the 3D shape reconstruction of the entire length of a catheter. However, to date, this technology has not been incorporated into clinical devices.

11.2.4.3 Catheter modelling

The shape of a catheter may also be reconstructed by modelling the mechanical properties of the device as well as its interaction with anatomical structures. This can provide an estimation of their current pose within the body [15, 20, 22, 37]. However, the use of mechanical modelling, such as finite element simulations, can be computationally expensive and difficult to implement for real-time processing.

The major advantage of these approaches, however, is the ability to provide a prediction on the effect of the catheter motion with respect to the vasculature. This can be particularly useful in situations where the interventionist wants to avoid particular areas of the vessel or assess beforehand the effect of a certain procedure. In addition, these models can be used to simulate the procedure and create a training environment for physicians.

11.3 IVUS for navigation

It is clear that there is a need for an improved navigation system for endovascular interventions and there is scope to achieve this through the use of intravascular imaging. To this end, we have proposed two separate frameworks for navigation for endovascular procedures based on endovascular imaging. The first method, combining IVUS imaging, catheter modelling and EM sensing, was initially proposed as part of the collaborative SCATh FP7 framework project [33] and then extended in the CASCADE FP7 framework project [7]. The second removes the need for explicit modelling and tracking, relying only on the IVUS imaging and a preoperative scan.

11.3.1 IVUS and EM sensing

Simultaneous localisation and mapping (SLAM) is a very popular approach in robotics [10] which aims to provide navigation capabilities to robots equipped with sensing capabilities (e.g. LiDAR, cameras, etc). In the SCATh project the concept of 'Endovascular SLAM' was introduced to provide a new navigation tool for catheter-based intervention based on information provided by EM and IVUS sensors integrated into a single catheter. The main motivation behind the proposed approach is to be able to obtain a 3D representation of the catheter shape and the vessel geometry which can be used by the surgeon to safely navigate the catheter within the vasculature without or with limited use of fluoroscopy.

11.3.1.1 Catheter design

In the SCATh project, a customised catheter was developed where an IVUS sensor and multiple EM sensors were integrated, as shown in figure 11.1.

The IVUS system from Volcano Corporation with a Visions® PV 8.2 catheter was used. An NDI Aurora EM tracking system (NDI, Ontario, Canada) was used with their sensors (9 × 0.5 mm, 5 degrees of freedom (DOF) and 9 × 1.8 mm 6 DOF) integrated with the IVUS catheter. Six 5 DOF sensors along the catheter and one 6 DOF at the tip of the catheter were employed to obtain information about the catheter position and orientation with respect to the EM reference system. In order

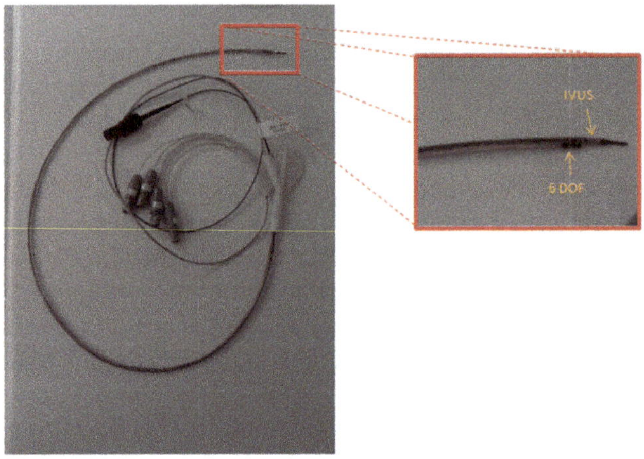

Figure 11.1. Custom made catheter, integrating IVUS and EM sensors, for the SCATh FP7 project.

to accurately track the catheter position and shape during the procedure, the 5 DOF sensors were placed at 125 mm intervals, with the first 80 mm from the 6 DOF sensor at the distal end of the catheter, to obtain better accuracy near the tip. The 3D catheter shape within the vessel could be reconstructed and mapped onto a 3D preoperative model to provide an effective and intuitive visualisation during the catheter insertion.

In order to cope with registration errors, vessel motion and deformation, the IVUS images were processed to extract the relative position of the catheter tip with respect to the vessel lumen.

11.3.1.2 Catheter shape estimation and vessel geometry reconstruction

The fusion of this information in a probabilistic framework and the 3D visualisation of catheter and vessel were introduced as a novel navigation approach for endovascular intervention.

The catheter was defined by a finite number of nodes

$$X_t = \{x_1, x_2, \ldots, x_n\}_t^T, \tag{11.1}$$

where $x_i = (x, y, z, \theta, \omega, \phi)$ represented the position and orientation at time t. The shape of the catheter was then estimated by a set of Catmull–Rom splines which were used to estimate the interconnection between the nodes.

In order to estimate the 3D position of the nodes a Kalman filter approach was used to integrate the information from the EM sensors and a physically based catheter simulation model based on real-time insertion length measures [11]. The catheter insertion simulation model provides the displacement of the nodes:

$$U_t = \{\delta x_1, \delta x_2, \ldots, \delta x_n\}_t^T, \tag{11.2}$$

that can be used as a prediction model in the Kalman filter, which is defined as

$$X_t = AX_{t-1} + BU_t + \omega_t, \qquad (11.3)$$

where A is an identity matrix and ω_t is the normally distributed process noise.

By considering the EM sensors as the catheter nodes, the EM tracking system provided the measurement for the Kalman filter.

The localisation and shape estimation of the catheter through this probabilistic framework offers useful cues for catheter navigation:

1. The reliability of the catheter position estimate can be assessed considering the covariance of the estimate.
2. The prediction model provides information to estimate in advance the position of the catheter as a consequence of its insertion of a certain magnitude.
3. The combination of EM measurement and the catheter insertion model compensates for the possible inaccuracy of the single elements.

In order to provide an online 'map' of the vasculature during the insertion and accurately estimate the position of the catheter tip with respect to the vessel wall, the IVUS images were processed to extract the vessel lumen (figure 11.2). The IVUS processing algorithm is represented in figure 11.3. Since the images were captured from the Volcano IVUS system using a frame-grabber, a pre-processing step was necessary to remove the grid marks on the images. Once the marks were removed, the image was transformed to polar coordinates and a flood fill algorithm was applied to identify the lumen area. The contour was then identified by transforming the image back to Cartesian coordinate system, applying a threshold on the flood

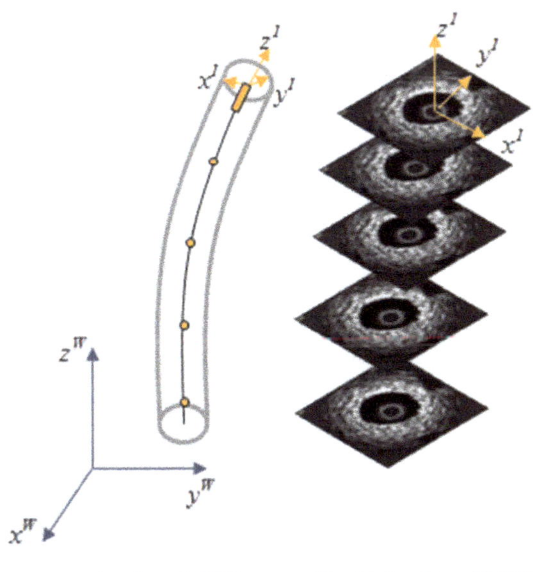

Figure 11.2. Catheter shape reconstruction via EM sensors. Combining this with IVUS images allowed for the reconstruction of the vessel geometry.

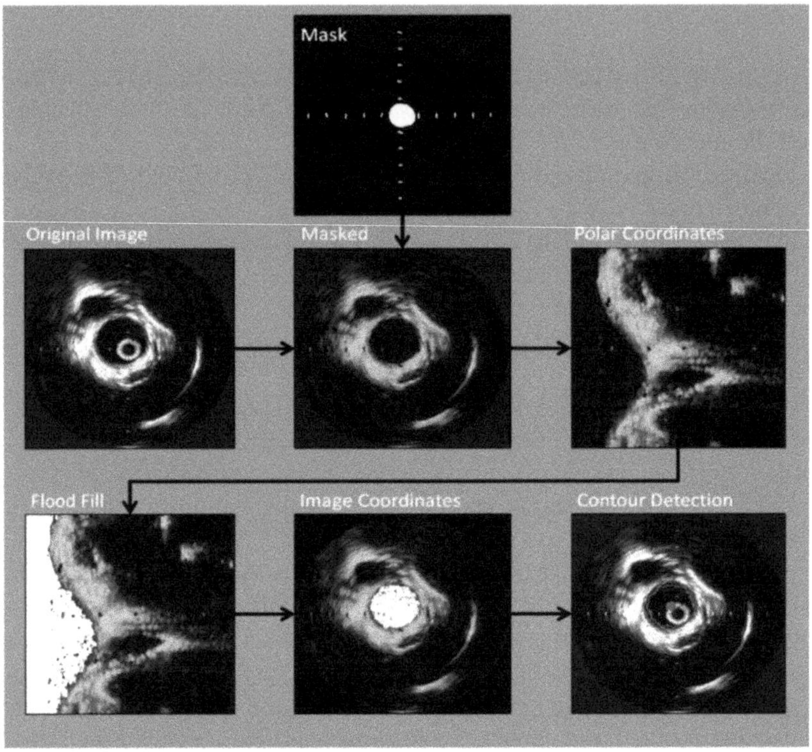

Figure 11.3. Workflow for IVUS image processing.

filled image and applying a contour detection algorithm. The centerline of the vessel was estimated by fitting an ellipse to the contour.

The 6 DOF EM sensor at the tip of the catheter was used to map the 2D IVUS-derived vessel lumen to a 3D representation. Each point of the contour in the 2D image coordinate system was then transformed to the 3D world coordinate system using the following transformations:

$$X_t^W = {}_I T_t^W X_t^I, \tag{11.4}$$

$${}_I T_t^W = {}_I T^E {}_E T_t^W, \tag{11.5}$$

where T is the transformation matrix, I is the IVUS image coordinate system, E is the EM tracker coordinate system, W is the world coordinate system and X_t^I is described in figure 11.4.

11.3.1.3 Results

The accuracy of the proposed algorithm for catheter shape estimation was validated in a 2D Plexiglas phantom created from an MRI scan of a patient aorta. A camera was used to record the catheter shape during the insertion and obtain the ground truth. The catheter is inserted into the aorta phantom with a constant velocity of

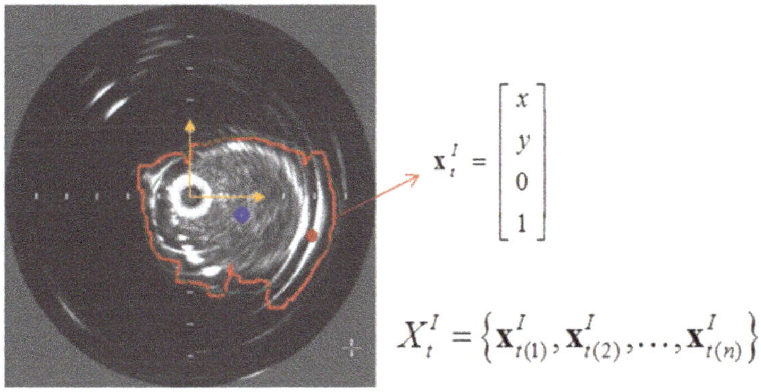

Figure 11.4. IVUS image point coordinates.

Table 11.1. Average position error (mm) computed on 20 catheter poses. S1 indicates the sensor at the catheter tip, S2 the sensor in the middle and S3 the sensor closer to the catheter distal end.

Sensor	EM tracking	Insertion model	Fusion
S1	2.5	3.0	1.8
S2	2.9	3.4	2.1
S3	3.5	3.2	2.3
∀S	3.0	3.2	2.1

10 mm s^{-1} by using an actuation mechanism. The results recorded in the experiments are shown in table 11.1.

The accuracy of the vessel shape reconstruction algorithm was also assessed *in vivo*. A porcine study was performed in The Intervention Centre, Rikshospitalet, Oslo, using a Volcano IVUS system and a Siemens Artis zeego interventional radiology system. To visualise the vessel in 3D within the animal, a contrast medium was also used during the dyna-CT scan. The animal was placed at different respiratory breath hold positions and catheter pullbacks were performed manually by the interventional radiologist, with the catheter withdrawal performed at a slow and consistent speed.

The errors of the generated centreline to the ground truth centreline can be seen in table 11.2.

An ongoing EU FP7 project (CASCADE) currently focusing on transcatheter aortic valve implantation (TAVI) is currently taking the research forward, with improved IVUS processing and integration with the preoperative model. The simultaneous catheter and environment mapping (SCEM) [35] improves on the image processing and model reconstruction. A RANSAC operator was used to improve the ellipse fitting in the absence of the entire contour and a full 3D model of the aortic arch has also been built. The research is being extended to dynamic models, with controlled simulations of the cardiac and respiratory cycles.

Table 11.2. The errors for the *in vivo* experiments at three different breath hold positions.

Breath hold	Mean error (mm)	Std dev error (mm)
Max inhalation	3.3	1.6
In between	3.9	1.8
Max exhalation	4.1	1.6

11.3.2 Vessel navigation and retargeting

While this previous approach for intra-operative navigation was based on the use of IVUS imaging along with another localisation technology, its use is limited to the clinical adoption of that technology, in this case, electromagnetic tracking. For example, to date, the NDI Aurora is not currently approved for clinical use. In addition, combining the localisation technology—in this case, a wired EM sensor—to the catheter or guidewire without constricting manoeuvrability is challenging.

To address these issues, we have recently proposed a framework to navigate through a patient-specific vasculature based only on IVUS imaging and a preoperative model [19]. The preoperative model can be derived from contrast-enhanced CT or MRI and provides a general map of the vasculature. This map is used to keep track of where the IVUS transducer is within the vasculature and is initialised with a single IVUS catheter pullback. This removes the need for intra-operative x-ray fluoroscopy and the introduction of any separate localisation technology. We introduce the proposed framework here, showing initial results on phantom data.

11.3.2.1 Image processing and segmentation

No localisation technology was required, only a Volcano© Visions® PV 8.2 Phased-Array IVUS Imaging Catheter was used with a Volcano© s5™ imaging system (Volcano, San Diego, CA, USA). The VGA output of the imaging system was connected to an Epiphan VGA2Ethernet frame-grabber, with that output fed to a PC via an Ethernet cable. For validation of the results, a 6 DOF EM sensor was attached just proximal to the ultrasound transducer; this sensor was connected to an NDI Aurora electromagnetic tracking system (NDI, Waterloo, ON, Canada).

Pullback sequences of this IVUS catheter were obtained within a rigid Plexiglas aorta phantom (figure 11.5) produced by Materialise (Leuven, Belgium); the phantom was submerged within water heated to approximately 37 °C. For each sequence recorded, the IVUS catheter was inserted to the aortic root (using a guidewire) and a manual pullback was obtained. Approximately 1200 images were collected for each pullback sequence.

For registration between the EM tracking coordinate system and the CT coordinate system, a set of five CT visible marks was mounted on the rigid phantom and the positions of these were collected in both systems. The ICP algorithm [5] was used to align these markers and provide the rigid transformation between the two coordinate systems.

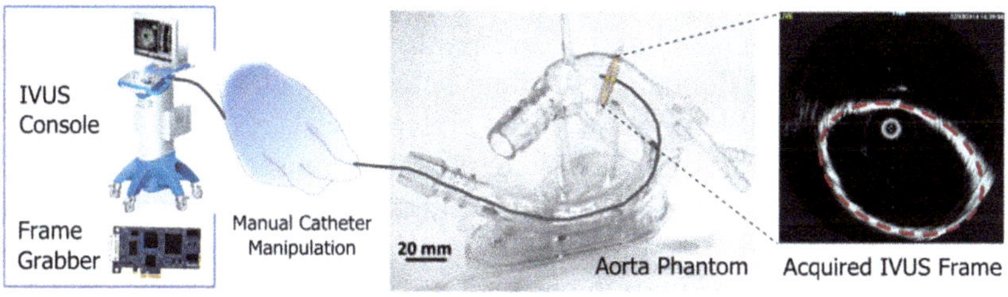

Figure 11.5. Full system workflow diagram.

The IVUS images required processing to enhance the appearance of the vessel lumen and to remove noise and labels. As a first step, a region of interest (ROI) was defined to reduce the size of the image to only the IVUS output. To remove the region defined by the catheter silhouette, appearing as a constant circle in the centre of the IVUS images, each image was transformed first to polar coordinates. A mask of minimum intensity (usually zero) pixels [21], of a width defined by the known catheter diameter, was then applied to the upper part of each polar image to remove this catheter artefact. The resulting image was then transferred back to Cartesian coordinates. To remove the grid markings in the IVUS images, a 6×10 neighbourhood median filter was applied at each point (known in advance).

IVUS images tend to be distorted by both speckle noise and modality-specific artefacts. To reduce speckle noise in the images, a global speckle reducing bilateral filter (SRBF) [4] was used. This incorporates local noise statistics to provide a full automated high-performance image despeckling and originates from classical bilateral filtering that takes into account both space- and intensity-oriented similarity in a specified region around the pixel. The filter combines both domain filtering, using pixel weights that decay as the distance to the central pixel rise, and range filtering, where pixel weights decrease when a dissimilarity-in-intensity measure increases. SRBF has been shown to demonstrate better results in ultrasound images, maintaining edge details, over other filters [36]. The filter is shown in the equations below:

$$f(i, j) = \frac{\sum_{s=1-n}^{i+n} \sum_{t=1-n}^{i+n} W_d(s,\, t) W_r(s,\, t) g(s,\, t)}{\sum_{s=1-n}^{i+n} \sum_{t=1-n}^{i+n} W_d(s,\, t) W_r(s,\, t)} \tag{11.6}$$

$$W_d(s,\, t) = e^{-\frac{(i-s)^2 + (j-t)^2}{2\sigma_d^2}} \tag{11.7}$$

$$W_r(s,\, t) = e^{-\frac{\|g(i,\, j) - g(s,\, t)\|^2}{2\sigma_r^2}}. \tag{11.8}$$

$g(i, j)$ is every pixel value of the input image and the filtered pixel is $f(i, j)$. The size of the window filter was $w = 7$ (an odd number for symmetry) and the span was

$n = 3$ ($w = 2n + 1$). d is an index corresponding to domain parameters while r is an index for range parameters. σ_d^2 and σ_r^2 are parameters (variances) that regulate the weight behaviour in the domain and range fields [42]. The choice of these values depends on the statistical features of noise; high values lead to edges loss while low values create a weak filter that is unable to eliminate noise. In our implementation, $\sigma_d^2 = \sigma_r^2 = 4$. Finally, to increase the contrast of the IVUS images, contrast stretching (histogram dynamic full range expansion) [32] was applied.

A number of IVUS segmentation methods have already been proposed and these can be divided into four main strategies: (1) edge detection techniques, (2) active contour methods, (3) statistical approaches and (4) multiscale analysis. Due to the absence of peripheral tissues and blood flow in our phantom and the structural homogeneity of the phantom vascular wall, a straightforward global thresholding strategy was implemented. Otsu's method [28] was chosen to distinguish between vessel wall and noise components. The method assumes that the pixel set of every image can be divided into two discrete classes: objects and background. The classification is performed through an optimisation problem which aims to detect an optimal threshold in the image histogram.

Finally, dilation and erosion were applied to the binary images. This was followed by a connect-component labelling (region labelling) whereby a graph-based process assigned a specific label to a set of pixels within a clearly bounded region. A two pass process was applied. In the first step, initial labels were assigned to the objects and label correspondences were recorded. In the second step, the algorithm substituted each previously specified label for the smallest of the corresponding class. For each region, a centre of mass was calculated and these values were used to estimate the main ring of image energy; this allowed for the safe application of vessel-specific geometrical constraints to further remove non-object (non-lumen) regions. First, regions of size below a certain threshold were removed. Geometric constraints on the size of the average human aorta were then used to remove regions that were too far away from the geometric centroid of all the regions.

It should be noted that the appearance of the IVUS images collected from the phantom currently does not resemble those from patients; however, *in vivo* data do exhibit the same kind of speckle noise that we encountered. For that reason, while the image processing steps presented here are not directly transferrable to *in vivo* sequences, many of the steps can be used.

11.3.2.2 Landmark detection

The detection of landmarks is a key step in the proposed IVUS-based navigation platform. In our platform, we cater for both anatomical and morphological landmarks. Morphological landmarks are structures which describe a specific shape, are present in all shapes of the same class, and are easily detected. Anatomical landmarks along the aorta may be as suggested by the ACCF/AHA (American College of Cardiology Foundation/American Heart Association) Task Force [17]; here the authors identified nine well-established anatomical landmarks to effectively describe the anatomy of a normal aorta. These include: the aortic sinuses of Valsalva, the sinotubular junction, the mid ascending aorta, the proximal aortic arch, the mid aortic arch, the proximal descending thoracic arch, the mid descending aorta, the aorta at diaphragm and the abdominal aorta at the coeliac axis origin.

As the landmarks used in the proposed framework must be effective descriptors of the vascular structures, some of these anatomical landmarks are unsuitable. For example, the mid aortic arch only refers to a length of the descending aorta, effectively a tube. For this reason, we only consider branches, being present in each artery, as well as morphological variations in the aorta, dilations and stenoses, representing the two main pathologies of the aorta, aneurysms and atherosclerotic lesions.

To detect these landmarks, two ellipses were fitted to the inner wall edge and outer boundary of the vessel in the processed IVUS frames. The ellipses were fitted using the direct least squares fitting approach by Fitzgibbon *et al* [13]. The method searches for an optimally fitted curve to a known set of scattered 2D data by minimising the sum value of the calculated residuals of the given points to the curve. A Cartesian quadratic representation of an ellipse was used:

$$a_1x^2 + b_1xy + c_1y^2 + d_1x + e_1y + f_1 = 0. \tag{11.9}$$

In addition to fitting the ellipses, the main ellipse parameters were calculated: the centre of each ellipse, semi-axis lengths and ellipse orientation. Subsequently, these parameters form the basis of the description of vessel morphology.

The absolute lengths of the major and minor axes of the ellipses defined the area covered by the ellipses and indicated the lumen area. Their relative lengths (calculating the eccentricity, defined by the ratio of major to minor lengths) describe the shape of the lumen. Finally, the absolute difference between the corresponding axes of the inner and outer ellipses described wall thickness.

A combination of these descriptors can be used to indicate the presence of landmarks along the aorta. It is challenging to identify certain landmarks in a single IVUS image in isolation but examining these parameters along the vessel axial dimension, i.e. along a series of IVUS images in a pullback sequence, it is possible to interpret the parameter fluctuations.

An aneurysm would be characterised by an increase and then a decrease in the inner or outer ellipse axes lengths. An atheromatic stenosis will be a decrease and then an increase. The presence of a branch would be indicated by a localised increase in the eccentricity of the inner ellipse.

11.3.2.3 3D IVUS–CT fusion

After detection of landmarks in the IVUS sequence, the landmarks must be matched to the equivalent landmarks detected in 3D. For this, we used a preoperatively obtained 3D surface mesh of the vessel. This was derived from a preoperative rotational-CT scan of the phantom obtained using a GE Innova 4100 interventional imaging suite. CT visible markers were attached to the phantom for registration purposes. ITK-SNAP [48] was used to segment the vessel from the images and a 3D surface mesh was produced.

To define the mesh skeleton (vessel centrelines), a mesh thinning algorithm was applied to the 3D surface mesh. Binvox [25, 27], followed by Thinvox [26, 29], was used for this purpose. Binvox first converts the 3D surface mesh to a voxel model while Thinvox is an iterative procedure that detects and removes boundary vessels until a single voxel curve is left. By taking the centroid of each of the voxels, the mesh skeleton was produced.

To find branch-points along the skeleton, all voxels along the initial voxel curve were examined. Each voxel could have up to 26 neighbouring voxels; however, as we are starting with a voxel curve, no voxel should have all 26 neighbours. Any voxel with a neighbouring voxel will either (1) share a common side (four common vertices), (2) share a common edge (two common vertices), or (3) share a single common vertex. After examining all neighbours of each voxel, it was determined that voxels with at least three neighbouring voxels were branch-points, i.e. were voxel junctions, and voxels with only one neighbouring voxel were end-points.

Subsequently, after all end-points and branch-points were identified along the vessel centreline, points along the centreline must be grouped, corresponding to each of the junctions. *K*-means clustering was used, with *k* set to the ideal number of junctions in the shape. After the lengths of centre points have been clustered together, the central axis of the aorta was determined using a Dijkstra-based directed path search algorithm. This sorted points within each junction and identified erroneous branch- and end-points. The total final output path was the centreline of the vessel, which was smoothed using a spline.

The final step was registration to the IVUS pullback sequence. For this, the start and end of the IVUS image sequence were registered to the end-points. Branches identified in the pullback were associated with the branch-points along the centreline. Images in between were linearly interpolated between these fixed points. As we currently do not have information on the orientation of the tip of the catheter, the IVUS images were oriented perpendicularly to the central axis.

11.3.2.4 Results

The image processing steps transforming each initial IVUS image to the final centralised binary frame are presented in figure 11.6.

Figure 11.7 depicts the main branch detection procedure. The three peaks of the inner ellipse eccentricity index plot along the vessel correspond to the three main branches of the aortic arch. The detection of other lesions is based on tracking other features of the fitted ellipses.

The calculated skeleton of the 3D CT model is presented in figure 11.8 along with the discretised vascular volume as well as the result of the IVUS–CT fusion procedure.

In figure 11.9 we present the results of our system in terms of navigation precision. This diagram provides a comprehensive comparison of the catheter tip points tracked by the EM system (red: ground truth) and the tip points calculated by our method (green). The point cloud of the 3D model (yellow points) as well as its smoothed central axis (blue curve) are also depicted. The absolute differences

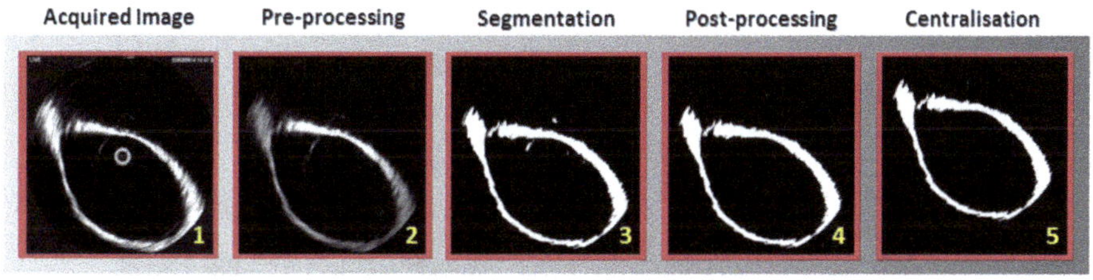

Figure 11.6. The processing stages transforming each raw image to the finally centralised frame.

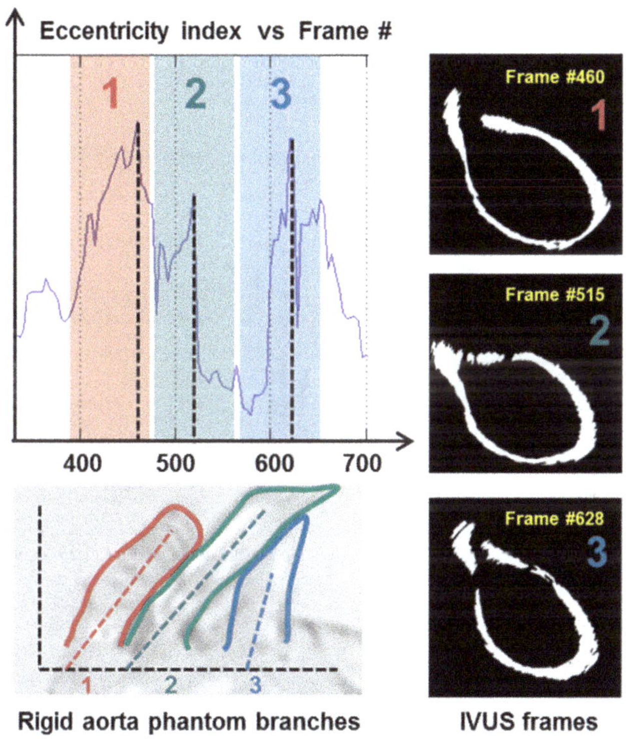

Figure 11.7. Branch detection and localisation based on eccentricity index of the inner fitted ellipse. Left: top—EI plot along the vascular structure; bottom—the three main branches of our aorta phantom. Right: the three branch-corresponding binary IVUS frames before the centralisation step.

between the tip point coordinates provided by the EM system and those estimated via our system are also given in the form of three supplementary boxplots.

The current implementation of the proposed programme is in MATLAB and can be seen in figure 11.10.

11.4 The future of intravascular imaging for navigation

There still remain a number of challenges to be addressed in the use of intravascular imaging for navigation and these remain the research priority areas for any potential

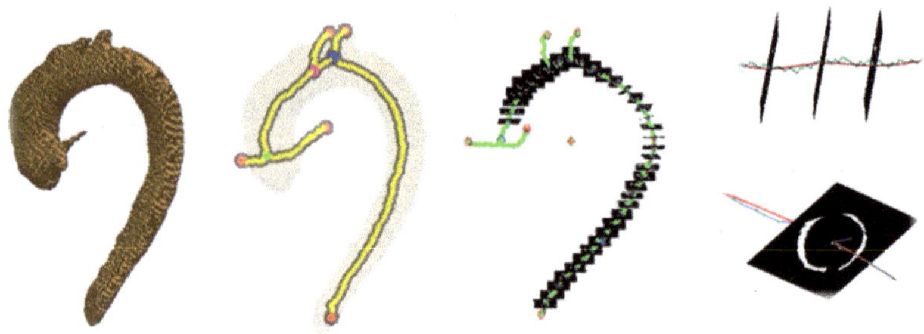

Figure 11.8. From left to right: Voxelised CT-derived vessel model, central axis with end- and branch-points and IVUS–CT data fusion.

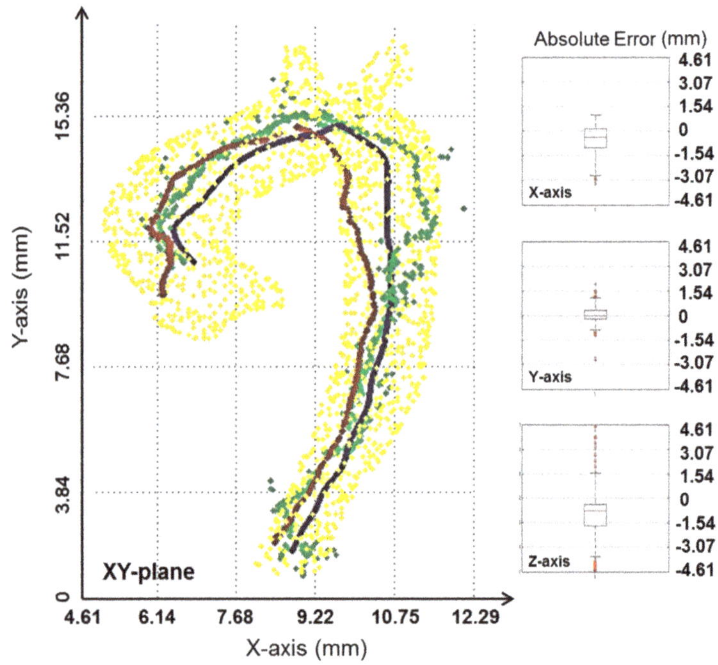

Figure 11.9. Precision results and absolute error in space. Yellow points: 3D model volume; red points: catheter tip tracked with EM system (ground truth); blue points: smoothed calculated central axis; green points: catheter tip according to the proposed method.

framework to enter clinical usage. The first is down to the limitations in vessel coverage using an imaging modality acquired at the tip of a catheter. The quality of the acquired image-sets may be degraded by unpredictable abrupt movements of the catheter tip (jumps) during the pullback scan due to localised bending, torsional stiffness and lumen irregularities. These events may create extended filling deficits of the vascular wall surface produced by the frame-sequence 3D repositioning. Furthermore, the relative position of the catheter and the wall at a cross section

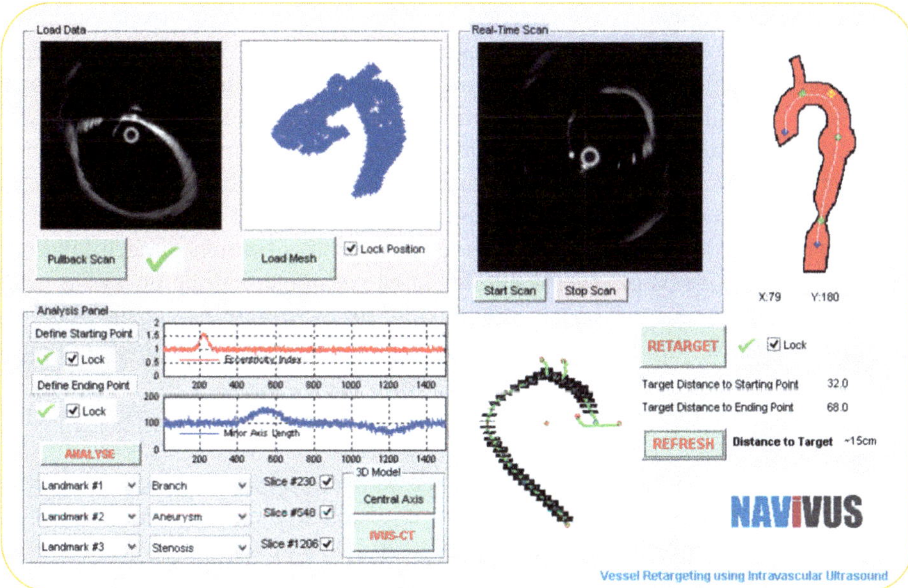

Figure 11.10. The graphical user interface for the proposed framework.

may cause an incomplete capture of the wall inner circumference in cases of large distances between the lumen and the frame centres; this is, in particular, possible in the aorta. This deficit may also extend several centimetres along the vessel, requiring rescanning. Scans conducted by using an automatic pullback device are more prone to these kinds of errors, while the manual steering of the catheter allows for better results. This way, the operator adapts the catheter configuration to the geometrical shape of the vascular structure by applying appropriate torque in a real-time model. However, multiple deficit regions may be present in the endovascular images due to imaging noise and artefacts and these may cause a loss of potentially valuable information that interferes with the different processing steps. As a solution we propose the implementation of a mechanism that detects the position and extent of the deficit and suggests a corrective rescanning of the corresponding vascular segment. This mechanism could be based on detecting discontinuities of the wall representation in a longitudinal mode, or tracking gaps in the wall region in polar coordinates.

For the use of a static 3D scan, such as a preoperative or intra-operative 3D model, co-registration is required. For example, in our framework, the detection of useful anchoring points that would serve as a reference pattern for this task is necessary on both IVUS and CT datasets, and consequently they must be matched. However, the lack of information on the exact diameter of the CT-derived model at every discrete cross section hinders the use of any point corresponding to a stenosis or an aneurysm limiting our landmark set to that containing only the branch- and end-points of the 3D model axis. One way to expand the usable landmark set could be the application of appropriate mesh-skeletonisation algorithms that would give feedback on the number of cycles (cropped voxels) needed to produce an ideal one-voxel central line. Furthermore, the use of a more sophisticated method of IVUS image segmentation could further enlarge the set of landmarks via embedding tissue characterisation features and, thus, allowing for the discretisation among different lesions of the same type and the creation of a plaque map. These improvements would increase navigation precision and get us one step further towards the fully automated detection of all landmarks. Our proposed system currently relies on a friendly graphical user interface which allows for the manual detection and classification of each landmark based on the fluctuations of several fitted-ellipses parameters along an IVUS image stack. The development of novel training algorithm strategies, which may also encompass statistical modelling data as well as anatomical and epidemiological information, should further facilitate this process.

The current commercial electromagnetic tracking systems provide excellent feedback on the position as well as the spatial orientation of the catheter tip (5 or 6 DOF sensors), as utilised in our first proposed system. However, the difficulties in incorporating EM sensing during arterial procedures are clear. While our second proposed framework provides independence from EM trackers, the system can only partially compensate for the loss of the 3D orientation of the catheter tip. Development of a strategy relying solely on IVUS image data that would resolve this limitation and lead to better precision results is thus an important research direction. The preliminary technique assumes a perfectly cylindrical model for the vessel under investigation, with a constant wall thickness. By using measured wall thickness, aided by an extension to *in vivo* data, it may be possible to determine the true angular orientation of the IVUS scanning plane. This would also provide clinicians with information about the current state of the catheter *in vivo*, without resorting to the use of fluoroscopy for confirmation.

The proposed methods also cannot depict the changes to the entire vessel structure caused by patient motion or the introduction of stiff endovascular devices during a procedure. With the first proposed method, it is possible to perform an extra IVUS pullback after deformation to reconstruct the new shape; however, the second method is only able to identify the location of an endovascular imaging device relative to a known map of the vasculature. The use of biomechanical modelling has a role here in the simulation of the shape of the vessels after deformation, in particular, with the use of limited intravascular imaging data to act as constraints. The current limitation in its use is, as reviewed earlier in this chapter, the computation time required.

In summary, while the benefits of using a safer and established intravascular imaging modality for navigation purposes are clear, there are still a number of challenging problems that require research to bring its application to clinical use.

11.5 Conclusion

We have presented here two intravascular navigation frameworks, both reliant on IVUS imaging. The first requires EM tracking for the reconstruction of the vasculature *in situ*, a technique able to compensate for any motion between the preoperative scan and the endovascular procedure. The second is based on image processing of intra-operative IVUS data and the use of a preoperative model, without the need for any external tracking equipment. This system aims to facilitate endovascular procedures and especially in providing the operator with the opportunity to tag a specific point of interest along a vessel and re-visit it in less time and with better precision.

While there remain issues to be addressed for the proposed frameworks to be accepted clinically, the use of endovascular imaging methods for navigation is a promising approach that limits the use of x-ray fluoroscopy and the accompanying contrast agents required to delineate the arteries.

Acknowledgements

Partial support of this research was provided by the FP7-EU Project 'Smart Catheterization (SCATh)'.

References

[1] Abi-Jaoudeh N, Glossop N, Dake M, Pritchard W F, Chiesa A, Dreher M R, Tang T, Karanian J W and Wood B J 2010 Electromagnetic navigation for thoracic aortic stent-graft deployment: a pilot study in swine *J. Vasc. Interv. Radiol.* **21** 888–95

[2] Alberti M, Balocco S, Gatta C, Ciompi F, Pujol O, Silva J, Carrillo X and Radeva P 2012 Automatic bifurcation detection in coronary IVUS sequences *IEEE Trans. Biomed. Eng.* **59** 1022–31

[3] Baert S A M, Viergever M A and Niessen W J 2003 Guide-wire tracking during endovascular interventions *IEEE Trans. Med. Imaging* **22** 965–72

[4] Balocco S, Gatta C, Pujol O, Mauri J and Radeva P 2010 SRBF: speckle reducing bilateral filtering *Ultrasound Med. Biol.* **36** 1353–63

[5] Besl P J and McKay N D 1992 A method for registration of 3-D shapes *IEEE Trans. Pattern Anal. Mach. Intell.* **14** 239–56

[6] Brost A, Wimmer A, Liao R, Hornegger J and Strobel N 2010 Catheter tracking: filter-based versus learning-based *Pattern Recognition* (*Lecture Notes in Computer Science* vol 6376) (Berlin: Springer) sect 30, pp 293–302

[7] Cascade. http://www.cascade-fp7.eu/

[8] Ciompi F, Balocco S, Caus C, Mauri J and Radeva P 2013 Stent shape estimation through a comprehensive interpretation of intravascular ultrasound images *Medical Image Computing and Computer-Assisted Intervention—MICCAI 2013* (*Lecture Notes in Computer Science* vol 8150) (Berlin: Springer) sect 43, pp 345–52

[9] Cochennec F, Riga C, Hamady M, Cheshire N and Bicknell C 2013 Improved catheter navigation with 3D electromagnetic guidance *J. Endovasc. Ther.* **20** 39–47

[10] Davison A J, Reid I D, Molton N D and Stasse O 2007 Monoslam: real-time single camera slam *IEEE Trans. Pattern Anal. Mach. Intell.* **29** 1052–67

[11] Dore A, Smoljkic G, van der Poorten E, Sette M, Sloten J V and Yang G Z 2012 Catheter navigation based on probabilistic fusion of electromagnetic tracking and physically-based simulation *IEEE/RSJ Int. Conf. on Intelligent Robots and Systems (IROS)* (Piscataway, NJ: IEEE) pp 3806–11

[12] Evans J L *et al* 1996 Accurate three-dimensional reconstruction of intravascular ultrasound data: spatially correct three-dimensional reconstructions *Circulation* **93** 567–76

[13] Fitzgibbon A, Pilu M and Fisher R B 1999 Direct least square fitting of ellipses *IEEE Trans. Pattern Anal. Mach. Intell.* **21** 476–80

[14] Froggatt M E, Klein J W, Gifford D K and Kreger S T 2011 Optical position and/or shape sensing *US patent* US20110109898 a1

[15] Gao B, Hu K, Guo S and Nan X 2013 Mechanical analysis and haptic simulation of the catheter and vessel model for the MIS VR operation training system *2013 IEEE Int. Conf. on Mechatronics and Automation (ICMA)* (Piscataway, NJ: IEEE) pp 1372–7

[16] Goldenberg I and Matetzky S 2005 Nephropathy induced by contrast media: pathogenesis, risk factors and preventive strategies *Can. Med. Assoc. J.* **172** 1461–71

[17] Hiratzka L F *et al* 2010 ACCF/AHA/AATS/ACR/ASA/SCA/SCAI/SIR/STS/SVM guidelines for the diagnosis and management of patients with thoracic aortic disease: a report of the American college of cardiology foundation/American heart association task force on practice guidelines, American association for thoracic surgery, American college of radiology, American stroke association, society of cardiovascular anesthesiologists, society for cardiovascular angiography and interventions, society of interventional radiology, society of thoracic surgeons, and society for vascular medicine *Circulation* **121** e266–369

[18] Kandarpa K 2013 Magnetic resonance imaging—guided endovascular interventions—are we there yet? *J. Vasc. Interv. Radiol.* **24** 891–3

[19] Karlas A and Lee S L 2015 Towards an IVUS-driven system for endovascular navigation *IEEE Int. Symp. on Biomedical Imaging* (Piscataway, NJ: IEEE) doi:https://doi.org/10.1109/ISBI.2015.7164119

[20] Langelaar M and Keulen F V 2004 Modeling of a shape memory alloy active catheter *Structures, Structural Dynamics, and Materials and Co-located Conf.* (Reston, VA: American Institute of Aeronautics and Astronautics) doi:https://doi.org/10.2514/6.2004-1653

[21] Lazrag H, Aloui K and Naceur M 2013 Automatic segmentation of lumen in intravascular ultrasound images using fuzzy clustering and active contours *Proc. Eng. Technol.* **1** 58–63

[22] Lenoir J, Cotin S, Duriez C and Neumann P 2006 Interactive physically-based simulation of catheter and guidewire *Comput. Graph.* **30** 416–22

[23] Liu H, Fu Y L, Zhou Y Y, Li H X, Liang Z G and Wang S G 2010 An *in vitro* investigation of image-guided steerable catheter navigation *Proc. Inst. Mech. Eng.* H **224** 945–54

[24] Manstad-Hulaas F, Tangen G A, Dahl T, Hernes T A N and Aadahl P 2012 Three-dimensional electromagnetic navigation versus fluoroscopy for endovascular aneurysm repair: a prospective feasibility study in patients *J. Endovasc. Ther.* **19** 70–8

[25] Min P B 3D mesh voxeliser http://www.cs.princeton.edu/min/binvox/ (Accessed: 8 September 2014)

[26] Min P B 3D voxel model thinning http://www.cs.princeton.edu/min/thinvox/ (Accessed: 8 September 2014)

[27] Nooruddin F S and Turk G 2003 Simplification and repair of polygonal models using volumetric techniques *IEEE Trans. Vis. Comput. Graph.* **9** 191–205

[28] Otsu N 1979 A threshold selection method from gray-level histograms *IEEE Trans. Syst. Man Cybern.* **9** 62–6

[29] Palágyi K and Kuba A 1999 Directional 3D thinning using 8 subiterations *Proc. of the 8th Int. Conf. on Discrete Geometry for Computer Imagery* (*Lecture Notes in Computer Science* vol 1568) (Berlin: Springer) sect 25, pp 325–36

[30] Rotger D, Radeva P and Bruining N 2010 Automatic detection of bioabsorbable coronary stents in IVUS images using a cascade of classifiers *IEEE Trans. Inf. Technol. Biomed.* **14** 535–7

[31] Saeed M, Hetts S W, English J and Wilson M 2012 MR fluoroscopy in vascular and cardiac interventions (review) *Int. J. Cardiovasc. Imaging* **28** 117–37
[32] Sahu S 2012 Comparative analysis of image enhancement techniques for ultrasound liver image *Int. J. Electr. Comput. Eng.* **2** 792–7
[33] Scath (2010-2012). http://www.scath.net/
[34] Schoonenberg G, Schrijver M, Duan Q, Kemkers R and Laine A 2005 Adaptive spatial–temporal filtering applied to x-ray fluoroscopy angiography *Proc. SPIE* **5744**
[35] Shi C, Giannarou S, Lee S L and Yang G Z 2014 Simultaneous catheter and environment modeling for trans-catheter aortic valve implantation *2014 IEEE/RSJ Int. Conf. on Intelligent Robots and Systems (IROS 2014)* (Piscataway, NJ: IEEE) pp 2024–9
[36] Shibin W, Qingsong Z and Yaoqin X 2013 Evaluation of various speckle reduction filters on medical ultrasound images *Conf. Proc. IEEE Eng. Med. Biol. Soc.* **2013** 1148–51
[37] Shoa T, Madden J D W, Munce N R and Yang V 2010 Analytical modeling of a conducting polymer-driven catheter *Polym. Int.* **59** 343–51
[38] Stephens D N *et al* 2006 5G-6 forward looking intracardiac imaging catheters for electrophysiology *Proc. IEEE Ultrasonics Symp.* (Piscataway, NJ: IEEE) doi:https://doi.org/10.1109/ULTSYM.2006.191
[39] Tangen G A, Manstad-Hulaas F, Brekken R and Hernes T A N 2013 Navigation in endovascular aortic repair aortic *Aneurysm—Recent Advances* (Rijeka: Intech) https://www.intechopen.com/books/aortic-aneurysm-recent-advances/navigation-in-endovascular-aortic-repair
[40] Tu S, Holm N R, Koning G, Huang Z and Reiber J H C 2011 Fusion of 3D QCA and IVUS/OCT *Int. J. Cardiovasc. Imaging* **27** 197–207
[41] Unal G, Gurmeric S and Carlier S G 2010 Stent implant follow-up in intravascular optical coherence tomography images *Int. J. Cardiovasc. Imaging* **26** 809–16
[42] Vanithamani R and Umamaheswari G 2014 Speckle reduction in ultrasound images using Neighshrink and bilateral filtering *J. Comput. Sci.* **10** 623–31
[43] Wahle A, Prause G P M, DeJong S C and Sonka M 1999 Geometrically correct 3-D reconstruction of intravascular ultrasound images by fusion with biplane angiography-methods and validation *IEEE Trans. Med. Imaging* **18** 686–99
[44] Wahle A, Prause G P M, Von Birgelen C, Erbel R and Sonka M 1999 Fusion of angiography and intravascular ultrasound *in vivo*: establishing the absolute 3-D frame orientation *IEEE Trans. Biomed. Eng.* **46** 1176–80
[45] Wang P, Ecabert O, Chen T, Wels M, Rieber J, Ostermeier M and Comaniciu D 2013 Image-based co-registration of angiography and intravascular ultrasound images *IEEE Trans. Med. Imaging* **32** 2238–49
[46] Wang Y, Chen T, Wang P, Rohkohl C and Comaniciu D 2012 Automatic localization of balloon markers and guidewire in rotational fluoroscopy with application to 3D stent reconstruction *Computer Vision—ECCV 2012* (*Lecture Notes in Computer Science* vol 7577) (Berlin: Springer) sect 31, pp 428–41
[47] Wood B J *et al* 2005 Navigation with electromagnetic tracking for interventional radiology procedures: a feasibility study *J. Vasc. Interv. Radiol.* **16** 493–505
[48] Yushkevich P A, Piven J, Hazlett H C, Smith R G, Ho S, Gee J C and Gerig G 2006 User-guided 3D active contour segmentation of anatomical structures: significantly improved efficiency and reliability *Neuroimage* **31** 1116–28

Section IV

Risk stratification in carotid and coronary artery

Chapter 12

A cloud-based smart IMT measurement tool for multi-center clinical trial and stroke risk stratification in carotid ultrasound

Luca Saba, Sumit K Banchhor, Harman S Suri, Narendra D Londhe, Tadashi Araki, Nobutaka Ikeda, Klaudija Viskovic, Shoaib Shafique, John R Laird, Ajay Gupta, Andrew Nicolaides and Jasjit S Suri

This study presents AtheroCloud™—a novel cloud-based smart carotid intima–media thickness (cIMT) measurement tool using B-mode ultrasound for stroke/cardiovascular risk assessment and its stratification. This is an anytime–anywhere clinical tool for routine screening and multi-center clinical trials. In this pilot study, the physician can upload ultrasound scans in one of several formats (DICOM, JPEG, BMP, PNG, GIF or TIFF) directly into the proprietary cloud of AtheroPoint from the local server of the physician's office. They can then run the intelligent and automated AtheroCloud™ cIMT measurements in point-of-care settings in less than five seconds per image while saving the vascular reports in the cloud. We statistically benchmark AtheroCloud™ cIMT readings against sonographer (a registered vascular technologist) readings and manual measurements derived from the tracings of the radiologist.

Scans of one hundred patients (75 M/5 F, mean age: 68 ± 11 years; institutional review board (IRB) approved, Toho University, Japan), of the left/right (L/R) common carotid artery (CCA; 200 ultrasound scans), were collected using a 7.5 MHz transducer (Toshiba, Tokyo, Japan). The measured cIMTs for the L/R carotid were as follows (in millimeters): (i) AtheroCloud™ (0.87 ± 0.20, 0.77 ± 0.20); (ii) sonographer (0.97 ± 0.26, 0.89 ± 0.29) and (iii) manual (0.90 ± 0.20, 0.79 ± 0.20), respectively. The coefficient of correlation (CC) between the sonographer and manual for L/R cIMT was 0.74 ($P < 0.0001$) and 0.65 ($P < 0.0001$), while between AtheroCloud™ and manual the CC was 0.96 ($P < 0.0001$) and 0.97 ($P < 0.0001$),

doi:10.1088/2053-2563/ab01fach12

respectively. We observed that 91.15% of the population in AtheroCloud™ had a mean cIMT error less than 0.11 mm compared to 68.31% for the sonographer. The area under the curve for receiving operating characteristics was 0.99 for AtheroCloud™ against 0.81 for the sonographer. Our Framingham risk score stratified the population into three bins as follows: 39% in low-risk, 70.66% in medium-risk and 10.66% in the high-risk bins. Statistical tests were performed to demonstrate the consistency, reliability and accuracy of the results. The proposed AtheroCloud™ system is a completely reliable, automated, fast (3–5 s depending upon the image size with an internet speed of 180 Mbps), accurate and intelligent web-based clinical tool for multi-center clinical trials and routine telemedicine clinical care.

12.1 Introduction

Cardiovascular diseases (CVDs) have been predicted as the main cause of morbidity globally. On an average, 7.4 million deaths were due to CVDs and 6.7 million were due to stroke [1]. It was found that over three-quarters of CVD deaths take place in low and middle-income countries. In particular, the South-East Asia region is showing a rapid increase of CVDs in the young and middle-aged population. Between 2000 and 2030, it is estimated that about 35% of all CVD deaths in India will occur among the 35–64 year age group [2]. Coronary artery disease and carotid artery disease are two primary examples of diseases caused by the build-up of atherosclerotic plaque that falls under the broader category of CVDs [3].

Atherosclerosis is a progressive process that damages the endothelium due to the deposition of plaque in the arteries [4, 5]. Atherosclerosis narrows the arteries, restricting the flow of oxygenated blood in the body [6]. As atherosclerosis progresses, the blockage can rupture, causing the clot to dislodge and travel downstream (figure 12.1) [7]. This results in myocardial infarction or stroke.

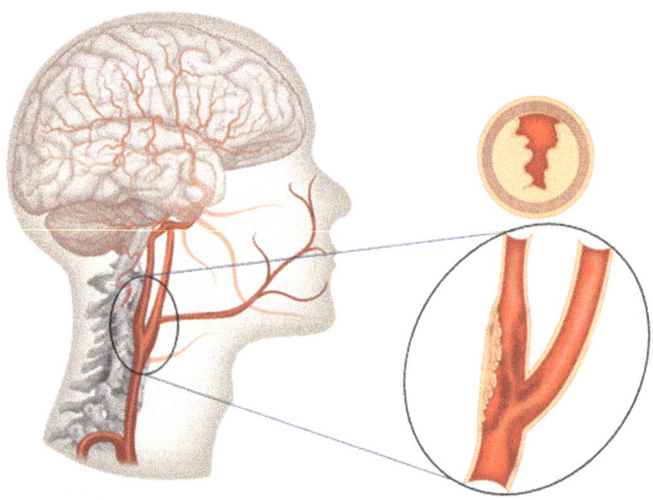

Figure 12.1. Illustration of plaque formation in the carotid artery. (Courtesy of AtheroPoint™, Roseville, CA, USA.)

People with cardiovascular disease or high cardiovascular risk may significantly benefit from early detection, monitoring and management [8, 9].

cIMT is one of the most popular methods for monitoring CVD and predicting the occurrence of major adverse cardiovascular events [10–22]. The prediction of CVD has been tied to cIMT in previous studies, with the aim of foreseeing cardiovascular events (CVE). Several studies have shown a relationship between threshold values of cIMT and CVD: (cIMT > 0.7 mm) [23], (cIMT > 0.85 mm) [24], (cIMT > 0.9 mm) [25, 26], (cIMT > 1.0 mm) [27] and (cIMT > 1.26 mm) [28]. Recent studies have also revealed a strong relationship between cIMT values and the severity of coronary artery disease (CAD) [8, 25, 26, 29]. The above studies have clearly shown that cIMT is a risk biomarker for CVEs.

In spite of the strong relationship between cIMT and CAD, clinicians have not routinely benefitted from automated processing of carotid ultrasound scans. Several studies [17–20] emphasized the need for an automated system for cIMT computation. This is mainly because current manual [19] or semi-automated systems [30] used by sonographers are subjective and associated with operator or observer bias. Current systems are not fully automated [30] and lack advanced image-based features for risk assessment [31, 32]. Often, these systems lack reliability, accuracy and reproducibility, and provide no comparative reference marker, which is needed for monitoring. Furthermore, there is no standardization towards clinical trials [33]. The lack of reproducibility is due to the methodology used to take the readings, such as (i) caliper-based and (ii) readings taken manually at a limited number of locations (positions) along the CCA [34]. We assume that a robust and validated automated system is more accurate and reliable compared to sonographer readings taken by a registered vascular technologist (RVT) in a vascular ultrasound laboratory. This assumption can be proven if the error between the automated AtheroCloud™ software based cIMT readings and the gold standard (manual tracings taken by the radiologist) is lower compared to the error between the sonographer's reading and the gold standard (manual).

Through automated systems, the operator variability and subjectivity can be controlled, but there are still challenges in stroke/cardiovascular risk monitoring, such as the ability to operate in remote areas of the world. The current methods for cIMT measurement use a cart-based ultrasound machine or portable machines which are bulky to carry, in contrast to pocket-sized machines [35], putting a strain on mobile-based infrastructure. Patients and doctors are physically confined to a machine and a clinical protocol cannot be executed if the patient, for example, is in a rural area without access to a physician [36]. The concept of home-healthcare [37] is not prevalent and the traditional approach lacks an 'anytime–anywhere' solution.

There are two major challenges in current cIMT system designs in cloud-based settings:

(i) The design of a two-pronged system, with a single (routine) mode and a batch (pharmaceutical) mode, that can recognize the far wall of the carotid artery [38] and detect the lumen–intima and media–adventitia interfaces [39, 40].

(ii) The design of a multicenter clinical tool which is completely automated (which can extract cIMT measurements over thousands of studies without interruption), which can handle the variability in image characteristics such as resolution, contrast, size, quality and formats, and be able to process images from different countries. A synopsis of previous techniques is presented in the discussion section.

The proposed patented system is 'smart' in the sense that intelligent cloud-computing is adapted for recognition of carotid anatomy in carotid scans (having multiple vascular beds) and computing the lumen–intima (LI)/media–adventitia (MA) (details discussed in the next section) interfaces along with the cIMT measurements. The system is intelligent in the sense that it is able to automatically recognize the far (posterior) wall of the carotid artery even in the presence of the near and far walls of the jugular vein [41].

In a cloud-based approach, the physician can upload ultrasound scans in one of several formats (DICOM, JPEG, BMP, PNG, GIF or TIFF) directly into the proprietary cloud of AtheroPoint from the local server of the physician's office, and then run the intelligent and automated AtheroCloud™ cIMT measurements in point-of-care settings in less than five seconds per image, while saving the vascular reports in the cloud. We then compare and validate AtheroCloud™ readings against a sonographer's measurements and manual (gold standard) readings by computing the precision-of-merit (PoM) and CC between these methods. The performance of the AtheroCloud™ system is then analyzed by computing the area under the curve (AUC) of the receiver operating characteristics (ROC) [42]. We also compare the Routine mode (a single image at a time) against the Pharmaceutical trial mode (a batch of images at a time without interruption) using the AtheroCloud™ software system, showing the reliability and reproducibility. Further, we benchmark AtheroCloud against the commercially available desktop-based systems such as AtheroEdge™ (AtheroPoint™, Roseville, CA, USA), that (i) previously has been benchmarked against original equipment manufacturer (OEM) vendors such as Siemens [43], (ii) is used for epidemiological studies [44] and (iii) is a 510(K) cleared medical device [45], establishing the standard for cIMT measurement [33], demonstrating the error difference which follows the criteria of acceptance under regulatory conditions.

12.2 Patient demographics and data acquisition

12.2.1 Patient demographics

Two hundred and four (204) patients underwent both (i) percutaneous coronary interventions using iMap (Boston Scientific®, Marlborough, MA) IVUS examination and (ii) B-mode carotid ultrasound scans. Both left and right CCA ultrasound scans (a total of 407 images, one patient had one image missing) were obtained from Toho University, Japan and retrospectively analyzed (ethics approved by the IRB). For this pilot study, due to cost and manual tracing constraints, we randomly selected 100 patients (200 CCA ultrasound scans) for this design study. No special criteria were adopted in choosing the 100 patients. There were 75 male and 25 female patients with a mean age 68 ± 11 ranging from 29 to 88 years. Of these, 53 patients had a proximal lesion location, 27 a middle location and 20 a distal location. These 100 patients have a mean HbA1c of 6.40 ± 1.2 mg dl^{-1}, mean low-density lipoprotein (LDL) cholesterol of 104.60 ± 30.4 mg dl^{-1}, mean high-density lipoprotein (HDL) cholesterol of 51.5 ± 15.9 mg dl^{-1} and total cholesterol of 179.40 ± 35.4 mg dl^{-1}. Thirty-nine of the pool of one hundred were smokers. These data were acquired from July 2009 to December 2010.

12.2.2 Ultrasound image data acquisition

All the patients were scanned using an ultrasound scanner (model: Aplio XV, Aplio XG, Xario) equipped with a 7.5 MHz linear array transducer from Toshiba, Inc., Tokyo, Japan. The same sonographer (with 15 years of experience) scanned all the patients. The American Society of Echocardiography Carotid Intima–Media Thickness Task Force protocol was used and high-resolution images of the CCA were acquired. First, the subjects were examined in the supine position and the head was tilted backward. The probe first located the carotid arteries using transverse scans (perpendicular to the blood flow) and then the probe was rotated by 90° to acquire the longitudinal carotid ultrasound scans. Two views were collected: anterior and posterior walls. The sonographer also acquired internal carotid artery (ICA) and carotid bulbs scans in addition to CCA images in order to calculate the plaque score (PS). This study does not use PS measurements and is discussed elsewhere. This study underwent a full ethics review by the IRB of Toho University Hospital and written informed consent was provided by all the patients. The average resolution factor for carotid ultrasound scans was 0.0529 mm/pixel.

12.2.3 Sonographer's cIMT readings

These are the measurements taken by the sonographer who is present in the vascular ultrasound laboratory during the digital acquisition of the ultrasound scan of the patient's carotid artery. A sonographer is a registered vascular technologist (RVT) and has a background in vascular ultrasound and is qualified enough to measure the cIMT in carotid ultrasounds. The sonographer uses the software integrated with the ultrasound scanning device for measuring the cIMT. The sonographer places two points manually: one along the lumen–intima (LI) interface and the second along the media–adventitia (MA) interface. The LI point is the transition point when going from the lumen region to the intima region. The MA point is the transition point when going from the media region to the adventitia region. The software then processes these points to compute the distance between them, which is called the cIMT. The sonographer places these points visually by looking at the plaque distribution in the carotid B-mode ultrasound scans. It is important to note that the sonographer places these points manually and uses his/her experience and judgment when placing these points.

Since experience and judgment can be different between different sonographers, the cIMT measurement can also differ between sonographers. That is why sonographer readings have larger variability. For this reason, there is a clear motivation to design an automated cIMT measurement system. It is also important to note that sometimes it is the physician who takes these measurements if the sonographer is not present. Several countries follow their own methodologies for cIMT measurements due to direct costs and overheads [46]. For example, in some European countries (excluding the United Kingdom and Ireland), it is the physician who takes these cIMT measurements. This places fewer financial burdens on the hospital or clinic. In Asia (especially in India), it is the sonologist who takes these measurements. A sonologist, who has a medical degree, is qualified to take these measurements. Our ultimate goal is to collect these measurements, taken either by a sonographer or a sonologist or the physician. Here we call these measurements sonographer readings.

12.2.4 Manual cIMT readings

For a performance evaluation of the AtheroCloud™ software system, the gold standard was created by manually tracing the LI/MA interfaces for the distal wall of the carotid artery in the ultrasound scan. We used a commercial software package ImgTracer™ (courtesy of AtheroPoint™, Roseville, CA, USA) for manual tracing of LI/MA interfaces. The LI/MA interface is the border between the lumen–intima (LI) and media–adventitia (MA). The carotid ultrasound image shows the carotid artery with a lumen at the center and walls on both sides of the lumen region. These walls are called the near (proximal) and far (distal) walls of the carotid artery. The carotid artery wall is surrounded by the lumen region on one side and the adventitia region on the other side, while the wall consists of the intima and media regions. The interface between the lumen and intima walls is called the LI interface or LI border. The interface between the media region and adventitia region is the MA interface or MA border. Between the LI and MA interface are found the plaque or athero-sclerotic diseased components. The mean distance between the LI border and the MA border is the cIMT or plaque burden. The greater the plaque burden, the larger is the cIMT measurement, and the AtheroCloud™ software system allows us to measure this plaque burden. A research scholar (SKB, the second author of this chapter), currently a doctoral candidate in the field of atherosclerosis imaging, traced the IM and MA interfaces. SKB was trained under the guidance of JSS (principal investigator on this project and corresponding author for this chapter), who is an expert in vascular ultrasound imaging, with experience of 25 years in imaging sciences. The gold standard tracings were finally checked and endorsed by LS (the first author of this chapter), a neuroradiologist with 15 years of experience in radiology and the author of over 100 international journal articles [47] in carotid ultrasound and radiology.

A sample view of ImgTracer™ is shown in figure 12.2. The top yellow line indicates the LI and the bottom yellow line the MA interface. The tracing protocol was adopted for all 100 patients, consisting of a total of 200 carotid scans. ImgTracer™ software has been installed at several geographical locations around the world such as India (NIT-Raipur), Malaysia (UTM Razak School of Engineering and Advanced Technology), Italy (University of Cagliari, Italy), Croatia (Department of Radiology and Ultrasound, Zagreb) and the USA

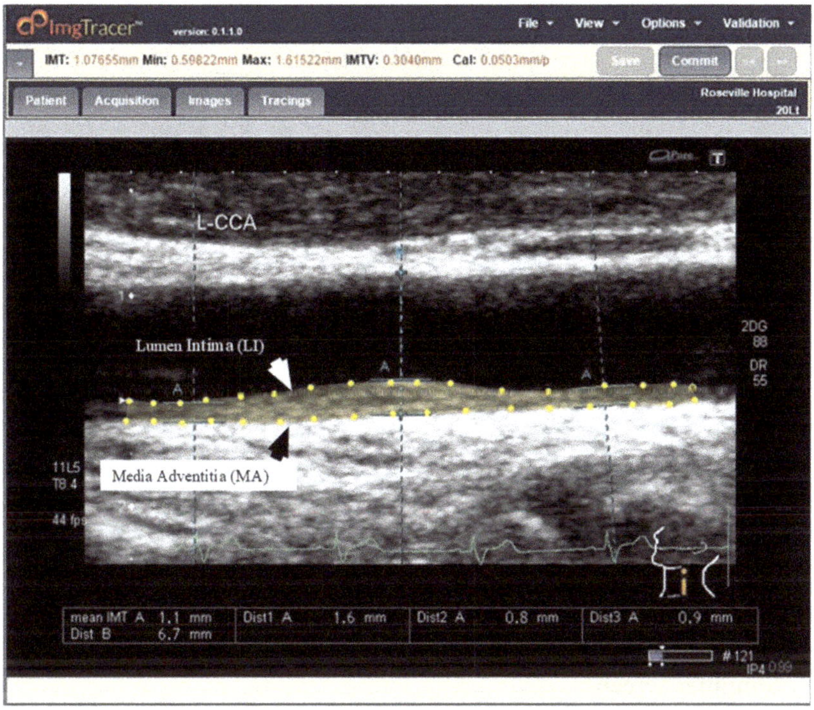

Figure 12.2. Manual tracings (yellow) of the carotid intima–media thickness region showing LI and MA borders using ImgTracer™. (Courtesy of AtheroPoint™, Roseville, CA, USA.)

(AtheroPoint, Roseville, CA), and has been successfully used for several anatomic applications.

12.3 Methodology and cloud-based workflow

AtheroCloud™ 1.0 (courtesy of AtheroPoint™, Roseville, CA, USA) is a cloud-based stroke monitoring software system which can be used in (a) completely automated or (b) user-interactive semi-automated modes for computing (i) intima–media thickness (IMT) and its variability (IMTV), (ii) lumen diameter (LD) and its variability (LDVar), and (iii) stenosis severity index (SSI) in carotid ultrasound scans.

12.3.1 Workflow architecture of the AtheroCloud™ 1.0 system

Even though there are automated desktop-based intelligent cIMT systems created by HSS (the principal investigator on this project) and his team [9, 11, 13, 14, 30, 48, 49], this study is the first of its kind in which cIMT is measured in carotid ultrasound scans through intelligent cloud-computing, with automated analysis occurring in the cloud-based settings. The workflow is shown in figure 12.3. It consists of a three-layer architecture:

(i) The *GUI layer*, where, the doctor can interact with the AtheroCloud™ software using a laptop or PC. This is mainly used for accessing ultrasound

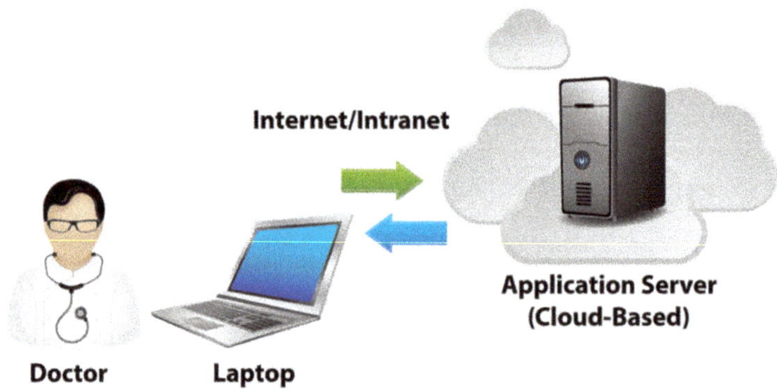

Figure 12.3. The workflow of AtheroCloud™ and its components. The tower represents a server in the cloud. The arrows represent the bidirectional flow of information. (Courtesy of AtheroPoint™, Roseville, CA, USA.)

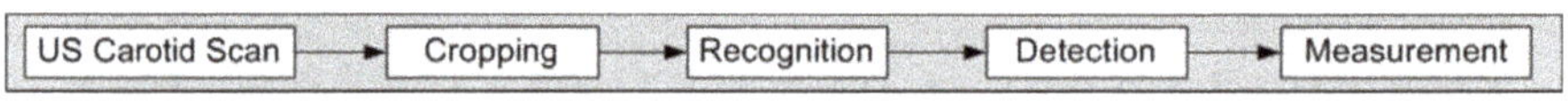

Figure 12.4. Block diagram for the overall engineering components of the design.

scans stored in the cloud-based server and displaying them on the local computer screen.

(ii) The *business logic layer*, which consists of scientific engines for measurement and is physically sitting in the cloud-based server. This layer receives the ultrasound scans, automatically computes the measurements and displays the measurements on the PC screen.

(iii) The *persistence or database layer*, is also present in the cloud-based application server and is used for the storage of digital measurements and images for later retrieval.

12.3.2 Engineering component design of the AtheroCloud™ 1.0 system

The main block diagram of the proposed system is shown in figure 12.4. The main components consist of (a) automated cropping, (b) the automated carotid artery recognition phase, (c) the automated LI/MA detection phase and (d) the automated cIMT measurement phase. Automated cropping is necessary to avoid interfering with the patient text information, any cardiac gating signals and peak systolic velocity waveforms [50, 51]. The second step consists of automated far wall recognition which is based on the hypothesis that far wall intensities are highest in the image [52]. This is combined with scale-space [13, 41, 53] for far wall region-of-interest (ROI) estimation all along the carotid artery. The detection step consists of LI/MA interface estimation using an edge operator [13, 41, 53]. The final LI/MA edges are then fed into the polyline distance method (PDM) for cIMT measurement (see appendix A) [39, 40].

12.3.3 General features of the AtheroCloud™ 1.0 system

AtheroCloud™ 1.0 helps in early diagnosis and monitoring of plaque build-up through its automated/semi-automated processing of ultrasound scans. The proposed system has the following main features: (i) the ability to measure cIMT in a reliable, accurate, reproducible and cost-effective manner; (ii) cloud-based cIMT/IMTV measurement of thin/thick carotid plaques in the Routine mode; (iii) cloud-based LD/LDVar/SSI measurement in a the Routine mode; (iv) fully automated or user-interactive (semi-automated by manually placing an ROI as a rectangular box); (v) the ability to monitor and compare measurement readings over follow-up time; (vi) the ability to interface with various commercial ultrasound scanners; (vii) the ability to import the following image formats: DICOM; JPEG, BMP, PNG, GIF and TIFF; (viii) an inbuilt database patient record system; (ix) reviewing of patient records/images/reports/; (x) the ability to e-mail a clinical report; (xi) instant screen/report printing capability; (xii) the ability to process a large number of ultrasound scans without human interaction for the Pharmaceutical Trials mode (batch-processing); (xiii) it can read carotid ultrasound image scans from a CD, local hard-drive, internal network server or external network cloud server. Overall, it provides a user-friendly means of saving, viewing, emailing and printing patient reports as well as carotid scans. After analyzing and processing carotid vascular scans, AtheroCloud™ 1.0 generates a PDF statistical report for each patient (one patient at a time) or produces a PDF statistical report for the Pharmaceutical Trial mode (consisting of cIMT readings taken from thousands of patients). Using the above features, AtheroCloud™ 1.0 can be adapted for advanced clinical applications.

12.3.4 Two application modes of AtheroCloud™: the Routine mode and Pharma mode

There are two major modes in which AtheroCloud™ can be used: (a) the Routine mode and (b) the Pharma Trial mode. In the Routine mode, the measurements are computed real-time during the patient's visit, one ultrasound scan at a time, and in the Pharma trial mode, the batch of carotid ultrasound scans are automatically processed in real-time one-by-one. Depending upon the physical space (gigabytes to terrabytes) and server RAM, the system can run large databases; however, we typically suggest up to a maximum of 10 000 images in the batch mode. An example of the Routine mode is shown in figure 12.5(a). Once the image is loaded in the Routine mode, with a click of the button 'Auto Trace', the LI/MA interface borders are computed and the IMT region representing the total plaque area is filled in with yellow (figure 12.5(a)). An example of the Pharma mode is shown in figure 12.5(b).

12.4 Results: measurements and visualization

12.4.1 Carotid intima–media thickness (cIMT) reading

There are two main factors which affect the speed of the system: (a) the size of the image to be processed in the cloud and (b) the downloading speed of the internet. For

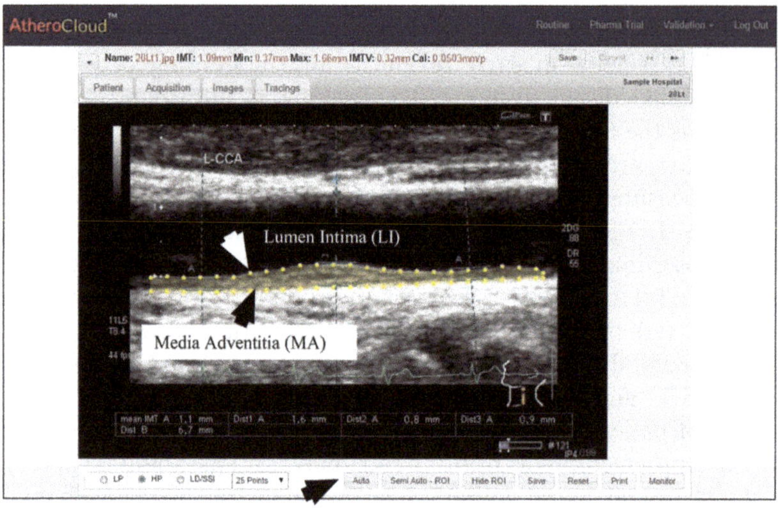

(a)

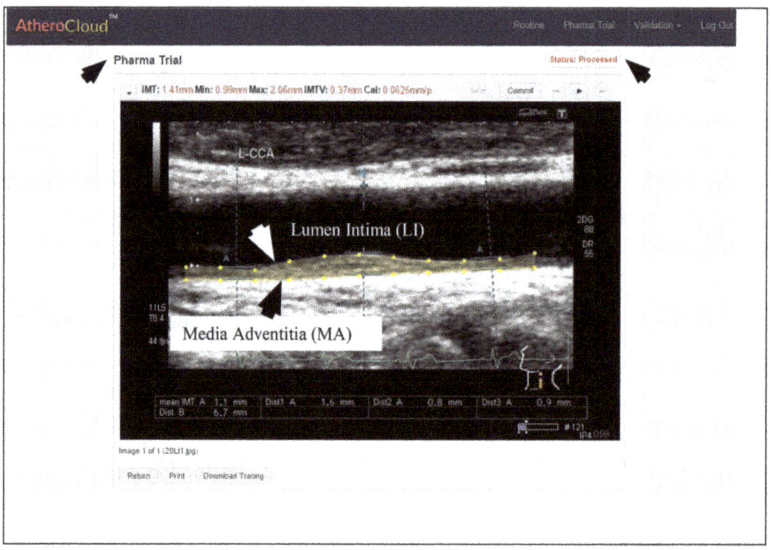

(b)

Figure 12.5. (a) Routine mode automated tracings (yellow) of the carotid intima–media thickness/variability region showing the LI and MA borders using AtheroCloud™. (b) Pharma Trial mode automated tracings (yellow) of the carotid intima–media thickness/variability region showing the LI and MA borders using AtheroCloud. A constant resolution factor of 0.0625 mm/pixel was adapted for this Pharma batch run. (Courtesy of AtheroPoint™, Roseville, CA, USA.)

factor (a), the size of the ultrasound image can vary from database to database. In our database, some images are smaller, e.g. 684 × 504 pixels, and took less than three seconds for downloading and processing, while for larger images, e.g. 1054 × 772 pixels, it took less than five seconds for downloading and processing. Our average scan dimension (W × H) over 200 images was 881 × 614 pixels. Our internet speed was

Table 12.1. cIMT using AtheroCloud™ (Routine mode versus Pharma Trial mode), sonographer readings and manual readings.

	AtheroCloud™ (mm)		Sonographer (mm)	Manual (mm)
Neck side	Routine mode	Pharma mode		
Left cIMT	0.87 ± 0.20	0.86 ± 0.20	0.90 ± 0.20	0.97 ± 0.26
Right cIMT	0.77 ± 0.20	0.77 ± 0.20	0.79 ± 0.20	0.89 ± 0.29

180 Mbps. The average time taken by our system is less than five seconds, which includes uploading the input ultrasound image to the cloud, processing the image in the cloud and displaying the result at the user's end.

Table 12.1 shows the mean and standard deviations of computed carotid intima–media thickness for 200 carotid scans using: (i) the automated AtheroCloud™ software (both in the Routine and Pharma Trial modes), (ii) sonographer readings and (iii) manual (gold standard) readings. Our observations show that the AtheroCloud™ mean cIMT readings for both the Routine and Pharma Trial modes were very similar. This clearly showed that AtheroCloud™ software can be used for clinical trials with very high reproducibility.

12.4.2 Display of LI/MA interfaces using AtheroCloud™ and manual methods

Using the 'Validation' button on the AtheroCloud™ front panel (top right corner), the user can upload the pair of LI/MA interfaces from AtheroCloud™ and corresponding manual tracings traced by the expert for comparison. Figure 12.6 shows LI/MA delineations using AtheroCloud™ software (solid line) and manual expert tracings (dotted line). As can be seen, the LI interface shows a bumper-to-bumper position with very slight deviations between AtheroCloud™ and manual tracings. A similar pattern can be seen for the MA interfaces. Cropped and zoomed images of AtheroCloud™ and the manual overlay image are shown in figure 12.7.

12.5 Performance evaluation of the AtheroCloud™ system

We evaluated the performance of the AtheroCloud™ system by computing a PoM that compares AtheroCloud™ readings against the manual (expert) readings. We used the polyline distance metric [39, 43] for evaluating the performance of the system. Details on the polyline distance metric can be found in appendix A. The following statistical analysis was performed between the three sets of readings (AtheroCloud™, sonographer and manual):

- PoM computation of (i) AtheroCloud™ and (ii) sonographer readings against manual.
- The CC among the three different methods.
- Bland–Altman plots among the three different methods.
- The CC between cIMT and the age of patients.

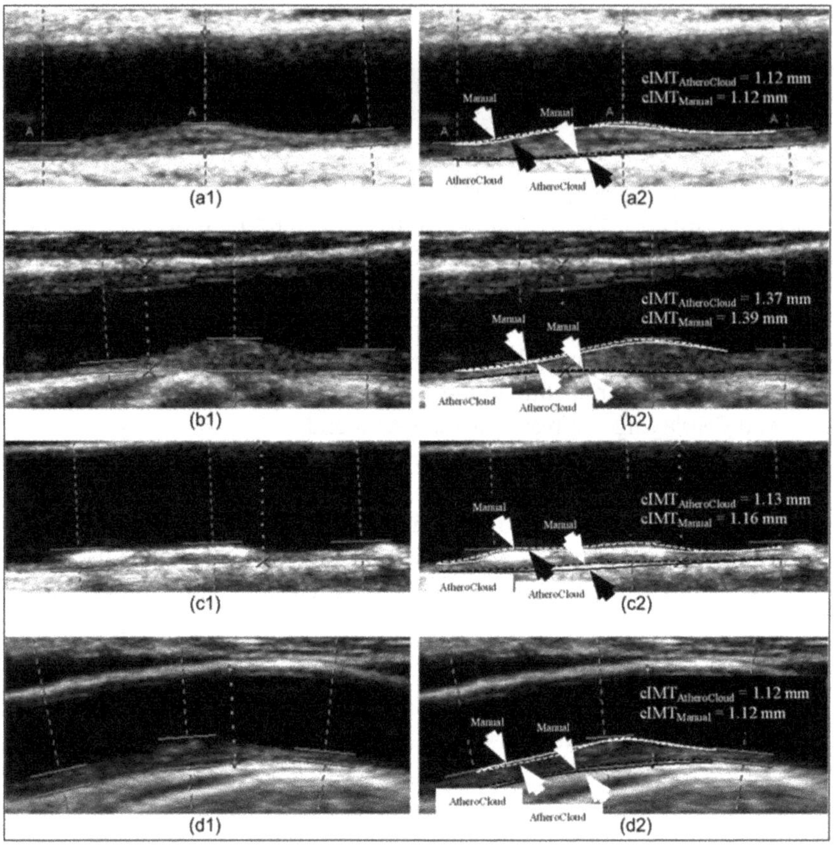

Figure 12.6. (a1), (b1), (c1) and (d1) original carotid artery images. (a2), (b2), (c2) and (d2) LI/MA overlays using AtheroCloud™ software (solid line) and manual tracings (dotted line), respectively. cIMT readings are the IMT values for AtheroCloud™ and manual tracings.

- Cumulative distribution of cIMT errors for AtheroCloud™ and sonographer readings.
- Statistical tests.

Once the AtheroCloud™ displays the final LI/MA borders, these borders undergo a three-step process. These processes are needed to match the final LI/MA borders from AtheroCloud™ with manual LI/MA borders traced by the physician. This is necessary for the performance evaluation of the system. The three-step process is as follows:

(i) *B-spline fitting*: We smooth the output results of the LI/MA borders using a B-spline technique. The LI/MA interfaces consist of 100 equal distance interpolated points after the B-spline smoothing of the LI/MA interfaces.

(ii) *Common support creation*: We ensure that the LI/MA automated boundaries and the LI/MA manual boundaries have the same starting and ending coordinates. For this, we apply a common support (the same length) on

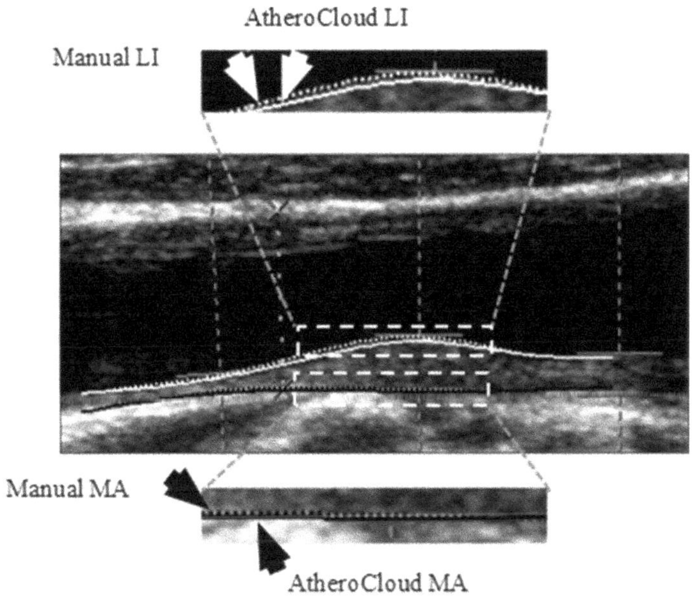

Figure 12.7. Cropped and zoomed images of AtheroCloud™ (solid line) and manual tracings (dotted line). LI—white; MA—black.

both the LI/MA boundaries. This ensures consistency between the measurements.

(iii) *Interpolation*: Finally, we interpolate the points so they are equidistant, i.e. the distance between the points is the same.

12.5.1 Precision-of-merit

The PoMs for AtheroCloud™ and sonographer readings were computed against the gold standard (manual readings). PoM computations were based on the basic concept of how close the AtheroCloud™ cIMT and sonographer cIMT readings are against the manual readings. cIMT was computed using the bidirectional concept of the PDM as shown by HSS [39, 43]. The final derivation of AtheroCloud™'s PoM is also shown in appendix A and is mathematically expressed as

$$\mathrm{PoM}_{\mathrm{AtheroCloud}}\,(\%) = 100 - \left[\left(\frac{|\overline{\mathrm{cIMT}}_{\mathrm{AtheroCloud}} - \overline{\mathrm{cIMT}}_{\mathrm{Manual}}|}{\overline{\mathrm{cIMT}}_{\mathrm{Manual}}}\right) * 100\right]. \tag{12.1}$$

Similarly, we can compute the sonographer's PoM as

$$\mathrm{PoM}_{\mathrm{Sono}}\,(\%) = 100 - \left[\left(\frac{|\overline{\mathrm{cIMT}}_{\mathrm{Sono}} - \overline{\mathrm{cIMT}}_{\mathrm{Manual}}|}{\overline{\mathrm{cIMT}}_{\mathrm{Manual}}}\right) * 100\right], \tag{12.2}$$

where $\overline{\mathrm{cIMT}}_{\mathrm{AtheroCloud}}$, $\overline{\mathrm{cIMT}}_{\mathrm{Manual}}$ and $\overline{\mathrm{cIMT}}_{\mathrm{Sono}}$ are the mean cIMTs using AtheroCloud™, manual and sonographer readings for the entire database as shown in equations (A.8) and (A.9). Note that the bars represent the absolute value.

Table 12.2. PoMs for left, right and combined cIMTs.

Parameters	Left cIMT	Right cIMT	Combined cIMT
AtheroCloud™ when compared against manual			
AtheroCloud™'s PoM	95.85%	97.24%	96.50%
Sonographer when compared against manual			
Sonographer's PoM	92.87%	87.31%	90.27%

Table 12.2 shows the PoMs between (i) AtheroCloud™ and manual and (ii) sonographer and manual for the (a) left, (b) right and (c) combined left and right cIMTs. We observe that the AtheroCloud™'s PoMs (95.85%, 97.24% and 96.50%) are much higher compared to the sonographer's PoMs (92.87%, 87.31% and 90.27%) for left cIMT, right cIMT and combined cIMT. The percentage improvements of PoMs for AtheroCloud™ over the sonographer were 2.98%, 9.93% and 6.23% for left, right and combined cIMTs. The PoMs between AtheroCloud™ and sonographer for the (a) left, (b) right and (c) combined left and right cIMTs are as shown in appendix B, table B1.

12.5.2 Coefficient of correlation between the three methods

The basic idea behind CC computation is to test the relationship and measure the strength of association between the two quantities. The corresponding CCs between these methods are shown in table 12.3. Our observations show a high degree of CC between AtheroCloud™ and manual (0.96 ($P < 0.0001$), 0.97 ($P < 0.0001$) and 0.97 ($P < 0.0001$)) for left, right and combined cIMTs, compared to sonographer versus manual (0.74 ($P < 0.0001$), 0.65 ($P < 0.0001$) and 0.69 ($P < 0.0001$)). The corresponding improvements in CC were 29.73%, 49.23% and 40.58%, respectively.

These CC scatter plots are shown in figure 12.8 between AtheroCloud™, sonographer and manual cIMT readings. There are three rows: Row 1 (a1 and a2) shows correlations between AtheroCloud™ and manual readings. Row 2 (b1 and b2) shows the correlations between sonographer and manual readings. Row 3 (c1 and c2) shows the correlations between the AtheroCloud™ and sonographer readings. The percentage improvements of CC for AtheroCloud™ over sonographer were 29.73%, 49.23% and 40.58% for the left, right and combined cIMTs. The CC between AtheroCloud™ and sonographer readings is as shown in appendix B, table B2.

12.5.3 Bland–Altman plots between the different methods

Bland–Altman plots show the average bias or the average of the differences between two readings. The bias can be in the positive difference direction or can be in the negative difference direction. Here, the differences between the two readings are plotted against the averages of the two readings. Three horizontal lines are drawn,

Table 12.3. CCs between the three methods for left, right and combined cIMTs.

Parameters	Left cIMT	Right cIMT	Combined cIMT
Method 1: AtheroCloud™ versus Manual			
CC	0.96	0.97	0.97
Method 2: Sonographer versus Manual			
CC	0.74	0.65	0.69

where the solid line represents the mean difference. The two dotted lines represent the limits of agreement, which are defined as the mean difference plus and minus 1.96 times the standard deviation of the differences. The average of the differences between two readings (i.e. average bias) can be higher in either the positive difference direction or the negative difference direction. The former represents that the first quantity readings are greater than the second quantity readings, and the latter represent that the first quantity readings are smaller than the second quantity readings.

The Bland–Altman plots of cIMT measurements using AtheroCloud™ software against (a) manual cIMT readings and (b) sonographer cIMT readings is shown in figure 12.9. This shows the average bias or the average of the differences between two cIMT readings. It can be observed that the bias is higher in the positive difference direction for AtheroCloud™ and manual reading. Higher bias in the positive difference direction shows that AtheroCloud™ cIMT readings are greater than the manual cIMT readings. We also observe that the bias is higher in the negative difference direction for AtheroCloud™ and sonographer cIMT measurements. Higher bias in the negative difference direction shows that AtheroCloud™ cIMT readings are smaller than the sonographer cIMT readings. The results show a high degree of agreement between AtheroCloud™ and manual readings compared to sonographer and manual cIMT readings.

12.5.4 Coefficient of correlation between age and cIMT

In this study, we have analyzed the relationship between age of the patient and cIMT using three different methods (AtheroCloud™, sonographer and manual). Figure 12.10 shows the scatter diagram showing a mild correlation between age and cIMT readings. Panels (a1), (b1) and (c1) show a correlation between age and left cIMT using the three methods and panels (a2), (b2) and (c2) show correlation between age and right cIMT using three methods, AtheroCloud™, manual and sonographer readings, respectively. The CC between age and left cIMT readings using AtheroCloud™, manual and sonographer readings were 0.27, 0.28 and 0.38, respectively. The correlation of age and right cIMT reading using AtheroCloud™, manual and sonographer readings were 0.30, 0.29 and 0.37, respectively. Thus, the CC was moderate and mild for both the left and right cIMTs, but right carotid was slightly higher compared to the left.

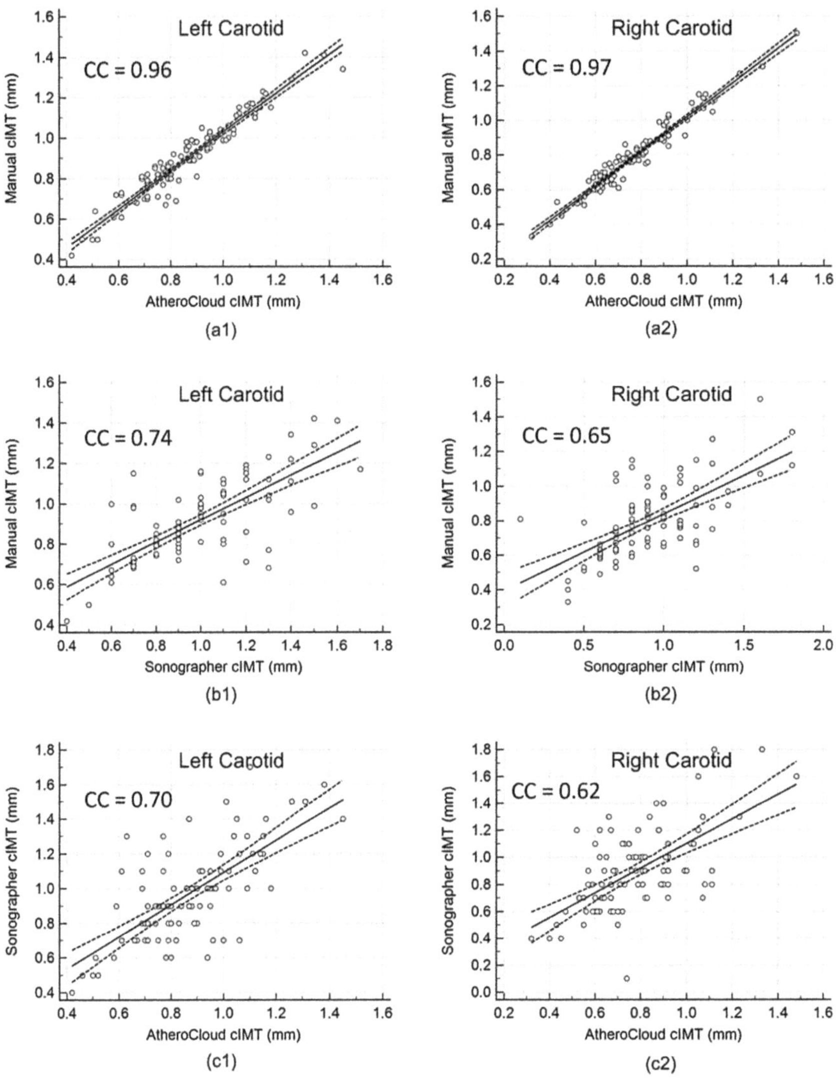

Figure 12.8. Scatter diagram showing a correlation between AtheroCloud, sonographer and manual cIMT readings. (a1), (b1) and (c1) show correlations between AtheroCloud™ and manual, sonographer and manual, and AtheroCloud™ and manual for left cIMT, and (a2), (b2) and (c2) show correlations for the above combinations for right cIMT readings, respectively.

12.5.5 Cumulative distribution of cIMT errors and LI/MA errors

The basic idea behind plotting cumulative distribution is to determine the percentage of the population that lies above (or below) a particular cIMT threshold value. The cumulative frequency is computed by adding each reading to the sum of its predecessor. Cumulative distribution plots show how well the system is behaving. The combined cumulative distributions of cIMT error curves for (i) AtheroCloud™ versus manual, (ii) sonographer versus manual, and (iii) AtheroCloud™ versus

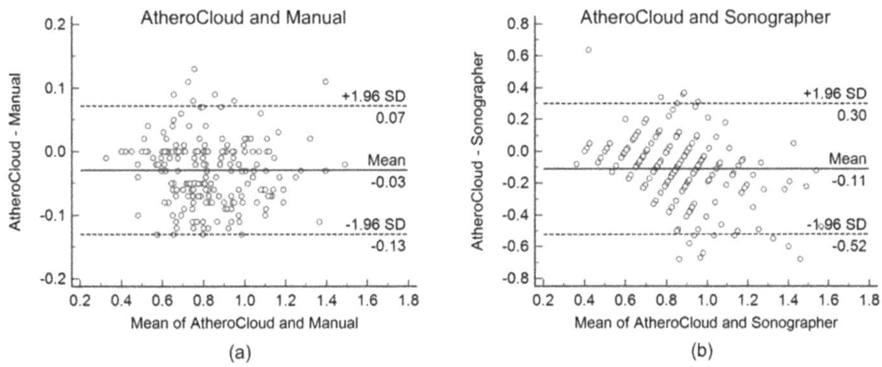

Figure 12.9. Bland–Altman plot of cIMT measurements using AtheroCloud™ software against (a) manual cIMT readings and (b) sonographer cIMT readings.

sonographer are shown in figure 12.11. Keeping the cIMT error threshold as 10% of the cIMT thickness (i.e. nearly 0.11 mm), we observed that 91.15%, 68.31% and 53.91% of the population met the error threshold criteria for three error curves. About 23% of the patients' cIMT was more accurate in AtheroCloud™ compared to the sonographer reading. The mean and standard deviation of the LI error and the MA error between AtheroCloud™ and manual readings were 0.0649 ± 0.0368 mm and 0.0673 ± 0.0362 mm, respectively.

12.5.6 Statistical tests

Statistical tests are performed to measure the reliability and stability of the system. It helps us to determine whether there is enough evidence to accept the null hypothesis. The null hypothesis is an assumption that the two readings are related to each other. All statistical analyses were performed using MedCalc software (Osteen, Belgium). The two-tailed *z*-test, chi-squared test and Mann–Whitney test with a standard normal distribution at the level of significance 0.05 were performed. The two-tailed *z*-test is generally used when there are more than 30 readings. The chi-squared test is used to determine whether there is a significant relationship between the two quantities. Finally, the Mann–Whitney test was used to identify the significance difference between the variables.

Table 12.4 shows the results of the two-tailed *z*-test, chi-squared test and Mann–Whitney test between AtheroCloud™ and manual for left (< 0.2888, < 0.0001 and = 0.1419) and right (< 0.4795, = 0.0002 and = 0.4321) cIMT, respectively. The results of the two-tailed *z*-test, chi-squared test and Mann–Whitney test between AtheroCloud™ and sonographer for left and right cIMT were (< 0.0023, < 0.0001 and = 0.0046) and (< 0.0001, < 0.0001 and = 0.0014), respectively. The negative *z*-score conveys that the corresponding raw result is below (less than) the mean. These statistical analyses were performed to demonstrate the positive relationships of AtheroCloud™ cIMT against manual and sonographer cIMT and were found to be statistically significant. The normality of each continuous variable group was further confirmed by the Kolmogorov–Smirnov (KS)-test.

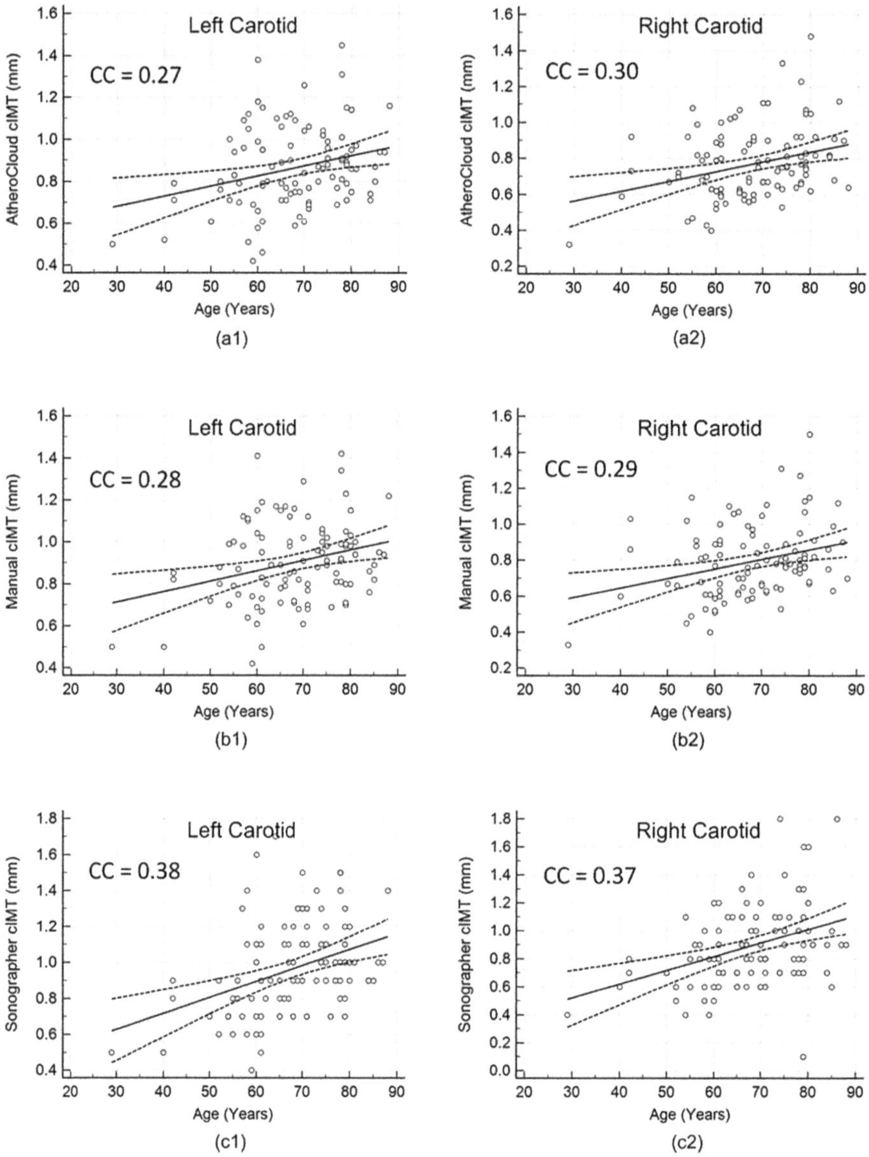

Figure 12.10. Scatter diagram showing a mild correlation between age and cIMT readings. Panels (a1), (b1) and (c1) show a correlation between age and left cIMT and panels (a2), (b2) and (c2) show a correlation between age and right cIMT using AtheroCloud™, manual and sonographer's readings, respectively.

12.5.7 Receiver operating characteristic (ROC)

The sensitivity and specificity are computed using the following four parameters: true positive (TP), true negative (TN), false positive (FP) and false negative (FN). TP is defined as the number of times cIMT correctly identified with respect to the manually computed cIMT for the cut-off risk threshold. FN is defined as the number

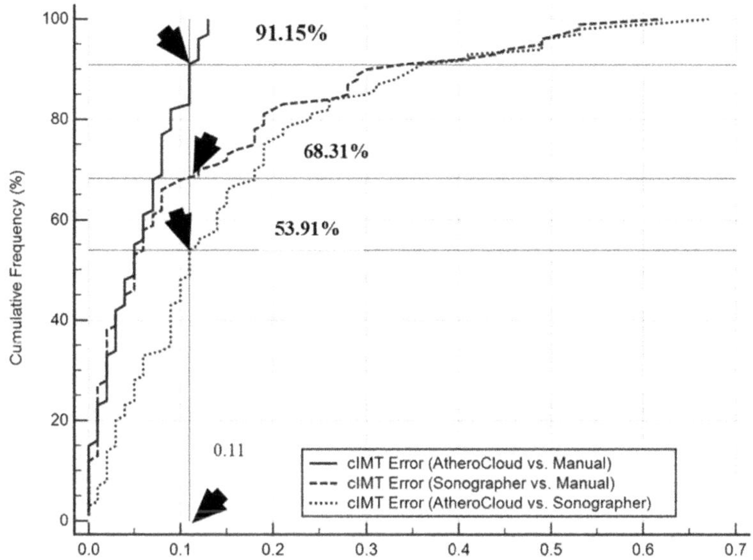

Figure 12.11. Combined cumulative distribution error curves for (i) AtheroCloud™ versus manual, (ii) sonographer versus manual and (iii) AtheroCloud™ versus sonographer.

Table 12.4. Statistical tests between AtheroCloud™, manual and sonographer cIMT readings.

	Two-tailed *z*-test		Chi-squared-test		Mann–Whitney
Combinations	*z*	*p*-value	Contingency coefficient	*p*-value	*p*-value
			Left cIMT		
AtheroCloud™ versus manual	−1.06	< 0.2888	0.984	< 0.0001	= 0.1419
Sonographer versus manual	−2.13	< 0.0328	0.950	< 0.0001	= 0.0976
			Right cIMT		
AtheroCloud™ versus manual	−0.71	< 0.4795	0.985	= 0.0002	= 0.4321
Sonographer versus manual	−2.84	< 0.0045	0.946	= 0.0002	= 0.0079

of times cIMT is incorrectly identified w.r.t the manually computed cIMT for the cut-off risk threshold. TN and FP are defined as the number of times cIMT is correctly or incorrectly identified for cut-off risk threshold, respectively. The sensitivity and specificity can be mathematically defined as

$$\text{Sensitivity} = \frac{\text{TP}}{(\text{TP} + \text{FN})} \text{ and Specificity} = \frac{\text{TN}}{(\text{TN} + \text{FP})}. \quad (12.3)$$

The ROC can be plotted by using two parameters: (i) the true positive rate (sensitivity) and (ii) the false positive rate (specificity). The area under the ROC curve (AUC) is the ability of the test to correctly classify readings into two diagnostic groups (diseased/normal). A higher AUC justifies the accuracy of the system. The ROC analysis was performed on the AtheroCloud™ and sonographer methods against the manual readings, as shown in figure 12.12.

As most of the previous clinical studies have shown that the cIMT cut-off risk threshold for cerebrovascular accident (stroke) or CVE (heart attack) is widely distributed, ranging from 0.7 mm [23] to 1.26 mm [28] with an average cut-off of 0.9 mm [25, 26], we, therefore, evaluate the AtheroCloud™ reading and sonographer's reading against the cIMT cut-off risk threshold of 0.9 mm. The difference in cIMT is due to variations in clinical demographics and focus of these studies. Clinical demographics include age, gender, ethnicity, body mass index, LDL, HA1c, the presence of CAD and family history for CVD. Using the cIMT cut-off risk threshold of 0.9 mm, the AUC for AtheroCloud™ and sonographer readings were: 0.99 and 0.81, respectively.

12.5.7.1 Operating point computation

Figure 12.13(a) and (b) shows the comparison plots of sensitivity and specificity for AtheroCloud™ and sonographer cIMT readings, respectively. These plots were computed by taking the manual cIMT readings with a cut-off of 0.9 mm. These were

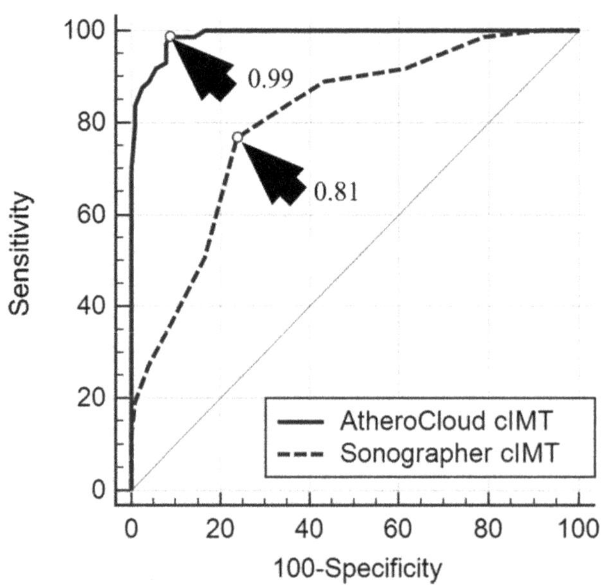

Figure 12.12. Receiver operating characteristic curve analysis for AtheroCloud™ versus sonographer cIMT readings. The AUCs are 0.99 and 0.81 for AtheroCloud™ and sonographer readings.

used to compute the operating point for both these methods. The operating point (also called equal error rate) is the point of maximum sensitivity and specificity for the system. Using the equal error rate concept, the operating point for AtheroCloud™ and sonographer cIMT readings were 0.83 mm and 0.9 mm, respectively. The corresponding specificity and sensitivity of AtheroCloud™ were 98.63% and 91.34%, while for the sonographer system they were 76.71% and 76.38%, respectively.

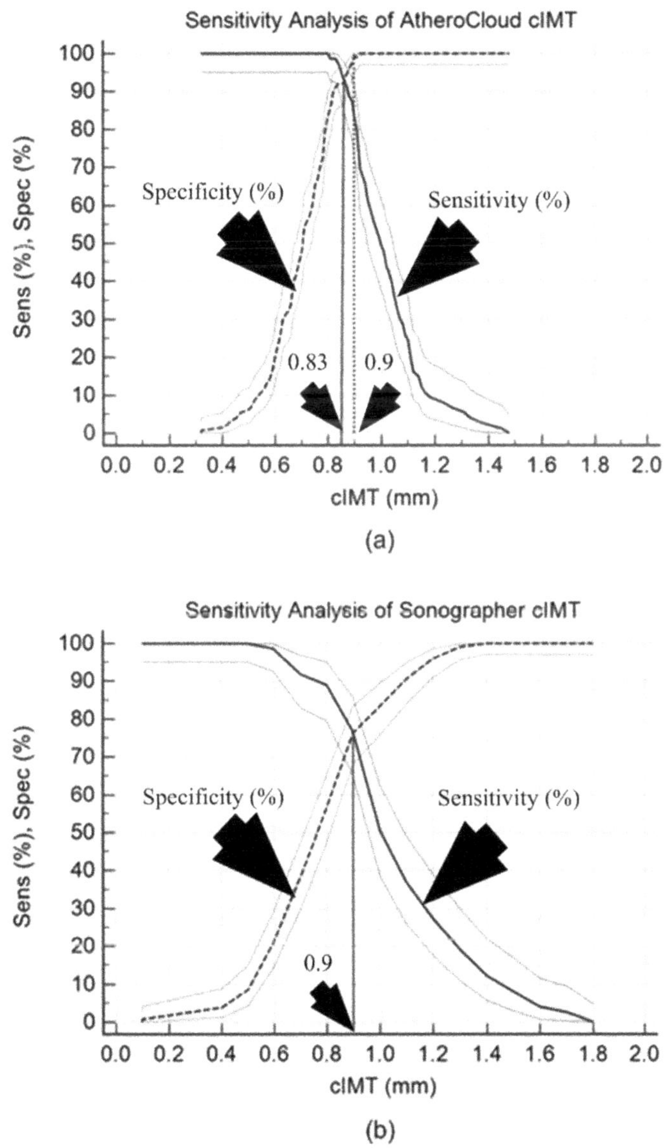

Figure 12.13. Sensitivity and specificity curves for (a) AtheroCloud™ and (b) sonographer cIMT and their respective operating points.

Figure 12.14(a) and (b) shows the interactive dot diagram for AtheroCloud™ and sonographer cIMT readings with reference to manual cIMT. An interactive dot diagram is a dual plot with a horizontal line showing the cut-off point with the best separation (minimum false negative and false positive results) between the two readings.

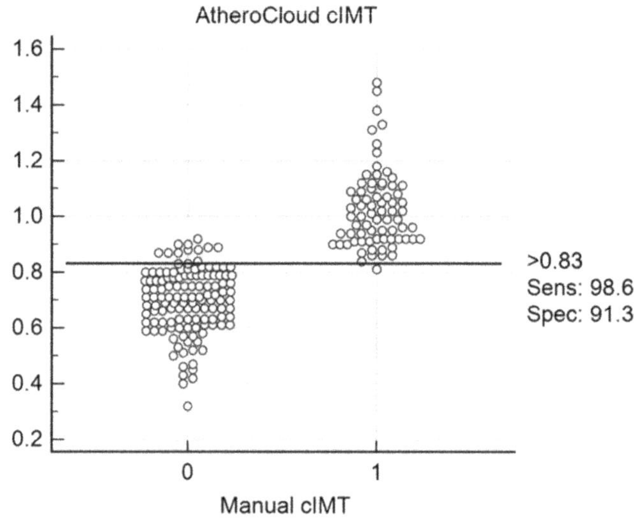

(a)

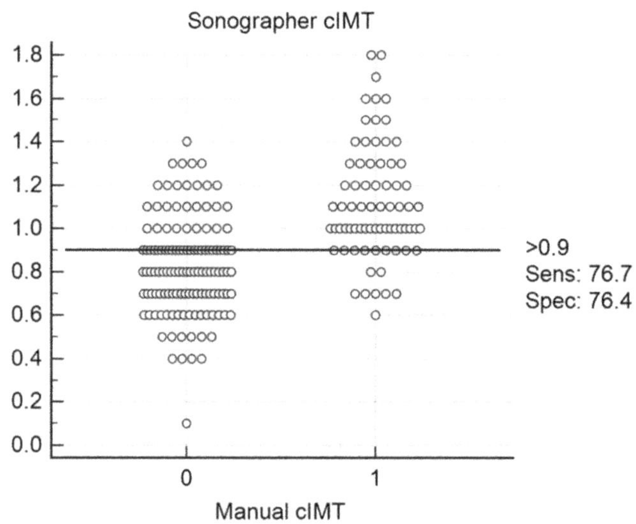

(b)

Figure 12.14. Interactive dot diagram for (a) AtheroCloud™ and (b) sonographer cIMT and their respective threshold, sensitivity and specificity. Classification of AtheroCloud and sonographer cIMT in high-risk and low-risk bins.

The data of the negative and positive groups are shown as dots on the two vertical axes. Figure 12.14(a) shows the AtheroCloud™'s two clusters corresponding to low- and high-risk represented by 0 and 1 in the plot with manual readings as a reference, with a cut-off of 0.83 mm. Figure 12.14(b) shows the sonographer's two clusters corresponding to low- and high-risk represented by 0 and 1 in the plot with manual reading as a reference, with a cut-off of 0.9 mm.

12.5.8 Risk stratification

Risk stratification is a tool to recognize high-risk patients for better management of carotid disease and stroke. It can identify and quantify differences and changes in the risk profiles of patients suffering from coronary artery disease [54]. In this study, we have used the conventional Framingham risk score (FRS) to stratify the population into low-, medium- and high-risk bins.

12.5.9 Framingham risk score

The role of the FRS is to identify the patient's chances of developing the cardiovascular disease in a specified period of time, typically between 10 to 30 years [55, 56]. Further, the FRS of the patient indicates if they are likely to benefit from risk prevention strategies such as early screening. The FRS has been slightly controversial because it does not take cIMT into account, but it has shown which individual patients are likely to benefit from which kinds of drugs.

A risk score is derived for each patient using the gender-specific prediction formulae proposed by Wilson [57], based on the following conventional cardiovascular risk factors: age, total cholesterol and HDL cholesterol, systolic blood pressure, diabetes and smoking status. The values adapted for these parameters were listed in the demographics section. For computing the FRS, we took all the parameters concerned except blood pressure, which was not available for all the patients during the retrospective study. At 10 years, the CHD risk for individuals with low Framingham risk is 10% or less, intermediate Framingham risk 10% to 20%, and high Framingham risk have 20% or more CHD risk. Previous studies [55] have shown that the FRS has been validated in the United States for both genders in both European Americans and African Americans. Even though there are studies which have claimed improvement via the FRS, but there is little evidence for improved prediction using the FRS [55]. We did not obtain any relationship between cIMT and FRS scores, but for the sake of relevance, we have computed FRS and given stratification ranges.

12.5.9.1 Risk stratification based on the FRS

Table 12.5 shows the 10 year mortality rate over the range of the FRS in both men and women. In men, 70.66%, 18.66% and 10.66% of the total population had FRS risk levels $<$ 10%, 10% to 19%, and $\geqslant$ 20%, respectively. For women, the entire population is under the 10% risk level.

Table 12.5. 10 year mortality rates in men and women by the FRS.

FRS	Men	Women
Low < 10%	14 (18.66%)	25 (100%)
Intermediate 10%–19%	53 (70.66%)	—
High ⩾ 20%	8 (10.66%)	—

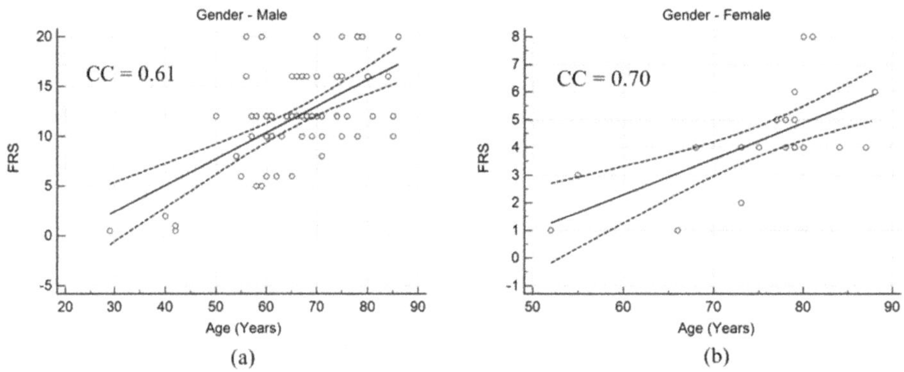

Figure 12.15. Scatter diagram showing a high correlation between age and FRS readings for (a) males and (b) females, respectively.

12.5.9.2 Age versus FRS

The scatter diagram of age versus FRS for males and females is shown in figure 12.15(a) and (b), respectively. We can observe a higher CC of female age with the FRS (0.70) compared to males (0.61). Although the CC was very high between age and FRS, there was no relationship between cIMT and FRS for this study.

12.6 Discussion

12.6.1 Our system

The main objectives of this pilot study were to:

- Propose (a) an automated and (b) user-interactive (semi-automated) cloud-based software system for cIMT measurements in ultrasound carotid scans using (i) Routine (single) mode and (ii) Pharmaceutical (batch) mode, intended for patient visit and clinical trials, respectively.
- Validate a cloud-based system against (a) manual tracings (gold standard) and (b) comparing Routine mode to Pharmaceutical mode for reproducibility evaluation for the entire database.
- Compare and contrast the cloud-based automated system against sonographer readings by performing exhaustive statistical analysis consisting of PoM, CC and ROC/AUC curve analysis compared to manual tracings.

- Benchmark the AtheroCloud™ software system for cIMT measurement against a desktop-based cIMT measurement system—AtheroEdge™ (AtheroPoint, Roseville, CA, USA) that has been previously benchmarked [33, 43–45].
- Establish the reliability of the AtheroCloud™ system through statistical tests such as the two-tailed paired Student's *t*-test, two-tailed *z*-test and Wilcoxon test.
- Risk assessment and stratification of the population using the FRS.
- Verification of the AtheroCloud™ software application against its functional requirements, such as automated cIMT report generation in the Routine and Pharmaceutical modes, and reproducibility between the Routine and Pharmaceutical modes.

This study shows the accuracy, reliability and functionality for the ultrasound-based AtheroCloud™ system, which can be adapted for multicenter clinical trials. Because our carotid scans did not have any bulbs, no reference point was chosen, and the cIMT was determined all along the carotid artery. We further demonstrated that mean cIMT readings were similar for the Routine mode and Pharmaceutical mode, even though the Pharmaceutical mode accepted the entire batch of carotid scans.

12.6.2 Benchmarking AtheroCloud™ against AtheroEdge™

As seen previously, our system measures cIMT, which is an automated, anytime–anywhere solution. We demonstrated that the AtheroCloud™ system is more accurate than sonographer readings. The system was capable of measuring cIMT ranging up to a 2.0–2.5 mm thickness (heavy plaque in the distal wall) based on advanced scale-space methods as developed by HSS's team [3, 11, 13, 54, 58–60]. In this study, we have compared our proposed AtheroCloud™ system against AtheroEdge™—a desktop-based commercial software (courtesy of AtheroPoint, Roseville, CA, USA). The results from a sample Pharmaceutical mode run are shown in figure 12.16.

We ran the same database pool using the AtheroEdge™ system and compared the results against the AtheroCloud™ system. The results can be seen in table 12.6. Column 'A' shows the output for the proposed AtheroCloud™ system and column 'B' shows the commercial desktop system AtheroEdge™. As shown in the table, the Pharma modes for cloud-based versus desktop-based showed nearly similar results: 0.86 ± 0.20 mm versus 0.88 ± 0.20 mm for left cIMT, and 0.77 ± 0.20 mm versus 0.80 ± 0.20 mm for right cIMT, respectively. There was a difference of 2.27% for the left artery and 3.75% for the right artery. Typically, a 5% error rule is adapted for regulatory settings and we showed that our system qualified under that benchmarking requirement. Furthermore, we showed that the results were reproducible. We matched our Pharmaceutical electronic batch reports between the AtheroCloud™ and AtheroEdge™ systems for all the patient ultrasound scans. The two-tailed paired Student's *t*-test, two-tailed *z*-test and Wilcoxon test demonstrated consistency

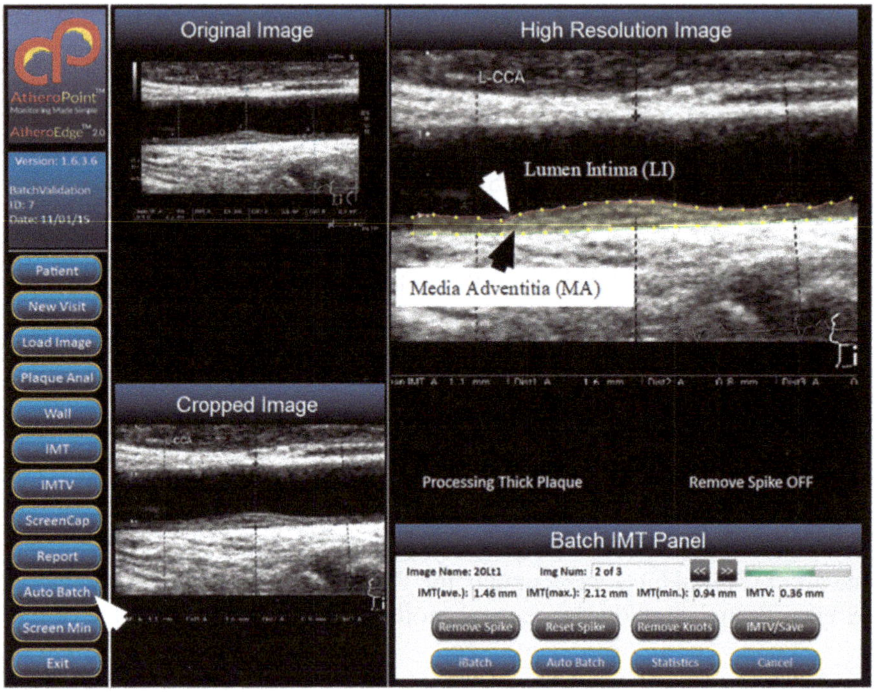

Figure 12.16. Pharmaceutical Trial mode automated tracings (yellow) of the carotid intima–media thickness region showing LI in red and MA in green using AtheroEdge™ software. (Courtesy of AtheroPoint™, Roseville, CA, USA.)

Table 12.6. Benchmarking of AtheroCloud™ (Routine and Pharmaceutical mode) against AtheroEdge™ (desktop-based system).

	AtheroCloud™ (cloud-based)		AtheroEdge™ (desktop-based)
Neck side	Routine mode	Pharma mode	Pharma mode
Left cIMT (mm)	0.87 ± 0.20	0.86 ± 0.20	0.88 ± 0.20
Right cIMT (mm)	0.77 ± 0.20	0.77 ± 0.20	0.80 ± 0.20

and reliability, making it the most practical and clinically adaptable system. To our knowledge, there is no existing pilot or commercial study of cloud-based cIMT measurements for stroke/cardiovascular applications, so we have used desktop-based comparisons.

12.6.3 A brief survey of previous techniques

In past years, many studies have proposed techniques to measure IMT in carotid ultrasound scans. In 2007, Delsanto *et al* [61] proposed a Completely User-independent Layer EXtraction algorithm based on signal approach (CULEXsa) for carotid artery segmentation in 2D ultrasound images. The snake-based technique was used and a segmentation error of less than one pixel was achieved. However, the algorithm suffers from noise and image artefacts.

In 2010, Molinari *et al* [13] proposed another automated algorithm called Completely Automated Layered EXtraction technique based on integrated approach (CALEXia) for IMT measurement and tried to eliminate the limitations of their previous work. CALEXia was based on an integrated approach of feature extraction, line fitting and classification. The IMT measurement error was equal to 0.87 ± 0.56 pixels for CALEXia and 0.12 ± 0.14 pixels for CULEXsa. Despite its limited performance in segmenting the LI interface, CALEXia outperformed CULEXsa in segmenting the MA interface. CALEXia also performed correctly in 95% of the tested images (against 92% of CULEXsa). The CALEXia technique was further validated by the same group on a large database of 200 images [14, 62]. The study proved CALEXia to be a robust technique for computer-based automated tracing of the CCA in longitudinal B-mode carotid ultrasound images. However, more work is needed to increase the performance of the IMT measurement.

In 2011, the groups led by HSS proposed a series of automated IMT measurement techniques, namely: (i) completely automated robust edge snipper (CARES) [63], (ii) the inter-greedy (IG) method [59], (iii) completed automated local statistics-based first-order absolute moment (CLASFOAM) [48], (iv) ultrasound double line extraction system using edge flow (CAUDLES-EF) [64] and (v) carotid artery intima layer regional segmentation (CAILRS) [38].

In the first technique, i.e. CARES [63], the authors used an integrated approach of intelligent image feature extraction and line fitting for automatically locating the carotid artery in the image frame. A Gaussian edge operator was then used for extracting the wall interfaces. Using 300 carotid ultrasound images, the study showed an IMT bias of 0.032 ± 0.141 mm. As compared to the IMT bias of their previously published method CALEXia, CARES improved the IMT accuracy by 67%, while increasing the standard deviation by 3%.

To remove their bias errors, in their second technique, i.e. the IG method [59], an IG approach was applied to the LI and MA boundaries traced by the three image segmentation techniques (namely, CALEXia, CULEXsa and Watershed transform (WS)). The validation was done against manual tracings on a large dataset of 200 images. With the IG method, an IMT error of 0.74 ± 0.75 pixels was observed, which showed an improvement of 44% against their previous proposed CULEXsa algorithm.

The third technique, i.e. CLASFOAM [48], was developed to overcome the limitations of a previously developed snake-based technique. The CALSFOAM technique consisted of two stages. Stage-I performs automatic recognition of the carotid artery system by using local statistics and by automatically tracing the profile of the distal adventitia in an image frame. Stage-II builds an ROI for distal wall segmentation by using a first-order absolute moment (FOAM) technique. CALSFOAM was validated against manual tracings on a 300 image multi-institutional dataset and showed an IMT measurement bias of 0.125 ± 0.103 mm. By fusing the boundaries from the two techniques, the bias was further reduced to 0.074 ± 0.068 mm, which demonstrated that the two techniques could be considered as complementary.

The fourth technique, i.e. CAUDLES-EF [64], can extract the far double line (i.e.LI and MA) in the carotid artery using an edge flow technique based on directional probability maps using the attributes of intensity and texture. CAUDLES-EF was validated against manual tracings on a large dataset of 300 longitudinal B-mode carotid images with normal and pathologic arteries. In comparison to previous techniques such as CULEXsa and CALEXia, CAUDLES-EF performed the best with a high figure-of-merit (FoM) of 94.8%.

The fifth technique, i.e. CAILRS [38], can automatically segment the intima layer of the far wall based on mean shift classification. CAILRS was validated against manual tracings on a large dataset of 300 longitudinal B-mode carotid images. CAILRS was benchmarked against a semi-automatic technique based on an FOAM edge operator. The proposed technique showed an IMT bias of −0.035 ± 0.186 mm. In comparison to all the previous techniques, such as CULEXsa, CALEXia, CALSFOAM and CAUDLES-EF, CAILRS showed the highest FoM of 95.6% compared to the other proposed techniques.

In 2012, Molinari *et al* proposed two more automated IMT measurement techniques: Completely Automated Multi-resolution Edge Snapper (CAMES) [53] and Carotid Measurement Using Dual Snakes (CMUDS) [65]. The first technique, CAMES [53], consists of two stages. Stage one consists of automated carotid artery recognition based on a combination of scale-space and statistical classification in the multi-resolution framework, and stage two targets IMT measurement by performing an automated segmentation of LI and MA interfaces for the far (distal) wall. By carrying out a study on 365 B-mode longitudinal carotid images, the study found an 8.4% increase in the FoM compared to their previous technique CALEXia. The study concluded that CAMES was a suitable and a validated clinical tool for automating and improving cIMT measurement in multicenter large clinical trials.

The second technique, CMUDS [65], used a snake-based approach for estimating the LI and MA borders. The technique used a novel first-order absolute moment-based external energy, which provides stable deformation. The dual snakes evolve simultaneously and are forced to maintain a regularized distance to prevent collapsing or bleeding. By carrying out a study on 665 B-mode longitudinal carotid images, the study produced a very high FoM of 98.4%. Wilcoxon and Fisher's test further proved its accuracy, making this system adaptable for large multi-center studies.

In 2013, Saba *et al* proposed the automated IMT measurement technique CARES 3.0 [66]. CARES 3.0 is an upgrade of CARES, proposed previously by Molinari *et al* [63] in 2011. After automated localization of the carotid artery, the LI/MA segmentation followed four stages: stage 1 consisted of the creation of the guided zone (i.e. ROI); in stage 2, edge enhancement was performed using the FOAM operator; stage 3 performed a heuristic search for locating the LI/MA peaks; finally, in stage 4, LI/MA regularization was performed. In a study on 250 patients, the results showed 80% of the images as having an IMT measurement bias ranging between −50% and +50%. The results outperformed previous CARES releases and showed high accuracy and reproducibility for IMT measurement.

A few months later, the same group [43] performed intra- and inter-observer variability analysis and computed the measurement error of their recently proposed completely automated IMT measurement software AtheroEdge™. The study was carried out on 200 carotid ultrasound images acquired from 50 asymptotic women patients. The intra- and inter-observer variability was tested using three readings. The measurement errors of AtheroEdge™ for the automated and semi-automated methods were −0.0004 ± 0.158 mm and 0.008 ± 0.157 mm, respectively, compared to the mean value of three expert readers. The FoMs were 99.9% and 98.9% compared to the mean value of the three expert readers and 99.8% and 99.9% compared to a commercial ultrasound scanner (using the automated and semi-automated method, respectively). The intra-class CC of the three independent users was 0.98. The proposed AtheroEdge™ software showed a diagnostic accuracy of 90%, proving its application in processing large datasets for CCA and avoiding subjectivity in cIMT measurements.

These systems were mainly research-based and did not allow for cross-institutional clinical trials [38, 43, 48, 53, 58, 59, 62–65]. To allow for the use of cIMT measurements to occur across institutions in a reproducible fashion, improving the uniformity and reliability of cIMT is critical. Therefore, we propose the use of cloud-based technology in order to allow for cross-institutional participation. The use of information technology to support clinical services is a major driver for the push to include cloud-based solutions in healthcare. Mobile or hand-held machines, such as the iPhone and iPad, have been rapidly accepted in many countries as point-of-care solutions, providing access to healthcare data and statistics in ways that were not previously conceivable [60]. Smartphones with faster processors, improved memory and smaller batteries, in concert with highly efficient operating systems, are affecting our personal and work environments [67]. The use of these pervasive technologies in healthcare provides an anytime–anywhere solution so patients and healthcare providers can both benefit from better atherosclerosis disease management.

12.6.4 A note on PoM, cross-correlation and ROC analysis

In this study, we computed the PoM for AtheroCloud™ and sonographer cIMT readings. The PoM computes the closeness of AtheroCloud™ and sonographer cIMT readings against the manual cIMT. Tables B3 and B4 clearly revealed the percentage improvement of the PoM and CC of AtheroCloud™ over sonographer readings, as shown in the appendix B. This proved our hypothesis that the error between the automated AtheroCloud™ software system and manual tracings (gold standard) was lower compared to the error between the sonographer readings and manual tracings. In this study, we also analyzed the correlation between age and left and right cIMT readings computed using AtheroCloud™, manually and by a sonographer. The CC is moderate and mild which showed an increase in the risk of a CAD with advancement in age. The combined cumulative distribution error curves of cIMT for (i) AtheroCloud™ versus manual, (ii) sonographer versus manual and

(iii) AtheroCloud™ versus sonographer are shown in figure 12.11. We observed that about 23% of the patients' cIMT was calculated more accurately in AtheroCloud™ compared to sonographer readings. The AUCs for the AtheroCloud™ and sonographer were 0.99 and 0.81, respectively, which further confirms the accuracy and reliability of our proposed system. Even though the automated system performs better compared to the manual readings and sonographer readings, there are subtle factors which we did not consider while designing this study. These include studying the effect of lighting conditions during the manual tracings [68], the attention of the sonographer while taking his/her readings, such as his/her mood, experience recording sonographer readings and type of image format (DICOM versus JPEG), as this can affect performance [69]. This is beyond the scope of this pilot study. We have, however, adapted a standardized software (ImgTracer™, AtheroPoint, Roseville, CA, USA), which has been applied to several studies in medical imaging [70–75].

12.6.5 Risk stratification

In the current analysis, we showed the risk stratification using the FRS. A risk score was derived for each patient using the gender-specific prediction formulae proposed by Wilson [57] based on the following standard conventional cardiovascular risk factors. Using the above technique, we stratified the population in low-, medium- and high-risk bins.

Table B5 clearly shows the percentage improvement of cIMT for left and right cIMTs for the cloud-based (AtheroCloud™) over the desktop-based (AtheroEdge™) system, as shown in appendix B. The percentage differences of AtheroCloud™ to AtheroEdge™ were 2.27% and 3.75% for left and right cIMTs, respectively.

12.6.6 Strengths, weaknesses and extensions

The proposed automated cloud-based system can be a very valuable tool for multi-center clinical trials and useful in the Routine mode to interface with OEM machines for cIMT computation. The proposed system is reliable, accurate, reproducible, cost-effective and fast (less than five seconds per image). The system is fully automated and can fall back on a user-interactive solution. Our pilot design has a multi-tenancy paradigm; hence multiple centers can use it at the same time. Further, the cloud servers can be changed to elastic, and therefore it is scalable depending upon usage. It can not only accept images from various ultrasound scanners, but also in various image formats. The system automatically computes the carotid SSI and the design has an inbuilt database of patient record systems that can be shared electronically or printed. This pilot study was performed in a private cloud, but can run in available public clouds such as IBM, Amazon or Hewlett Packard (HP). Batch-processing further improves the processing speed and provides a reproducible feature needed for pharmaceutical trials and can be used as a teaching tool. Thus, the proposed system is a fully automated 24/7 system (anytime–anywhere solution) with multiple features that bring more user-friendliness compared to a sonographer's manual methods. Even though the proposed system is fully automated and very fast, it offers certain challenges and limitations:

(a) The processing speed of AtheroCloud™ depends on the speed of the WIFI or land-line connection. If the internet speed is slow, it can be challenging for the physician to load imaging and process images.
(b) The cloud's cost can also increase over time, but as cloud-based technologies evolve, we expect the systems to become more economical [76] for hospital and clinic-based settings.

Finally, since our local server is Windows-based, all the encryption is performed using Microsoft bit blocker device encryption and these details are outside the scope of this pilot study. All the transfer and storage is performed by the Microsoft server. This is a pilot research study, so no cost analysis was attempted. This is being adopted as a service model and it can be used in a service setting. Current reports are produced in PDF, Word or Excel-sheet formats. It can be converted to HTML format (H7 format) for universal usage. Under the information technology framework, more work can be accomplished as part of future research studies, but the current results are truly encouraging.

12.7 Conclusion

We presented AtheroCloud™—a completely automated, cloud-based, point-of-care system for ultrasound carotid intima–media thickness measurement. AtheroCloud™ cIMT readings were compared against sonographer readings and showed superior performance. AtheroCloud™ showed its usability in the Routine and Pharmaceutical modes when benchmarking against the desktop-based AtheroEdge™ (AtheroPoint™, Roseville, CA) system, which was previously benchmarked against a Siemens system. Comprehensive statistical analyses were performed demonstrating its reliability. Although more tests need to be performed for this pilot study, current results show that the system can be adopted in the clinical setting for the clinical Routine mode or multicenter Pharmaceutical Trial mode.

Acknowledgments

Reprinted from Saba L, Banchhor S K, Suri H S, Londhe N D, Araki T, Ikeda N, Viskovic K, Shafiquc S, Laird J R, Gupta A, Nicolaidcs A and Suri J S 2016 Accurate cloud-based smart IMT measurement, its validation and stroke risk stratification in carotid ultrasound: a web-based point-of care tool for multicenter clinical trial *Comput. Biol. Med.* **75** 217–34, with permission from Elsevier.

Funding

This research did not receive any specific grant from funding agencies in the public, commercial, or not-for-profit sectors.

Conflicts of interest

The authors declare no conflict of interest.

Appendix A Polyline distance metric and precision-of-merit for AtheroCloud™ cIMT measurements

This section presents a brief derivation for the computation of the PoM for AtheroCloud™ cIMT measurements. Section A.1 presents the mathematical derivation for the polyline distance method (PDM) used for the measurement of AtheroCloud™ cIMT [39, 40] and section A.2 presents the derivation of the PoM [63].

A.1. Polyline distance metric

The PDM is used to measure the cIMT. It measures the changes of the contours of the far wall LI interface and MA interface. Let the first contour LI be denoted by C_1 and a reference point on this contour be (p_0, q_0). Let the second contour MA be denoted by C_2 and the two consecutive points on C_2 be (p_1, q_1) and (p_2, q_2), forming a line segment s. Next $d(v, s)$ is obtained, which is the distance between the reference point $v(p_0, q_0)$ on C_1 and the line segment formed by the two points on C_2. Let the distances between the reference point (p_0, q_0) and the two consecutive points be d_1 and d_2. Let λ be the distance of the reference point v towards the line segment s. The perpendicular distance between the line segment s and the reference point v is given by $d^{\perp}$. Using the calculus, one can derive the value of λ and $d^{\perp}$ as follows:

$$\lambda = \frac{(q_2 - q_1)(q_0 - q_1) + (p_2 - p_1)(p_0 - p_1)}{(p_2 - p_1)^2 + (q_2 - q_1)^2} \tag{A.1}$$

$$d^{\perp} = \frac{(q_2 - q_1)(p_1 - p_0) + (p_2 - p_1)(q_0 - q_1)}{\sqrt{(p_2 - p_1)^2 + (q_2 - q_1)^2}}. \tag{A.2}$$

The distance $d(v, s)$ between the vertex v and the line segment s can be mathematically given as

$$d(v, s) = \begin{cases} \min\{d_1, d_2\} & \lambda < 0, \lambda > 1 \\ |d^{\perp}| & 0 \leqslant \lambda \leqslant 1 \end{cases}. \tag{A.3}$$

The process to obtain $d(v, s)$ is repeated for the rest of the points of the contour C_1 and is given by

$$d(C_1, C_2) = \sum_{i=1}^{N} d(v_i, C_2), \tag{A.4}$$

where n is the number of points in the contour C_1, and S_{C2} is the segment on contour C_2. Second, the algorithm above is repeated where C_2 now becomes the reference contour and C_1 becomes the segment contour S_{C1}. The reverse can be represented by $d(C_2, C_1)$. Lastly, combining both $d(C_1, C_2)$ and $d(C_2, C_1)$ will yield the equation below which is the PDM:

$$D_S(C_1 : C_2) = \frac{d(C_1, C_2) + d(C_2, C_1)}{(\#\ \text{vertices}\ \epsilon C_1 + \#\ \text{vertices}\ \epsilon C_2)}. \tag{A.5}$$

In this study, we have used the term PDM which is a more convenient expression for equation (A.5). We will use equation (A.5) for computation of AtheroCloud™ cIMT and PoM in section A.2.

A.2 Precision-of-merit for AtheroCloud™ cIMT measurements

Given that $LI_{AtheroCloud}$ and $MA_{AtheroCloud}$ are the interfaces computed using the AtheroCloud™ automated method, we compute the AtheroCloud™ cIMT using the PDM equation (A.5) and it is given as

$$\text{cIMT}_{\text{AtheroCloud}} = \text{PDM}\ (\text{LI}_{\text{AtheroCloud}},\ \text{MA}_{\text{AtheroCloud}}). \tag{A.6}$$

Similarly, using the definition of PDM, we can compute the cIMT measurements using manual tracings using equation (A.5), given as

$$\text{cIMT}_{\text{Manual}} = \text{PDM}\ (\text{LI}_{\text{Manual}},\ \text{MA}_{\text{Manual}}). \tag{A.7}$$

Let AtheroCloud™ cIMT_i be the cIMT value automatically computed by the proposed system, AtheroCloud™, on the ith image of the database of N patients. If a database of N images is considered, then the overall mean AtheroCloud™ cIMT estimate can be defined as

$$\overline{\text{cIMT}}_{\text{AtheroCloud}} = \frac{1}{N}\sum_{i=1}^{N}\text{cIMT}_{\text{AtheroCloud}_i}. \tag{A.8}$$

Correspondingly, if manual cIMT_i is the cIMT value computed from the radiologist's traced manual measurements, the mean manual cIMT for the manual is given as

$$\overline{\text{cIMT}}_{\text{Manual}} = \frac{1}{N}\sum_{i=1}^{N}\text{cIMT}_{\text{Manual}_i}. \tag{A.9}$$

The overall system's performance can be computed using PoM in percentage as

$$\text{PoM}_{\text{AtheroCloud}}\ (\%) = 100 - \left[\left(\frac{|\overline{\text{cIMT}}_{\text{AtheroCloud}} - \overline{\text{cIMT}}_{\text{Manual}}|}{\overline{\text{cIMT}}_{\text{Manual}}}\right) * 100\right]. \tag{A.10}$$

Appendix B Tables

Table B1. PoM for left, right and combined cIMTs.

Parameters	Left cIMT	Right cIMT	Combined cIMT
AtheroCloud™ when compared to sonographer			
AtheroCloud™ PoM	89.47%	86.29%	87.94%

Table B2. CC between the three methods for left, right and combined cIMTs.

Parameters	Left cIMT	Right cIMT	Combined cIMT
Method 3: AtheroCloud™ and sonographer			
CC	0.70	0.62	0.66

Table B3. Percentage improvement of PoM for left, right and combined cIMTs.

% Improvement of AtheroCloud™ over sonographer			
Parameter	Left cIMT	Right cIMT	Combined cIMT
PoM	2.98%	9.93%	6.23%

Table B4. Percentage improvement in CC for left, right and combined cIMTs.

% Improvement of AtheroCloud™ over sonographer			
Parameter	Left cIMT	Right cIMT	Combined cIMT
CC	29.73%	49.23%	40.58%

Table B5. Percentage difference between AtheroCloud™ and AtheroEdge™ systems for left cIMT and right cIMT.

% Difference between AtheroCloud (cloud-based) and AtheroEdge™ (desktop-based)		
Parameter	Left cIMT	Right cIMT
cIMT	2.27%	3.75%

References

[1] WHO CVD website, http://who.int/mediacentre/factsheets/fs317/en/ (Accessed: 20 Sep 2018)

[2] Leeder S, Raymond H and Greenberg H 2004 *A Race Against Time: The Challenge of Cardiovascular Disease in Developing Countries* (New York: Columbia University)

[3] Araki T *et al* 2014 Link between automated coronary calcium volumes from intravascular ultrasound to automated carotid IMT from B-mode ultrasound in coronary artery disease population *Int. Angiol.* **33** 392–403

[4] Ross R 1995 Cell biology of atherosclerosis *Annu. Rev. Physiol.* **57** 791–804

[5] Libby P, Ridker P M and Hansson G K 2011 Progress and challenges in translating the biology of atherosclerosis *Nature* **473** 317–25

[6] Sobieszczyk P and Beckman J 2006 Carotid artery disease *Circulation* **114** 244–7

[7] Arroyo L H and Lee R T 1999 Mechanisms of plaque rupture: mechanical and biologic interactions *Cardiovasc. Res.* **41** 369–75

[8] Araki T *et al* 2015 A comparative approach of four different image registration techniques for quantitative assessment of coronary artery calcium lesions using intravascular ultrasound *Comput. Methods Programs Biomed.* **118** 158–72

[9] Suri J S, Kathuria C and Molinari F 2010 *Atherosclerosis Disease Management* (Berlin: Springer)

[10] Saba S, Pedro and Suri J S 2012 *Advanced Atherosclerosis in Diagnosis and Therapy using MR, CT, Ultrasound* (Berlin: Springer)

[11] Saba L *et al* 2013 Association of automated carotid IMT measurement and HbA1c in Japanese patients with coronary artery disease *Diabetes Res. Clin. Pract.* **100** 348–53

[12] Sanches M J, Laine A and Suri J S 2011 *Advanced Ultrasound Imaging* (Berlin: Springer)

[13] Molinari F, Zeng G and Suri J S 2010 Intima–media thickness: setting a standard for a completely automated method of ultrasound measurement *IEEE Trans. Ultrason. Ferroelectr. Freq. Control* **57** 1112–24

[14] Molinari F, Zeng G and Suri J S 2010 A state of the art review on intima–media thickness (IMT) measurement and wall segmentation techniques for carotid ultrasound *Comput. Methods Programs Biomed.* **100** 201–21

[15] Suri J S and Laxminarayan S 2003 *Angiography and Plaque Imaging: Advanced Segmentation Techniques* (Boca Raton, FL: CRC Press)

[16] Amato M *et al* 2007 Carotid intima–media thickness by B-mode ultrasound as surrogate of coronary atherosclerosis: correlation with quantitative coronary angiography and coronary intravascular ultrasound findings *Eur. Heart J.* **28** 2094–101

[17] Bots M L *et al* 2007 Carotid intima–media thickness and coronary atherosclerosis: weak or strong relations? *Eur. Heart J.* **28** 398–406

[18] Polak J F *et al* 2010 Associations of carotid artery intima–media thickness (IMT) with risk factors and prevalent cardiovascular disease comparison of mean common carotid artery IMT with maximum internal carotid artery IMT *J. Ultrasound Med.* **29** 1759–68

[19] Polak J F *et al* 2011 Associations of edge-detected and manual-traced common carotid intima–media thickness measurements with Framingham risk factors the multi-ethnic study of atherosclerosis *Stroke* **42** 1912–6

[20] Ikeda N *et al* 2014 Ankle–brachial index and its link to automated carotid ultrasound measurement of intima–media thickness variability in 500 Japanese coronary artery disease patients *Curr. Atheroscler. Rep.* **16** 1–8

[21] Liao H, Hong H and Wang H 2014 Relation between carotid stenosis severity, plaque echogenicity characteristics and IMT assessed by ultrasound in the community population of Southern China *Open Access Library J.* **2** e2014
[22] Nezu T *et al* 2015 Carotid intima–media thickness for atherosclerosis *J. Atheroscler. Thromb.* **23** 18–31
[23] Lacroix P A, Aboyans V, Espaliat E and Cornu E 2003 Carotid intima–media thickness as predictor of secondary events after coronary angioplasty *Int. Angiol.* **22** 279
[24] Geroulakos G A, O'gorman D J, Kalodiki E, Sheridan D J and Nicolaides A N 1994 The carotid intima–media thickness as a marker of the presence of severe symptomatic coronary artery disease *Eur. Heart J.* **15** 781–5
[25] Ikeda N *et al* 2013 Impact of carotid artery ultrasound and ankle–brachial index on prediction of severity of SYNTAX score *Circulation* **77** 712–6
[26] Araki T *et al* 2015 Shape-based approach for coronary calcium lesion volume measurement on intravascular ultrasound imaging and its association with carotid intima–media thickness *J. Ultrasound Med.* **34** 469–82
[27] Amato M, Montorsi P, Ravani A, Oldani E, Galli S, Ravagnani P M and Baldassarre D 2007 Carotid intima–media thickness by B-mode ultrasound as surrogate of coronary atherosclerosis: correlation with quantitative coronary angiography and coronary intravascular ultrasound findings *Eur. Heart J.* **28** 2094–101
[28] Elias-Smale S E *et al* 2012 Carotid intima–media thickness in cardiovascular risk stratification of older people: the Rotterdam Study *Eur. J. Prev. Cardiol.* **19** 698–705
[29] Ikeda N *et al* 2015 Improve the correlation between the carotid and coronary atherosclerosis SYNTAX score using automated ultrasound carotid bulb plaque IMT measurement *Ultrasound Med. Biol.* **41** 1247–62
[30] Molinari F *et al* 2012 Ultrasound IMT measurement on a multi-ethnic and multi-institutional database: our review and experience using four fully automated and one semi-automated methods *Comput. Methods Programs Biomed.* **108** 946–60
[31] Sharma A M *et al* 2015 A review on carotid ultrasound atherosclerotic tissue characterization and stroke risk stratification in machine learning framework *Curr. Atheroscler. Rep.* **17** 1–13
[32] Saba L *et al* 2016 Carotid inter-adventitial diameter is more strongly related to plaque score than lumen diameter: an automated and first ultrasound study in Japanese diabetic cohort *J. Clin. Ultrasound* **44** 210–20
[33] Molinari F, Zeng G and Suri J S 2010 Intima–media thickness: setting a standard for completely automated method for ultrasound *IEEE Trans. Ultrason. Ferroelectr. Freq. Control* **57** 1112–24
[34] McCloskey K *et al* 2014 Reproducibility of aortic intima–media thickness in infants using edge-detection software and manual caliper measurements *Cardiovasc. Ultrasound* **12** 18
[35] Sicari R *et al* 2011 The use of pocket-size imaging devices: a position statement of the European Association of Echocardiography *Eur. J. Echocardiogr.* **12** 85–7
[36] Switzer J A, Levine S R and Hess D C 2009 Telestroke 10 years later—'telestroke 2.0' *Cerebrovasc. Dis.* **28** 323–30
[37] Acharya R U *et al* 2011 *Distributed Diagnosis and Home Healthcare (D2H2)* (Valencia, CA: American Scientific)
[38] Meiburger K M *et al* 2011 Automated carotid artery intima layer regional segmentation *Phys. Med. Biol.* **56** 4073–90

[39] Suri J S, Haralick R M and Sheehan F H 2000 Greedy algorithm for error correction in automatically produced boundaries from low contrast ventriculograms *Pattern Anal. Appl.* **3** 39–60
[40] Saba L *et al* 2012 What is the correct distance measurement metric when measuring carotid ultrasound intima–media thickness automatically? *Int. Angiol.* **31** 483–9
[41] Molinari F *et al* 2012 Carotid artery recognition system: a comparison of three automated paradigms for ultrasound images *Med. Phys.* **39** 378–91
[42] Saba L *et al* 2012 Comparison between manual and automated analysis for the quantification of carotid wall by using sonography. a validation study with CT *Eur. J. Radiol.* **81** 911–8
[43] Saba L *et al* 2013 Inter-and intra-observer variability analysis of completely automated cIMT measurement software (AtheroEdge™) and its benchmarking against commercial ultrasound scanner and expert readers *Comput. Biol. Med.* **43** 1261–72
[44] Molinari F *et al* 2012 Automated carotid IMT measurement and its validation in low contrast ultrasound database of 885 patient Indian population epidemiological study: results of AtheroEdge™ software *Int. Angiol.* **31** 42–53
[45] AtheroEdge 510(K) clearance for desktop application: http://accessdata.fda.gov/cdrh_docs/pdf12/K122022.pdf (Accessed: 20 Sep 2018)
[46] Hertzberg B S *et al* 2000 Physician training requirements in sonography: how many cases are needed for competence? *Am. J. Roentgenol.* **174** 1221–7
[47] BioMed Central: http://nvijournal.biomedcentral.com/ (Accessed: 1 June 2016)
[48] Molinari F *et al* 2011 CALSFOAM-completed automated local statistics based first order absolute moment' for carotid wall recognition, segmentation and IMT measurement: validation and benchmarking on a 300 patient database *Int. Angiol.* **30** 227–41
[49] Saba L *et al* 2014 *Multi-Modality Atherosclerosis Imaging and Diagnosis* (New York: Springer)
[50] Mari G *et al* 2005 Middle cerebral artery peak systolic velocity technique and variability *J. Ultrasound Med.* **24** 425–30
[51] Molinari F *et al* 2009 Automated computer-based tracings (ACT) in logitudinal 2-D ultrasound imaging using different scanners *J. Mech. Med. Biol.* **9** 481–505
[52] Molinari F *et al* 2012 Hypothesis validation of far-wall brightness in carotid-artery ultrasound for feature-based IMT measurement using a combination of level-set segmentation and registration *IEEE Trans. Instrum. Meas.* **61** 1054–63
[53] Molinari F *et al* 2012 Completely automated multiresolution edge snapper—a new technique for an accurate carotid ultrasound IMT measurement: clinical validation and benchmarking on a multi-institutional database *IEEE Trans. Image Process.* **21** 1211–22
[54] Chhabra B, Kiran S and Thakur A 2002 Risk stratification in anaesthesia practice *Indian J. Anaesth.* **46** 347
[55] D'Agostino R B *et al* 2008 General cardiovascular risk profile for use in primary care the Framingham Heart Study *Circulation* **117** 743–53
[56] Tzoulaki I, Liberopoulos G and Ioannidis J P 2009 Assessment of claims of improved prediction beyond the Framingham risk score *J. Am. Med. Assoc.* **302** 2345–52
[57] Wilson P W *et al* 1998 Prediction of coronary heart disease using risk factor categories *Circulation* **97** 1837–47
[58] Saba L *et al* 2013 Automated analysis of intima–media thickness analysis and performance of CARES 3.0 *J. Ultrasound Med.* **32** 1127–35

[59] Molinari F, Zeng G and Suri J S 2011 Inter-greedy technique for fusion of different segmentation strategies leading to high-performance carotid IMT measurement in ultrasound images *J. Med. Syst.* **5** 905–19

[60] Franko O I and Tirrell T F 2012 Smartphone app use among medical providers in ACGME training programs *J. Med. Syst.* **36** 3135–9

[61] Delsanto S, Molinari F, Giustetto P, Liboni W, Badalamenti S and Suri J S 2007 Characterization of a completely user-independent algorithm for carotid artery segmentation in 2-D ultrasound images *IEEE Trans. Instrum. Meas.* **56** 1265–74

[62] Molinari F, Zeng G and Suri J S 2010 An integrated approach to computer-based automated tracing and its validation for 200 common carotid arterial wall ultrasound images a new technique *J. Ultrasound Med.* **29** 399–418

[63] Molinari F *et al* 2011 Completely automated robust edge snapper for carotid ultrasound IMT measurement on a multi-institutional database of 300 images *Med. Biol. Eng. Comput.* **49** 935–45

[64] Molinari F *et al* 2011 CAUDLES-EF: carotid automated ultrasound double line extraction system using edge flow *J. Digital Imaging* **24** 1059–77

[65] Molinari F *et al* 2012 Fully automated dual-snake formulation for carotid intima–media thickness measurement a new approach *J. Ultrasound Med.* **31** 1123–36

[66] Saba L *et al* 2013 Automated analysis of intima–media thickness: analysis and performance of CARES 3.0 *J. Ultrasound Med.* **32** 1127–35

[67] Ozdalga E, Ozdalga A and Ahuja N 2012 The smartphone in medicine: a review of current and potential use among physicians and students *J. Med. Internet Res.* **14** e128

[68] Suri J *et al* 2005 Image quality assessment via segmentation of breast lesion in x-ray and ultrasound phantom images from Fischer's full field digital mammography and ultrasound (FFDMUS) system *Technol. Cancer Res. Treat.* **4** 83–92

[69] Kim S W *et al* 2014 DICOM-based intravascular ultrasound signal intensity analysis. Echoplaque medical imaging bench study *Coron. Artery Dis.* **25** 236–41

[70] Noor N M *et al* 2015 Automatic lung segmentation using control feedback system: morphology and texture paradigm *J. Med. Syst.* **39** 1–18

[71] Araki T *et al* 2015 A new method for IVUS-based coronary artery disease risk stratification: a link between coronary and carotid ultrasound plaque burdens *Comput. Methods Programs Biomed.* **124** 161–79

[72] Araki T *et al* 2016 Reliable and accurate calcium volume measurement in coronary artery using intravascular ultrasound videos *J. Med. Syst.* **40** 1–20

[73] Saba L *et al* 2011 Evaluation of carotid wall thickness by using computed tomography and semiautomated ultrasonographic software *J. Vasc. Ultrasound* **35** 136–42

[74] Saba L *et al* 2012 Analysis of carotid artery plaque and wall boundaries on CT images by using a semi-automatic method based on level set model *Neuroradiology* **54** 1207–14

[75] Saba L *et al* 2013 Semiautomated and automated algorithms for analysis of the carotid artery wall on computed tomography and sonography a correlation study *J. Ultrasound Med.* **32** 665–74

[76] Suri J S *et al* 2005 Economic impact of telemedicine: a survey *Stud. Health Technol. Inf.* **114** 140–56

IOP Publishing

Vascular and Intravascular Imaging Trends, Analysis, and Challenges, Volume 1
Stent applications
Petia Radeva and Jasjit S Suri

Chapter 13

Stroke risk stratification and its validation using ultrasonic echolucent carotid wall plaque morphology: a machine learning paradigm

Tadashi Araki, Pankaj K Jain, Harman S Suri, Narendra D Londhe, Nobutaka Ikeda, Ayman El-Baz, Vimal K Shrivastava, Luca Saba, Andrew Nicolaides, Shoaib Shafique, John R Laird, Ajay Gupta and Jasjit S Suri

Stroke risk stratification based on grayscale morphology of the ultrasound carotid wall has recently been shown to have promise in the classification of high-risk versus low-risk plaques or symptomatic versus asymptomatic plaques. In previous studies, this stratification has been mainly based on analysis of the far wall of the carotid artery. Due to the multifocal nature of atherosclerotic disease, plaque growth is not restricted to the far wall alone. This chapter presents a new approach for stroke risk assessment by integrating assessment of both the near and far walls of the carotid artery using grayscale morphology of the plaque. Further, this chapter presents a scientific validation system for stroke risk assessment. Both these innovations have never been presented before.

The methodology consists of an automated segmentation system of the near wall and far wall regions in grayscale carotid B-mode ultrasound scans. Sixteen grayscale texture features are computed and fed into the machine learning system. The training system utilizes the lumen diameter to create ground truth labels for the stratification of stroke risk. A cross-validation procedure is adapted in order to obtain the machine learning testing classification accuracy through the use of three sets of partition protocols: *K*5, *K*10 and Jack Knife.

The mean classification accuracies over all sets of partition protocols for the automated system in the far and near walls are 95.08% and 93.47%, respectively. The corresponding accuracies for the manual system are 94.06% and 92.02%, respectively. The precisions-of-merit (PoMs) of the automated machine learning system compared to the manual risk assessment system are 98.05% and 97.53% for the far and near walls, respectively. The receiver operating characteristic (ROC) of the risk assessment system for the far and near walls is close to 1.0, demonstrating high accuracy.

13.1 Introduction

Stroke is the fifth leading cause of death in the United States. On average, someone in the United States has a stroke every 40 s [1]. The WHO estimates that these cerebrovascular accidents (CVA), or strokes, account for the loss of 6.7 million lives per year [2]. One of the leading causes of these strokes is carotid artery disease (CAD) [3–5], which occurs when the carotid arteries become blocked (so called 'stenosis'). When carotid artery stenosis occurs, there is a risk that oxygenated blood may not be available to the brain because of either reduced perfusion pressure from the narrowed carotid artery or because of a rupture plaque that blocks a downstream blood vessel in the brain. This stenosis of the carotid arteries, as depicted in figure 13.1, is most commonly caused by atherosclerosis [6]. Atherosclerosis is caused by to the accumulation of fatty deposits known as plaque along the innermost layer of the arteries (causing stenosis), where blood normally flows.

13.1.1 Small changes in the wall leading to cIMT

The biology of atherosclerotic disease leads to the formation of different plaque components in the carotid arterial wall over time [6]. An atherosclerotic plaque has

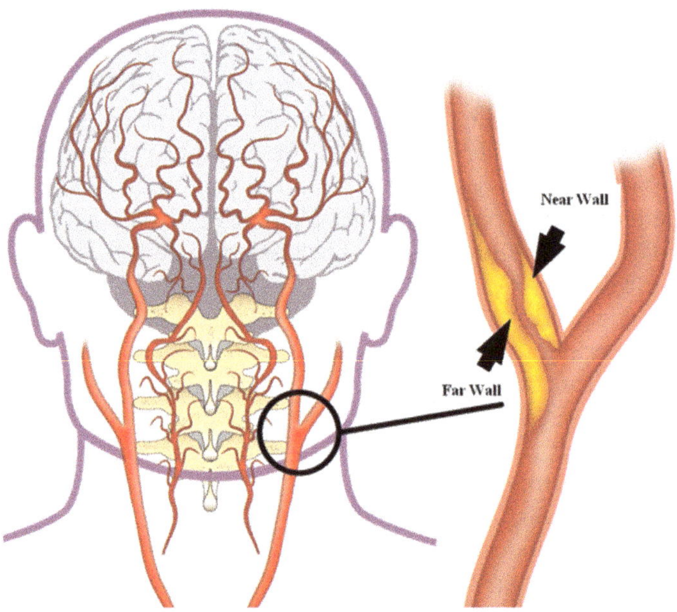

Figure 13.1. Carotid anatomy (left) and carotid atherosclerotic plaque formation in the near and far walls (right).

multiple components such as plaque hemorrhage (PH), thrombus (T), lipids, necrotic cap thickness (NCT), intima thickness, calcium, fibrosis cap (FC) and smooth muscle cells (SMCs) [7, 8]. There are two biological changes emerging out of this formation: (a) small changes in the intima and media walls [9] and (b) aggressive changes in the arterial wall leading to stenosis [10]. These small changes in the walls of the carotid artery bring an increase in thickness, which is measured as the carotid intima–media thickness (cIMT). Scientists have used *c*IMT as a biomarker for predicting the occurrence of major adverse cardiovascular events [11, 12]. Several studies have shown a relationship between varying *c*IMT thresholds and cardiovascular disease (CVD) [13–15]: (cIMT > 0.8 mm) [10], (cIMT > 0.9 mm) [13, 14], (cIMT > 1.1 mm) [16], (cIMT> 1.15 mm) [17] and (cIMT > 1.26 mm) [18].

13.1.2 The role of the lumen diameter

Multifocal and aggressive changes in the arterial wall cause a drastic change in the lumen diameter (LD), and are referred to as stenosis. Previous research [12, 19] has shown a link between LD and CVE. In 2011, Polak *et al* [20] hypothesized that an increase in the internal diameter of the common carotid artery (CCA), also known as the LD, is associated with age, gender and echocardiographically estimated left ventricular (LV) mass. Recent studies have shown that the carotid arterial diameters also have a better predictive power for CAD [11, 12, 21–23]. We infer that LD offers a method for characterization of high and low stroke risk [24–27]. It is important to note here that these measurements are of great value and must be calculated without subjectivity, and further can be utilized as a building block for risk assessment based on machine learning.

13.1.3 The role of grayscale morphological-based tissue characterization

As plaque matures with age in a carotid artery, the number of plaque components increases in the plaque [28]. This is shown to change the echolucency in ultrasound scans [29]. These plaques can be symptomatic or asymptomatic [30–32]. In general, studies have shown that symptomatic plaques may be predominantly hypo-echoic in nature, while asymptomatic plaques are less bright and relatively hyper-echoic, although there is significant variability across individual patients [29]. Due to the multifocal nature of the disease, it has been seen that hypo-echoic plaque regions can be surrounded by hyper-echoic regions [33]. It is therefore challenging to characterize the plaque visually and thus it is necessary to have a morphological-based tissue characterization protocol for stroke risk assessment. We assume that the plaque components in ultrasound scans can be used to assess the risk based on tissue morphology, along with the carotid LD measurements, which can act as a label for high or low risk. This can be accomplished using machine learning and this study adapts such a model. In order to classify the risk posed by different levels of plaque build-up in the carotid artery, a technique of tissue characterization is used which qualitatively analyzes the different statistical features that compose the plaque in the carotid artery [34–38]. Note that the risk assessment based on LD alone is not sufficient. This is because the grayscale information corresponding to different plaques (such as lipids, macrophages, fibro fatty tissue and calcium) in the wall region is not utilized during the risk assessment [39–41].

13.1.4 The importance of near wall and tissue characterization

The study of ultrasound tissue characterization relies on the results from B-mode ultrasound [9] in order to characterize the difference between high- and low-risk patients based on the values of statistical features [42]. This process is repeated in the near wall, far wall and combined wall of the carotid artery in order to determine a holistic method of risk assessment, while at the same time comparing the error obtained from two different places of interaction within an ultrasound image. This is of unique value because the near wall of the carotid artery is thought to be of little historical importance [14] in risk assessment and is thus the main contribution of this study. The reason for this is the low intensity contained in ultrasound images corresponding to the near wall. However, as there is an equal likelihood for the development of plaque build-up on this side of the carotid artery, this current study aims to develop a machine learning based stroke risk assessment system (sRAS) so that the visual (manual) error from the low intensity of the near wall does not affect the reliability of the overall results.

13.1.5 A sRAS for the near and far walls using a machine learning paradigm

The machine learning approach [39] adapted in this study aims to provide a more comprehensive solution to the problems in manual risk assessment, in particular when the combined grayscale wall (near and far) of the carotid artery ultrasound scan is taken into consideration. By first segmenting the desired wall region in ultrasound scans, then extracting its grayscale features along with measurements of LD, we were able to train the machine learning system and obtain the high- and low-risk coefficients [43]. This information was then given to the system along with the test segmented wall region and its corresponding grayscale statistical features [44] to categorize the carotid disease risk into low-risk or high-risk categories. This process was done for $K = 5$ partitions to begin with, where the system would separate 80% of the patient sample size for learning and 20% for testing. In the testing phase, when the input of high- or low-risk is not given to the system and using the information it has learned from the 80% of the data along with the segmented grayscale statistical features from the remaining 20%, we can predict a decision of high- or low-risk carotid plaque. Similarly, this was done for $K = 10$ (where 90% of the data were used for learning and 10% for testing) and $K = N$ (Jack Knife or JK) (where 99% of the data were used for learning and 1% for testing). In order to determine the error in the machine learning system, the results from the testing phase were compared with manual results, which were taken as the ground truth for risk assessment. Because the manual results of the near wall risk assessment are likely to have greater error than the machine learning system (due to the low intensity quality of the ultrasound images from the near wall), the accuracy of the system will be principally evaluated against the manual risk assessment in the far wall category.

The goal of this study is to propose a machine learning based sRAS. The main innovations in this study are: (i) building a morphological-based risk assessment system using all three kinds of walls: far, near and combined far and near; (ii) utilizing the LD stenosis as a ground truth for training the tissue characteristic based system; (iii) embedding of automated recognition and segmentation of wall regions with the risk assessment system; (iv) validating the risk assessment using manual-traced wall regions and computing the PoM; (v) optimization of the best kernel during the classification paradigm; and (vi) understanding the size of the dataset needed for developing a generalization versus memorization approach.

13.2 Demographics, data acquisition and data preparation

This section consists of the following subsections: section 13.2.1 discusses the patient demographics; section 13.2.2 presents the data acquisition; section 13.2.3 presents the ground truth data preparation; and the stratification of the ground truth into high-risk and low-risk is presented in section 13.2.4.

13.2.1 Patient demographics

Two hundred and four (204) patients' left and right CCA artery B-mode ultrasound images were obtained from Toho University, Japan, and retrospectively analyzed (with ethics approval from the institutional review board (IRB)). One patient had only one image of the right CCA artery, therefore, the total number of images was 407. The patient demographics are shown in appendix B, table B1.

13.2.2 Data acquisition

In this study, a Japanese scanner (Aplio XV, Aplio XG, Xario, Toshiba, Inc., Tokyo) with a probe frequency of 7.5 MHz linear array transducer was used for carotid scanning by our sonographer, who had 15 years' experience. The acquisition was adapted as per the recommendations and standards of the American Society of Echocardiography Common Carotid Intima–Media Thickness Task Force. A full ethics review by the IRB was approved along with written informed consent from the patients. During the acquisition, the subjects were asked to lie in the supine position with their head tilted backwards. Once the carotid arteries were detected in the transverse view, the transducer was rotated 90° to acquire the anterior and posterior views along the long axis view of the CCA (the blood flow direction). For this database, the image resolution was 0.05 ± 0.01 mm. Figure 13.2 shows the sample raw images of B-mode ultrasound.

13.2.3 Ground truth data preparation

For machine learning based stroke risk assessment, the training system requires the ground truth information. We considered the LD as a gold standard for tracing of the lumen–intima (LI) borders for the near (proximal) and the far (distal) walls in B-mode carotid ultrasound scans. ImgTracer™ (courtesy of AtheroPoint™, Roseville, CA, USA)—a commercial software package—was used for manual tracings of the LI borders for the near/far walls of CCA. These delineated LI borders were then carefully examined and endorsed by a neuroradiologist (author LS), with 15 years' experience.

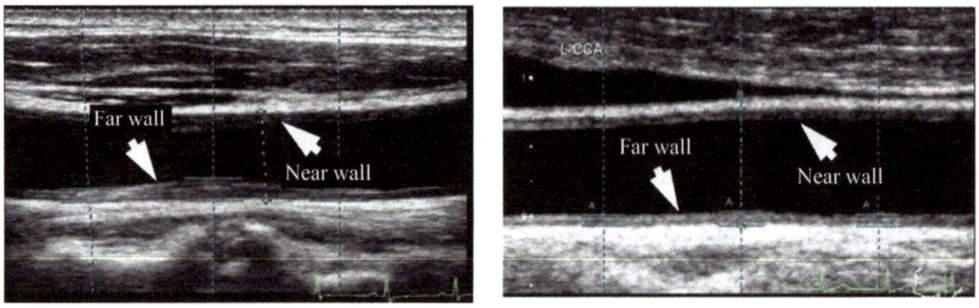

Figure 13.2. Sample raw images of B-mode ultrasound corresponding to high risk (left) and low risk (right) on the basis of the lumen diameter alone.

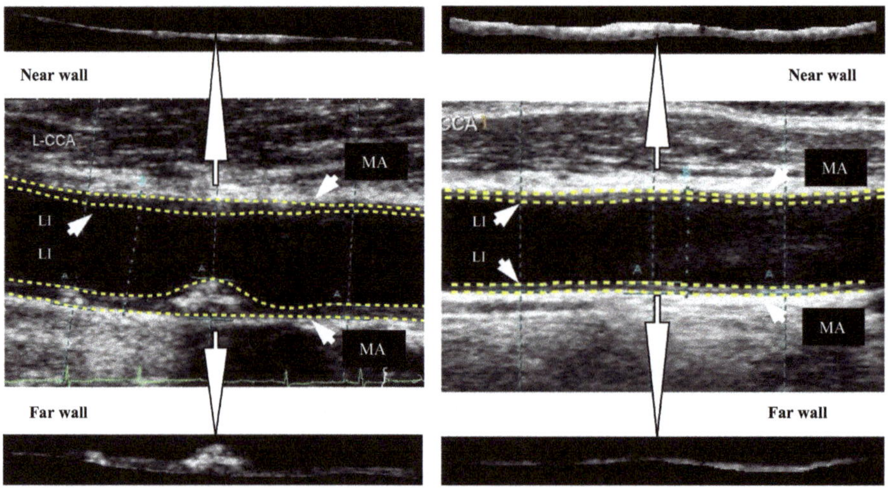

Figure 13.3. Ground truth tracing by an expert on high-risk (left) and low-risk (right) carotid scans.

A sample view of ImgTracer is shown in figure 13.3 for a high-risk (left) and low-risk (right) patient. Each image has near and far walls showing the LI and media–adventitia (MA) borders. The top dotted line for the wall indicates the LI interface and the bottom dotted line indicates the MA interfaces, corresponding to the near wall and far wall of the carotid artery. The region between the LI/MA walls is the wall strip shown as the near wall strip and far wall strip, which were utilized for grayscale feature extraction and risk stratification using the machine learning system. The tracing protocol was adopted for all 204 patients, consisting of a total of 407 carotid scans.

13.2.4 Stratification of manual LD into high risk and low risk

There are two reasons why we need the manual or ground truth LDs:

(i) to understand the distribution of manual LDs in our population. This will help in designing the automated sRAS as a threshold criterion can be developed for stratification.

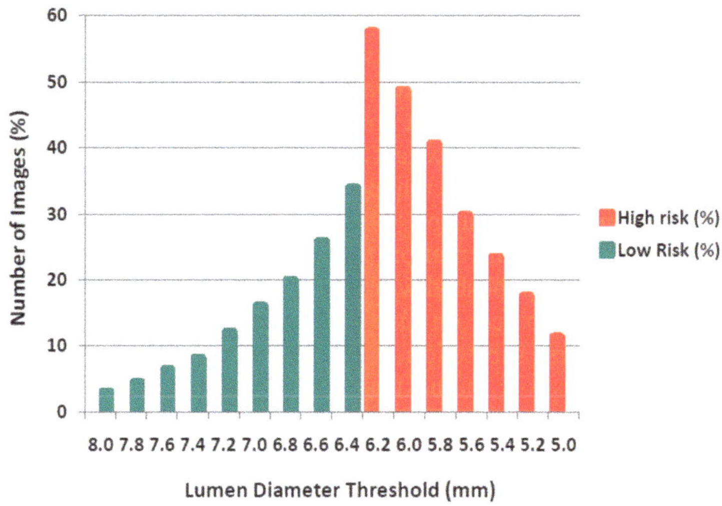

Figure 13.4. Stratification of ground truth population into high- and low-risk on the basis of LD.

(ii) To validate the sRAS, we need to design a manual risk assessment system (mRAS). For this mRAS, we need the manual LDs.

Figure 13.4 shows the percentage distribution of our population into high-risk and low-risk bins on the basis of the manual LDs changing from a maximum LD of 8 mm to a minimum LD of 5 mm in an interval of 0.2 mm, thus leading to 16 sets of LDs. Red represents the high-risk patients and green represents the low-risk patients. As the LD decreases from 8 mm to 5 mm with an interval of 0.2 mm, the number of patients in the high-risk pool decreases, while the number in the low-risk pool increases. Note that the distribution resembles a bell-shaped curve with the highest population consisting of 6.2–6.4 mm. Appendix B, table B2 shows the distribution of high-risk (HR) and low-risk (LR) patients in our population based on LD threshold (LDT). Thus, depending upon the choice of LDT, one can stratify the patients into high-risk and low-risk category.

13.3 Methodology

The fundamental concept in stroke risk stratification is to utilize the power of grayscale texture features combined with the stenosis severity of the carotid artery. Since plaque growth is multifocal in nature and never concentrated at one place, it is therefore necessary to consider the hyper- and hypo-echoic distribution of grayscale contrast all along the carotid arterial wall. Further, since the plaque growth has been attributed to a complex disease consisting of internal factors, such as genetics, lipid formation and blood pressure, and external factors, such as dietary conditions and daily physical activity, there is no fixed plaque growth pattern and it leans toward the class of randomness behavior [28]. Such randomness can be considered as chaotic in nature which can be modeled in a fractal paradigm in computer models. We thus model the grayscale wall contrast as a tissue characterization problem which, when combined with blockage severity, can be used for automated identification of high-risk and low-risk patients.

Note that the above grayscale features are computed in the wall region only. Since the atherosclerotic plaque is present in the wall, we thus need an automated segmentation protocol which can extract the IMT wall region for tissue characterization. Here onwards, we will interchangeably use the terms IMT wall region or IMT wall strips, or simply 'wall strips'. Thus our entire system consists of two major steps: (a) automated wall segmentation for the near and far wall which has been adapted from our recently published work [40] and (b) a risk assessment system for stroke risk stratification based on tissue characterization in combination with stenosis severity. The first subsection briefly discusses the technique adapted for automated wall segmentation; the next subsection discusses the main blocks of the sRAS, as shown in figure 13.5; finally, the last subsection presents the feature extraction system.

13.3.1 Wall segmentation

The objective of the wall segmentation is to automatically delineate the LI and MA borders for the near and far wall of the carotid artery. The overall system for wall segmentation is composed of two stages: the global stage to extract the region-of-interest (ROI) and MA borders for the near/far wall, and the local stage for extraction of LI borders for the near and far wall.

During the global stage, we adopt a dependency approach where the goal is to identify the adventitia region based on the physics of image reconstruction, which hypothesizes that this region is brightest [45–50]. To detect these far adventitial edges, a higher order derivative of a Gaussian filter is convolved with nearly the same width as the carotid intima–media thickness (say, close to 16 pixels). Using this as an origination point, we use a sweeping method along each column of the image region and analyze the spectral signal to detect the peaks which corresponds to the

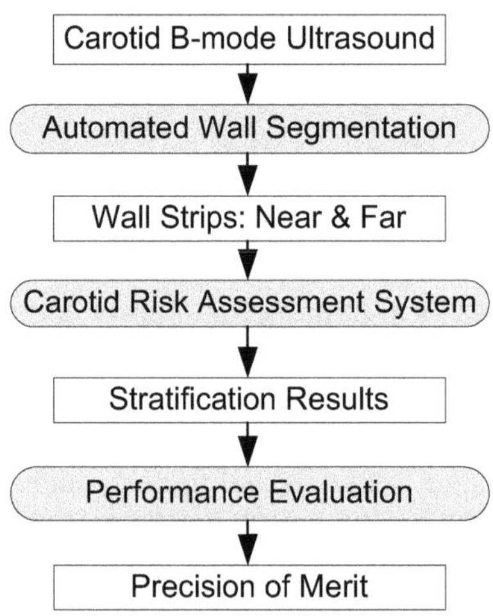

Figure 13.5. Global pipeline design for the sRAS and its validation.

MA of the near wall. Thus the MA of the near and far wall constitute the ROI of the carotid region. The distance between the near/far MA walls constitute the IAD (inter-adventitial distance). The local stage consists of LI extraction in the ROI region. This is computed by first adapting the constant class model and extracting the lumen region using a pixel-classifier approach. Here, we hypothesize that the blood intensity in the lumen region is constant. In the post-binary region of the lumen, one can obtain the edges of the LI for the near/far walls. LD is then estimated by taking the mean distance between the near/far walls of the LI using the polyline distance method [49]. Figure 13.6 shows the far wall strips of high-risk (left) and low-risk (right) patients. Similarly figure 13.7 shows the near wall strips of the high-risk (left) and low-risk (right) patients. The role of wall segmentation is shown in an overall block diagram in figure 13.5.

13.3.2 Stroke risk assessment system (sRAS)

Figure 13.8 shows the machine learning system, the sRAS, that consists of offline and online phases based on morphology-based tissue characterization. The offline system comprises the training paradigm where the grayscale texture-based features are computed, namely: (i) the gray-level co-occurrence matrix (GLCM), (ii) the gray-level run length matrix (GLRLM) and (iii) chaotic features, totaling 16 features. The offline system uses the LD labels corresponding to high risk and low risk, the morphology-based grayscale features and the support vector machine (SVM)-training classifier [51–53] to generate the offline parameters. The online system consists of risk prediction labels which consist of the transformation of online

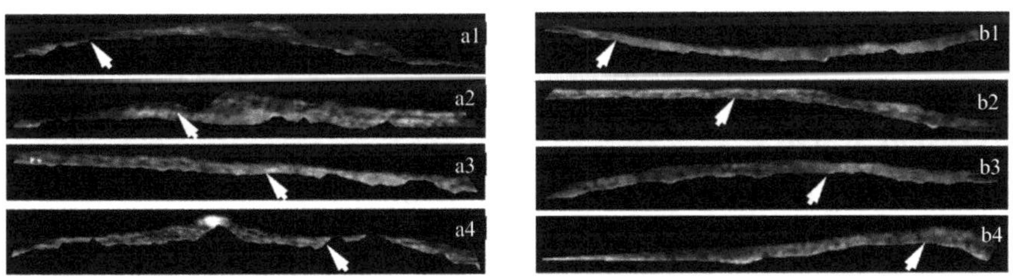

Figure 13.6. Far wall strips of high-risk and low-risk patients. Left: high-risk patients shown in images (a1), (a2), (a3) and (a4). Right: low-risk patients shown in images (b1), (b2), (b3) and (b4).

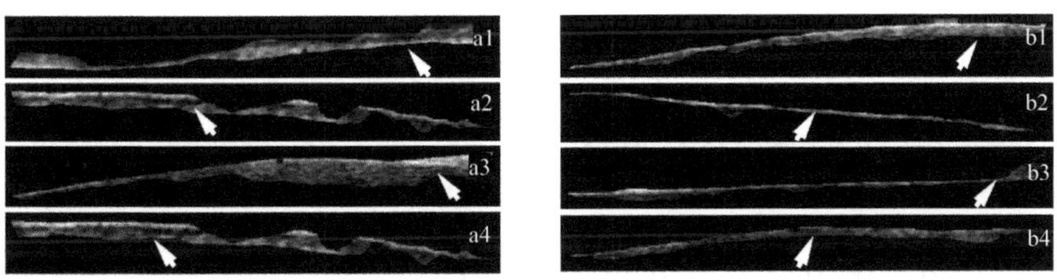

Figure 13.7. Near wall strips of high-risk and low-risk patients. Left: high-risk patients shown in images (a1), (a2), (a3) and (a4). Right: low-risk patients shown in images (b1), (b2), (b3) and (b4).

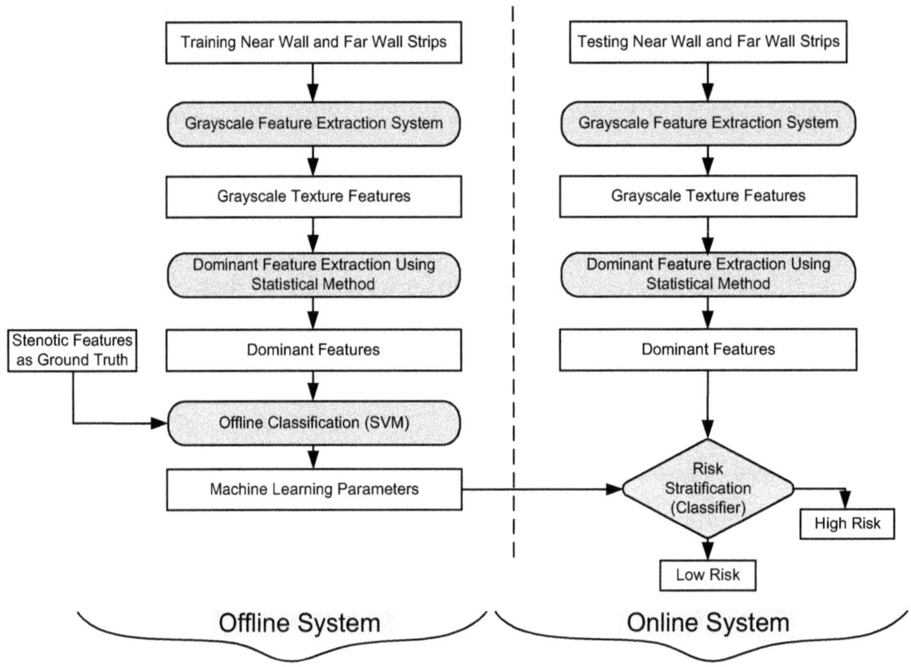

Figure 13.8. Carotid disease risk assessment system for the near wall and the far wall.

morphological features by the offline training parameters. Thus the basic model uses the cross-validation approach for computing the accuracy, sensitivity and specificity of the sRAS using three kinds of protocols: *K*5, *K*10 and JK. This will be discussed in the experimental protocol section.

13.3.3 Texture features

13.3.3.1 Gray-level co-occurrence matrix (GLCM)

Using the statistical tool, one can use GLCM for extracting textural information of the ultrasound image by considering the neighborhood pixel relationship [54, 55]. Considering the grayscale 2D image to be represented by $\boldsymbol{I}$ having the gray levels $(0, 1, \ldots, L_g - 1)$,one can compute the GLCM matrix M_x of order L, where, the $P_d(i, j)$th entry of M_x represents the probability of the number of occasions a pixel with intensity i is adjacent to a pixel with intensity j. Dividing each element of M_x by the total number of co-occurrence pairs in M_x will yield the normalized co-occurrence matrix. One can compute the adjacency by taking any specified direction such as horizontal, vertical, right, left and diagonal. Finally, the texture features were computed by taking the average of the chosen direction of the co-occurrence matrix. We extracted four kind of features, shown in appendix A, table A1.

13.3.3.2 Gray-level run length matrix (GLRLM)

Run length is defined as a set of collinear pixels having the same gray level in a particular direction [56]. Given the reference pixel, one can compute GLRLM and this measures the gray intensity pixel in a particular direction. GLRLM is a 2D matrix in which element $p(x, y)$ gives the total number of consecutive runs of length y at gray level x. A total of 11 features were extracted using GLRLM, as shown in appendix A, table A2. Note that M represents the number of gray levels and L represents the maximum run length.

13.3.3.3 Chaotic features

The fractal dimension (FD) feature is a well known feature which measures the chaotic pattern. The FD is measured by computing the irregularity over multiple scales [57]. The FD feature is relevant since the plaque's pattern has randomness and is multifocal. Thus, one can apply FD computation for stratification of plaque into high-risk and low-risk bins. For a given self-similar object of N parts scaled by a ratio r from the whole, its FD is given by

$$\frac{\mathrm{FD} = \log Nr}{\log\left(\frac{1}{r}\right)}. \tag{13.1}$$

13.3.3.4 Classification using SVM

SVM is the most fundamental classifier strategy for separating data points into different classes [58]. In our scenario, we utilize a two-class problem, i.e. high risk and low risk. The objective is to find the best hyper-plane which stratifies the two classes with the largest margin. This margin defines the maximal width of the two slabs parallel to the hyper-plane having no interior data points. Appendix A shows the working of SVM in detail, where different kernels are being used such as: linear-, polynomial- and radial-basis functions [59, 60].

13.4 Experimental protocol

This section presents three sets of experimental protocols adapted for optimization of machine learning parameters, understanding the effect of dominant features on classification accuracy for risk assessment, and understanding the effect of a change in data size on machine learning performance.

13.4.1 Experiment 1: Kernel optimization during machine learning training phase

Experiment 1 is focused on choosing the best kernel for the SVM classifier during the training and testing phases. Once the best kernel is selected, we use this kernel for the other two experimental protocols. For the selection of the best kernel, we run the machine learning system using five sets of kernels: Linear, RBF, Poly-1, Poly-2 and Poly-3. The optimization is executed using a cross-validation protocol by taking a particular partition (K) and a particular LDT and studying the effect of classification accuracy for risk assessment with respect to a change in dominant features. The kernel which yields the highest classification accuracy over all the dominant features is selected.

13.4.2 Experiment 2: The effect of dominant features on classification accuracy

Experiment 2 is merely an extension of experiment 1, where the cross-validation protocol is implemented by taking the exhaustive combinations of all three partitions, all LDTs ranging from 5 mm to 8 mm (16 sets) and all dominant features (from $D = 1$ to $D = 16$). During the automated set-up, the training component of the machine learning system utilizes the automated grayscale IMT wall region along with the automated LD measurements, which act as a gold standard (ground truth) for the training phase. Such a cross-validation paradigm is repeated for all three walls: the near wall, far wall and combined wall. These IMT wall regions correspond to experiments 2(a), 2(b) and 2(c), respectively.

13.4.3 Experiment 3: The effect of data size on machine learning performance

Experiment 3 evaluates the effect of an increase in data size on the classification accuracy for risk assessment using the machine learning paradigm. In this experiment, the image data sampling size is made to increase by 10% to study the effect on classification accuracy. It starts from a minimum number of patients (say 40, selected empirically) and is made to increase at a rate of 10%. This protocol is run for the optimal kernel, as obtained in experiment 1. Similar to experiment 2, experiment 3 is also conducted for the automated and manual protocols. This paradigm for increasing data size is repeated for all three walls, the near wall, far wall and combined wall, labeled as experiments 3(a), 3(b) and 3(c), respectively. Since the machine learning is characterized by a combination of population size, types of grayscale features, types of thresholds for ground truth, types of kernels in the classification paradigm during the training and testing phases, and the types of associated risks, we therefore adopted three different kinds of cross-validation protocols (*K*5, *K*10 and JK).

13.5 Results

13.5.1 Experiment 1—Results: Kernel optimization during the machine learning training phase

Using the cross-validation protocol for kernel optimization (experiment 1) on $N = 407$ images, the resultant plot can be seen figure 13.9 and the corresponding table can be seen in appendix B, table B3. The general tendency of the sRAS shows an increase in stratification accuracy with an increase in dominant features (D). The plot further shows that Poly-2 has the highest accuracy for each of the three partition protocols ($K = 5$, $K = 10$, $K =$ JK) and thus is selected as the best kernel for our automated stratification based on characterization of tissue morphology. Note that in appendix B, table B3, the values in the table represent the mean values of all the dominant features within each batch of kernels.

13.5.2 Experiment 2—Results: The effect of dominant features on classification accuracy

This experiment shows the cross-validation accuracy by taking: (a) all three protocols ($K = 5$, $K = 10$, $K =$ JK); (b) all LDT ranges from 5 mm to 8 mm

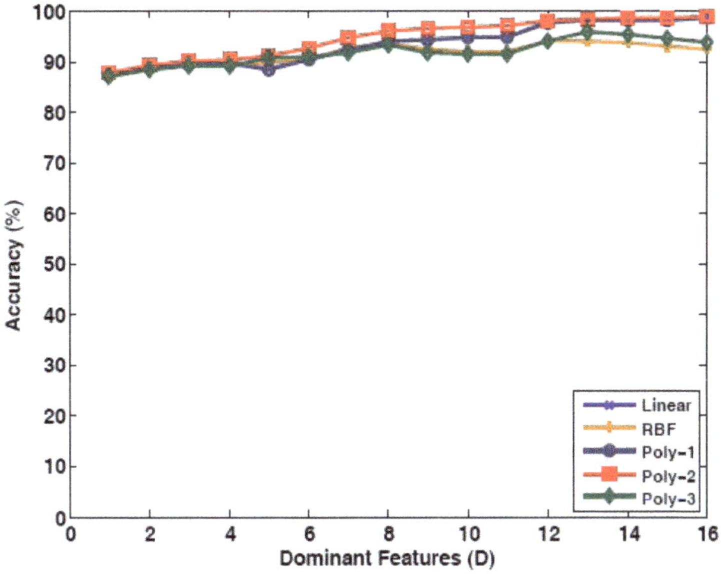

Figure 13.9. Plot of accuracy versus dominant features for fixed data size (N) of 407 images using five kernels: linear, RBF, Poly-1, Poly-2 and Poly-3.

(16 sets); (c) an increase in dominant features (from $D = 1$ to $D = 16$); and (d) all three kinds of carotid wall,: far, near and combined. The three kinds of walls correspond to the three different combinations shown in figures 13.10–13.12, respectively. Figure 13.10 corresponds to the far wall experiment, while figures 13.11 and 13.12 correspond to the near wall and combined wall experiments, respectively. Each figure has 2×3 matrices consisting of six plots: two rows corresponding to the automated sRAS versus the mRAS and three columns corresponding to the three sets of protocols: $K = 5$, $K = 10$ and $K =$ JK. In figure 13.10 (the far wall experiment), the columns for the automated sRAS are labeled as (a1), (a2) and (a3) while the columns for the mRAS are labeled as (b1), (b2) and (b3). In figure 13.11 (the near wall experiment), the columns for the automated sRAS are labeled as (c1), (c2) and (c3) while the columns for the mRAS are labeled as (d1), (d2) and (d3). In figure 13.12 (the combined wall experiment), the columns for the automated sRAS are labeled as (e1), (e2) and (e3) while the columns for the mRAS are labeled as (f1), (f2) and (f3). The classification accuracy corresponding to nine automated sRASs is shown in appendix B, table B4. The percentage stratification accuracy for different feature combinations (D) and for different partition protocols ($K = 5$, $K = 10$ and $K =$ JK) for $T = 20$ trials are computed using

$$\eta_w^{\text{auto}}(k) = \frac{\sum_l^L \sum_d^D \sum_t^T \eta_w^{\text{auto}}(l, d, t)}{L \times D \times T} \tag{13.2}$$

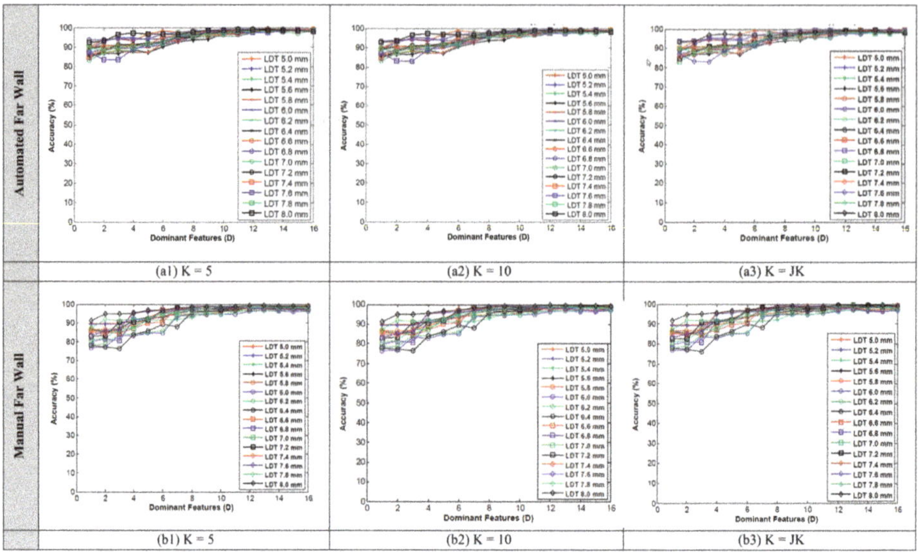

Figure 13.10. Experiment 2(a): Accuracy versus dominant features for the automated sRAS (top row) versus the manual mRAS (bottom row) corresponding to the far wall using the three partition protocols: $K = 5$ (first column), $K = 10$ (second column) and K = JK (third column).

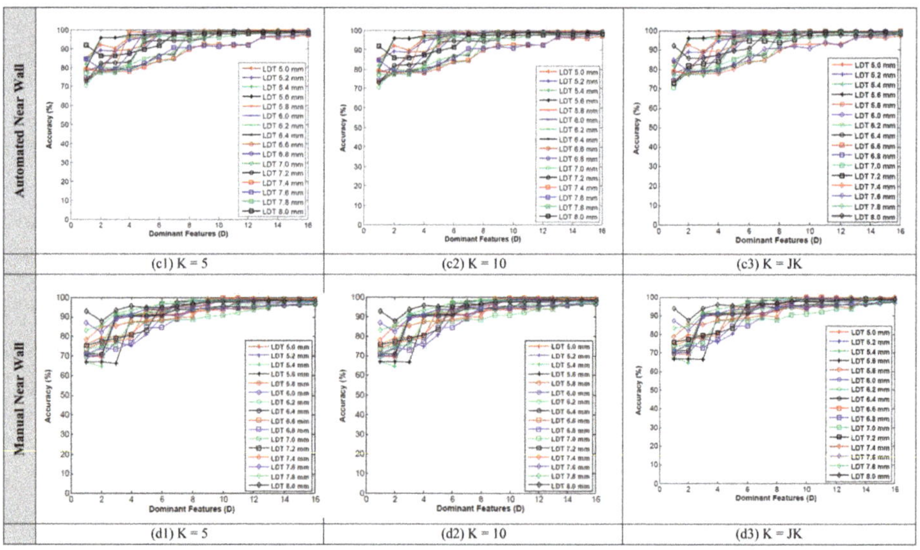

Figure 13.11. Experiment 2(b): Accuracy versus dominant features for the automated sRAS (top row) versus the manual mRAS (bottom row) correponding to the near wall using the three partition protocols: $K = 5$ (first column), $K = 10$ (second column) and K = JK (third column).

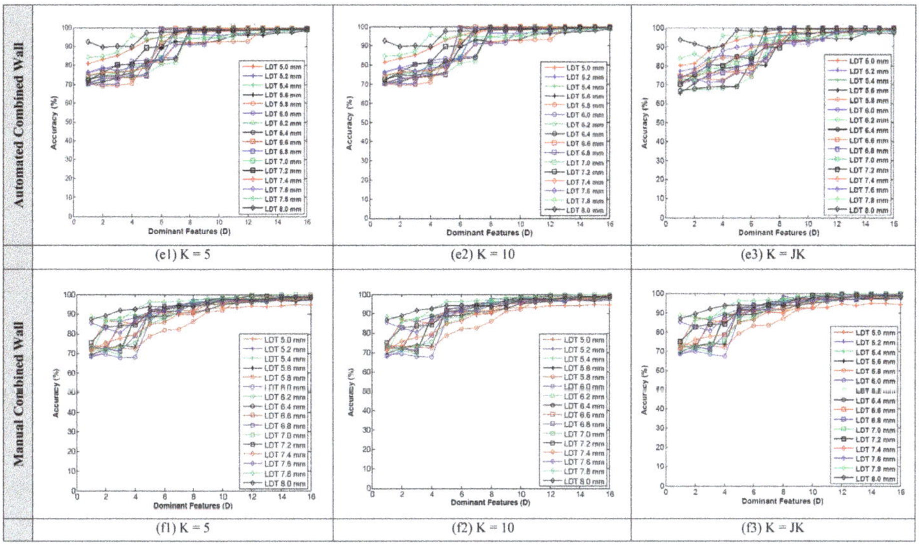

Figure 13.12. Experiment 2(c): Accuracy versus dominant features for the automated sRAS (top row) versus the manual mRAS (bottom row) correponding to the combined wall using the three partition protocols: $K = 5$ (first column), $K = 10$ (second column) and $K =$ JK (third column).

$$\eta_w^{\text{man}}(k) = \frac{\sum_l^L \sum_d^D \sum_t^T \eta_w^{\text{man}}(l, d, t)}{L \times D \times T}, \tag{13.3}$$

where $\eta_w^{\text{auto}}(l, d, t)$ is the accuracy using the automated method for wall type w, lumen diameter l, dominant feature d and trial number t. Correspondingly, $\eta_w^{\text{man}}(l, d, t)$ is the accuracy using the manual method for wall type w, lumen diameter l, dominant feature d and trial number t. Using the above equations, the mean accuracies are calculated and are shown in appendix B, table B5 for automated LD and manual LD. All nine plots of figures 13.10–13.12 demonstrate the increase in accuracy with the increase in the number of dominant features used for the training and testing of the machine learning system. There are 16 lumen diameter thresholds in each of the nine plots, corresponding to stenosis severity, which ranges from 5 mm to 8 mm in intervals of 0.2 mm. We observed that even when the LDT decreases from 8 mm (normal artery) to 5 mm (severe artery), the behavior of the machine learning system is consistent in the cross-validation protocol and generalizes as the number of dominant features increases. For each LDT selected, the order of dominant features changes, which is shown in appendix B, table B6, taken as an example for the far wall at LD = 6.4 mm. Even though the behavior of the near wall, far wall and combined wall is similar when dominant features are increased, the far wall accuracy curves are more clustered together compared to the near and combined walls. This behavior is attributed to accurate media wall detection in the far wall region compared to the near wall during the B-mode acquisition. As the number of dominant feature combinations increases beyond 6, the classification accuracy stabilizes to nearly 99%, converging to 100%

when D is 16. This behavior is consistent for all three walls, as can be seen in figures 13.10–13.12. The corresponding mean accuracies for automated (sRAS) versus manual (mRAS) for the three different protocols ($K = 5$, $K = 10$ and $K =$ JK) using $N = 407$ images is shown in appendix B, table B3, which is consistent with the plots in figures 13.10–13.12, respectively.

13.5.3 Experiment 3—Results: The effect of data size on machine learning performance

This experiment shows the effect of an increase in data size on the classification accuracy of the machine learning system corresponding to the far wall, near wall and combined wall in figures 13.13–13.15, respectively. Each figure has two plots corresponding to the automated sRAS (left) and manual mRAS (right). Each plot of the far wall has three protocols corresponding to three partitions, $K = 5$, $K = 10$

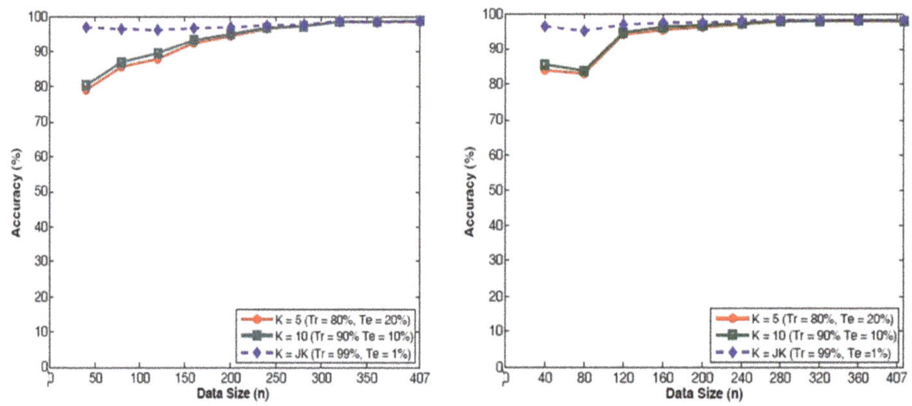

Figure 13.13. Experiment 3(a)—the effect of increase in data size: automated (left) versus manual (right) in the far wall for the $K = 5$, $K = 10$ and $K =$ JK protocols.

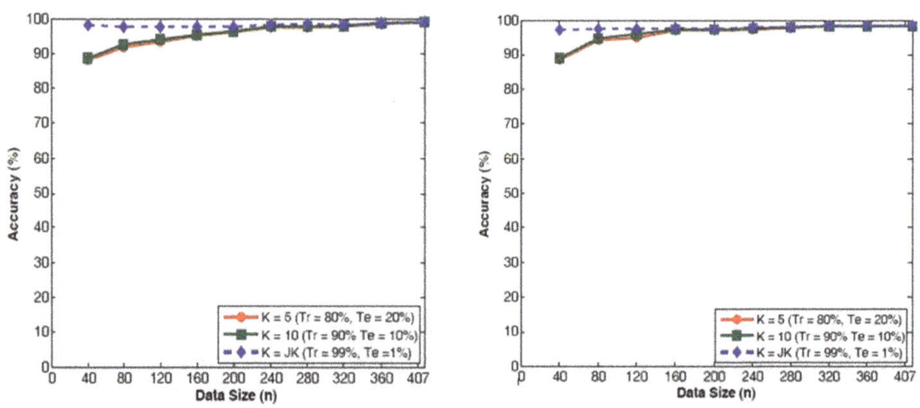

Figure 13.14. Experiment 3(b)—the effect of increase in data size: automated (left) versus manual (right) in the near wall for the $K = 5$, $K = 10$ and $K =$ JK protocols.

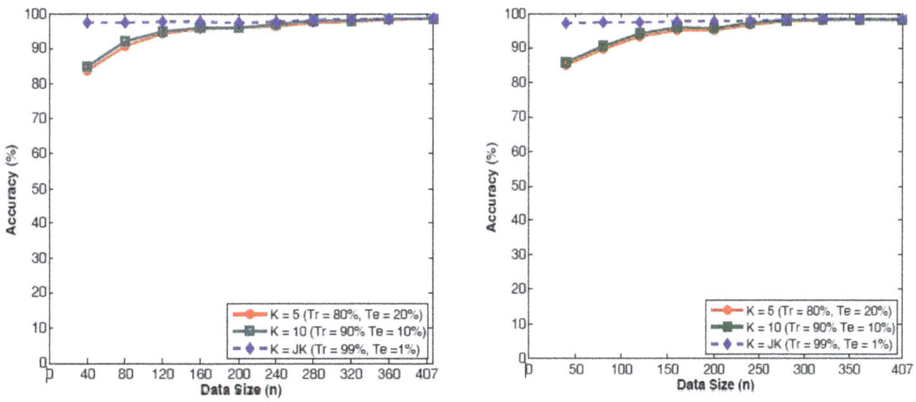

Figure 13.15. Experiment 3(c)—the effect of increase in data size: automated (left) versus manual (right) in the combined wall for the $K = 5$, $K = 10$ and $K =$ JK protocols.

and $K =$ JK shown in red, green and blue, respectively. Thus, there are a total of six plots in this experiment shown as 3(a), 3(b) and 3(c), corresponding to the far, near and combined walls. For all six plots, as the data size increases during the machine learning protocol, the classification accuracy increases until it eventually reaches nearly 100%. When the data size is 40 images (empirically selected), the accuracy is close to 80%. As the number of patients in the training set gradually increases, the machine learning classification accuracy increases and stabilizes to the point of diminishing returns and beyond this point there is no further change in the accuracy. The point at which the curve starts to show no more change is the point where learning changes to generalization during the machine learning phase. Our population shows that this occurs at around $n = 200$ for the automated system and $n =$ 240 for the manual system. Such a behavior is seen in both the automated sRAS and manual mRAS. Appendix B, table B7 shows the increase in accuracy with the increase in the number of patients during the training phase. Note that this is the mean accuracy over all the LD thresholds.

13.6 Performance evaluation

13.6.1 Precision-of-merit (PoM) analysis

The performance or PoM of the machine learning system is evaluated by replacing the automated grayscale IMT wall strips region with a manual segmented grayscale IMT wall strip region. Similarly, we replaced the automated LD with manual LD during the training phase of the machine learning system. The protocols adapted during the validation of our machine learning system are exactly similar in nature to the automated and real set-up. This means there are three kinds of partition protocols: $K = 5$, $K = 10$ and $K =$ JK. We replicate these protocols for all three sets of walls: the far wall, near wall and combined walls. Mathematically, the PoM is given as follows:

$$\mathrm{PoM}_w(k) = 100 - \left(\frac{\left| \eta_w^{\mathrm{auto}}(k) - \eta_w^{\mathrm{man}}(k) \right|}{\eta_w^{\mathrm{man}}(k)} \right) \times 100, \qquad (13.4)$$

where $\mathrm{PoM}_w(k)$ is the PoM for the wall type w with partition protocol k, $\eta_w^{\mathrm{auto}}(l, d, t)$ is the accuracy using the automated method for wall type w, lumen diameter l, selected dominant feature d and trial number t, and is computed using equation (13.2). Correspondingly, $\eta_w^{\mathrm{man}}(l, d, t)$ is the accuracy using the manual method for wall type w, lumen diameter l, dominant feature d and trial number t and is computed using equation (13.3).

Figure 13.16 (g1), (g2) and (g3) (the left column) shows that the probability of the PoM values for the far wall is greater than that of the near wall for given accuracy values within 5% tolerance (ε) for three kinds of protocols: $K = 5$, $K = 10$ and $K = \mathrm{JK}$. Similarly, figure 13.16 (h1), (h2) and (h3) (the right column) shows that the probability of the PoM values for the far wall is greater than of the combined wall within 5% tolerance (ε) for given accuracy values for the three kinds of protocol: $K = 5$, $K = 10$ and $K = \mathrm{JK}$. Note that our stratification of probability curves utilizes three bins: mild (or low), moderate (or medium) risk and severe (or high) risk, and their computed LD ranges were: mild (low) risk—7.4 mm to 8.0 mm; moderate (or medium) risk—6.4 mm to 7.2 mm; and severe (or high) risk—5.0 mm to 6.2 mm. Further, it is clear from figure 13.16 that a PoM of 95% is achieved when D is greater than or equal to ten dominant features. We therefore selected $D = 10$ as a threshold for seeing the overall PoMs.

Appendix B, table B8 shows the PoM values for the far, near and combined walls for three partition protocols: $K = 5$, $K = 10$ and $K = \mathrm{JK}$, and total trials (T) = 20 for three different dominant feature (D) conditions. The mean PoM for all the walls and all three protocols are computed on the basis of $D < 10$ or $D > 10$ or all D included. As can be seen, when $D > 10$ the PoM increases compared to when $D < 10$, which is intuitive and consistent with the behavior.

13.6.2 ROC analysis

After choosing the optimized kernel, i.e. a polynomial of order 2, we computed the ROC curve for all three partition protocols, i.e. $K = 5$, $K = 10$ and $K = \mathrm{JK}$, and for the automated sRAS and manual mRAS using the far wall, near wall and combined wall. The results in appendix B, table B9 show the mean sensitivity, mean specificity and AUC for the far, near and combined walls for the $K = 5$, $K = 10$ and $K = \mathrm{JK}$ partition for 16 values of LD ranging from 5.0 mm to 8.0 mm in the interval of 0.2 mm. The mean AUC value for the whole wall is close to unity which indicates the high accuracy of our system.

13.7 Discussion

13.7.1 Our system

In this study, we present an automated sRAS using morphology-based tissue characterization of plaque build-up in the carotid arterial wall. The sRAS is a

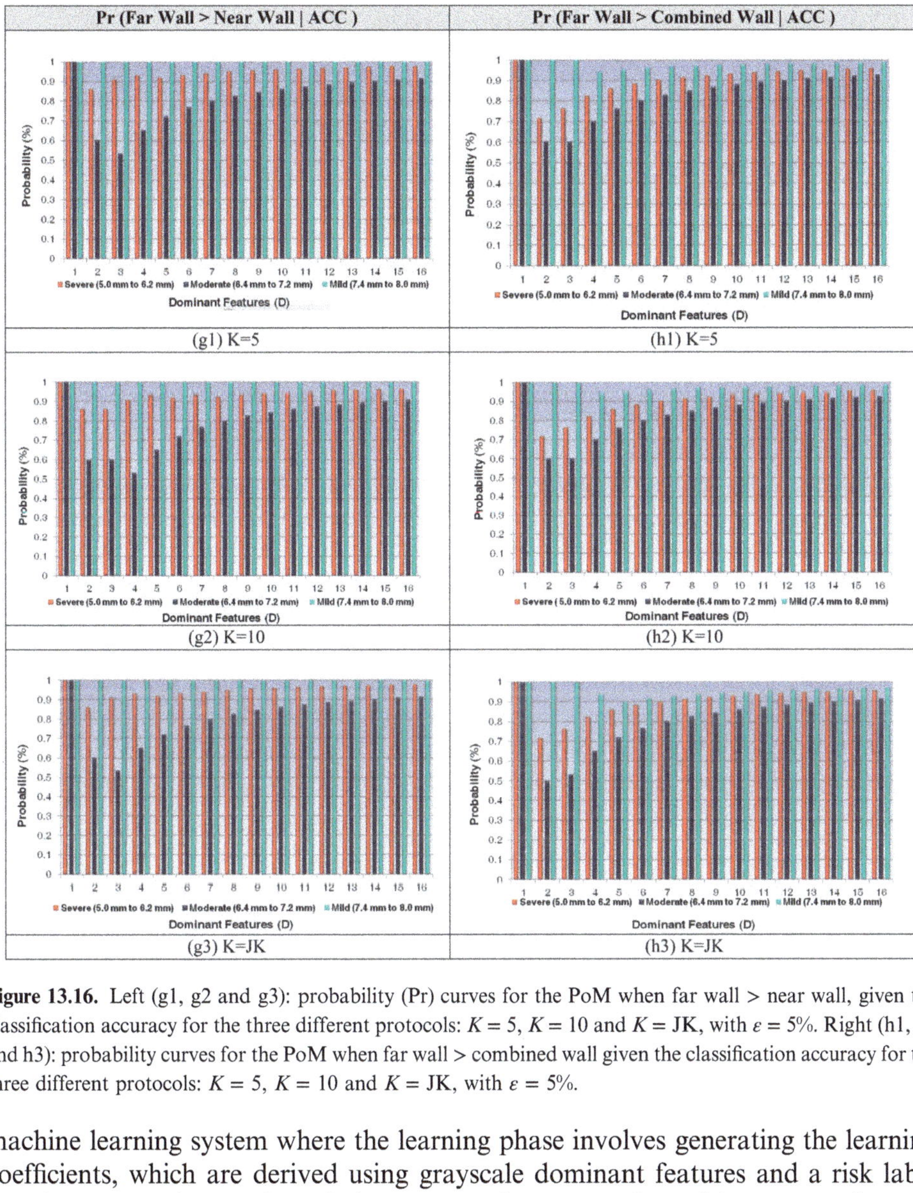

Figure 13.16. Left (g1, g2 and g3): probability (Pr) curves for the PoM when far wall > near wall, given the classification accuracy for the three different protocols: $K = 5$, $K = 10$ and $K =$ JK, with $\varepsilon = 5\%$. Right (h1, h2 and h3): probability curves for the PoM when far wall > combined wall given the classification accuracy for the three different protocols: $K = 5$, $K = 10$ and $K =$ JK, with $\varepsilon = 5\%$.

machine learning system where the learning phase involves generating the learning coefficients, which are derived using grayscale dominant features and a risk label based on stenosis severity of the artery. Three sets of partition protocols were adopted and online stratification accuracy was measured using a cross-validation paradigm. This scheme was applied to the three wall types in the carotid artery: the near, far and combined walls. Even though the far wall proved to have superior performance, the near wall also performed well (see appendix B, table B6). This proves our hypothesis that the near wall carries an equal risk of atherosclerotic disease and should be taken into consideration for stroke risk assessment. We, however, think more analysis needs to be performed on this aspect in the future.

13.7.2 Parameters of the machine learning system

We studied the sensitivity of the partition protocols for $K = 5$, $K = 10$ and $K = \text{JK}$. Certainly, with an increase in training sets during machine learning, the classification accuracy improved. We also optimized the choice of kernel for the SVM-based classifier during the training and testing phases. Of all the kernels, Poly-2 performed the best. We also exhaustively studied the effect of increasing data size on the classification accuracy (see appendix B, table B7), while keeping the number of dominant features constant. Our observations show that as the data size increases, the classification accuracy also increases under all stratification conditions (LD varying from 5 mm to 8 mm).

13.7.3 A note on wall segmentation validation

In order to evaluate the inter-observer variability [49], the manual tracings are obtained from the trained observer twice, traced over a period of two weeks. The observer was not given access to his previous tracings. The observer manually delineated the lumen as well as adventitia borders using ImgTracer™, commercial software from AtheroPoint™ (Roseville, CA, USA) [3, 5, 32, 44, 61, 62]. The borders are delineated by choosing 15–25 edge points proximal to the bulb depending upon the length of the carotid artery [10]. The observer had the ability to zoom in on an image in the wall region for better visualization. The output of the ImgTracer™ is the ordered set of traced (x, y) coordinates. The mean Auto LD and IAD measurements were 5.86 mm and 8.00 mm, respectively. A reduction in the Auto LD can be observed due to plaque growth in the far wall region and hence a decrease in the Auto LD.

13.7.4 Tissue characterization for risk assessment

The key aspect in tissue characterization is in understanding the linear and non-linear behavior of the plaque characteristics using a combination of the following texture feature categories: intensity histogram (IH), gray-level run length matrix (GLRLM) and gray-level co-occurrence matrix (GLCM).

GLCM features: 1—entropy; 2—energy; 3—contrast; 4—homogeneity; GLRLM features: 5—short run emphasis (SRE); 6—long run emphasis (LRE); 7—gray-level non-uniformity (GLN); 8—run length non-uniformity (RLN); 9—run percentage (RP); 10—low gray-level run emphasis (LGRE); 11—high gray-level run emphasis (HGRE); 12—short run low gray-level emphasis (SRLGE); 13—short run high gray-level emphasis (SRHGE); 14—long run low gray-level emphasis (LRLGE); 15—long run high gray-level emphasis (LRHGE); and 16—FD feature.

13.7.5 Benchmarking

Several authors have presented stroke risk assessment based on tissue characterization, including work our group has previously performed [31, 34, 36, 37]. The table of comparison between these techniques and the proposed method is shown in appendix B, table B10.

Seven attributes were chosen to compare the previous methods against the proposed method. They are the following: year of publication, algorithm type, data size, features adapted, classifier(s) used, cross-validation accuracy, whether or not ground truth validation was performed, and system performance evaluation.

Acharya *et al* (2011) in [63] used machine learning based on tissue characterization with three features for symptomatic versus asymptomatic plaque classification. The authors used an SVM-based classifier for training and testing, resulting in a classification accuracy of 83.77%. The ROI was manually segmented unlike this study where everything was automated. The same authors perform a research, in [38], with the same configuration, except that tissue characterization was performed using 32 texture features. Their accuracy was 90.66%. Also, another paper was published with the same purpose, however, the authors adapted two different sets of data (plaque and far wall data), for their risk stratification [34]. Eight and four features were used in this approach, respectively. LBP_{18}Ent, LBP_{18}Ene, LBP_{216}Ent, LBP_{216}Ene, LBP_{324}Ene, LTE_5Ene, LTE_6Ene and LTE_8Ene were the plaque features, while LBP_{324}Ene, LTE_2Ene, LTE_8Ene and $IMTV_{poly}$ were the wall features. The accuracy for the plaque region was 83%, while the accuracy for the far wall region was 89.5%. In 2013, Acharya *et al* [64] demonstrated another combination of features for the Atheromatic™ (trademarked by AtheroPoint, CA, USA) system to classify symptomatic versus asymptomatic plaques. Seven features were used in this study, three of which were texture features, two were discrete wavelet transforms (DWTs) and two were higher order spectral (HOS) features. The accuracy achieved in their results was 91.77%. In [37], Acharya *et al* adapted the same approach with two sets of data, 346 and 146 images, consisting of machine learning with 16 and 12 features, respectively. Their accuracy in this study was 85.3% and 93.1% for both datasets, respectively. In 2014, Pedro *et al* developed a risk stratification strategy [33] that had a similar motivation to Acharya's work, but addressed the vulnerability of plaque rupture, using a tissue characterization approach (AtheroRisk™, trademarked by AtheroPoint, CA, USA). The system using a total of the following 16 features: Rayleigh parameter (4th, 5th, 6th), GLCM, wavelet, percentile (10, 50), degree of stenosis, echogenic cap, appearance, mean, skewness, mixture components and plaque disruption. Their classifier was an enhanced activity index based on the Bayes factor. The accuracy for their results was 77%. Our group's prior best accuracy using his Atheromatic™ system was published in 2015, in which a value of 99.1% was obtained [43]. A combination of non-linear HOS features and two wall features under four different classifiers allowed these results to be achieved. However, the system did not demonstrate any evidence of performance evaluation and system validation, nor did it discuss machine learning systems for the near wall or combined near and far wall.

The fundamental novelties of the proposed method compared to previous methods are:

(i) The proposed study combines the use of automated segmentation of both the near and far walls for stroke risk assessment, while previous methods have evaluated stroke risk without the use of automated segmentation.

(ii) None of the past methods have explored the role of tissue characterization for the near wall of the common carotid artery.
(iii) In addition to feature estimation, we also optimize the criteria for feature selection.
(iv) The demonstration of stroke risk assessment by jointly taking into consideration the near and far walls of the common carotid artery.
(v) Comprehensive design of an online cascaded system, consisting of a far and near wall segmentation block and stroke risk assessment via a tissue characterization block.
(vi) Comprehensive validation of the cascaded system through comparison to the manual strategy.

We believe that one of the most remarkable results of our study is the extremely high cross-validation accuracy achieved under the proposed method. Such high accuracy is obtained through the optimization of the feature selection process. In machine learning, feature selection determines the thought process of the machine. Optimization of the features which are given to the machine avoids the selection of noisy and redundant features, which would likely decrease the accuracy [42]. In the proposed method, dominant features are determined using the differences between the mean values of each feature of the two classes (high risk and low risk). The larger the difference between these mean values, the higher the dominance level of the feature. The features are then arranged in descending order of their dominance level. In this way, a total of 16 feature combinations are constructed from highest dominant feature to lowest dominant feature with the increment of one feature in each feature combination.

13.7.6 Strengths and weaknesses

A sRAS is presented based on tissue characterization of the near, far and combined walls. Our results show that the near wall is equally important for stroke risk assessment compared to the far wall. Additionally, the tissue characterization system gave the highest cross-validation accuracy, compared to previous published results, with all three partition protocols: $K = 5$, $K = 10$ and $K = \text{JK}$. These results are consistent with the current literature. The online system is completely automated, where the near and far walls are automatically segmented in carotid scans.

In the validation of our risk assessment system, a histological approach would have yielded more accurate validation. However, this is very tedious and expensive, and therefore was not feasible for this study. Our approach for validation is the standard in machine learning, and gave encouraging results. Even though the results are encouraging, more sophisticated feature selection techniques such as principal component analysis (PCA) or functional data analysis (FDA) can be adopted. Further, intra- and inter-observer studies can be conducted on manual tracings of the LD and labeling of the ground truth risks.

13.8 Conclusions

In this study, a system for comprehensive stroke risk assessment based on tissue characterization of the near, far and combined walls is designed and developed. This system consists of (i) automated segmentation of near and far walls followed by (ii) a machine learning paradigm with three partition protocols. The selected features are optimized based on their statistical distribution. Three different kinds of experiments are conducted: first, the selection of the best kernel in the SVM-based classifier; second, studying the effect of dominant features on classification accuracy; and third, to study the effect of data size on this cross-validation accuracy. All these experiments are independently conducted for the near, far and combined walls to understand the relative risk of plaque in the carotid walls. The system shows consistent, stable and reliable results throughout. The system is fully novel and adds value to the field of stroke risk assessment.

Conflict of interest

Dr Jasjit S Suri has a relationship with AtheroPoint™ (Roseville, CA, USA) which is dedicated to atherosclerosis disease management, including stroke and cardiovascular imaging.

Contributions

Tadashi Araki, MD: Support in image data collection.
Pankaj K Jain, MTech: Statistical plots, analysis and programming.
Harman S Suri: Understanding and writing the original draft of the machine learning manuscript.
Narendra D Londhe, PhD: Advice and support in arranging IT resources.
Nobutaka Ikeda, MD, PhD: Support in clinical demographics collection.
Ayman El-Baz, PhD: Physics of vascular imaging protocols.
Vimal K Shrivastava, MTech: Support in programming.
Luca Saba, MD: Clinical discussions, manual tracings and validations.
Andrew Nicolaides, PhD: Clinical discussions on carotid imaging.
Shoaib Shafique, MD: Clinical application and risk scores.
John R Laird, MD: Clinical discussions on the link between the carotid and coronary.
Ajay Gupta, MD: Support in clinical writing of the manuscript.
Jasjit S Suri, PhD, MBA, Fellow AIMBE: Principal Investigator of the project.

Acknowledgements

Reprinted from Araki T, Jain P K, Suri H S, Londhe N D, Ikeda N, El-Baz A, Shrivastava V K, Saba L, Nicolaides A, Shafique S and Laird J R 2017 Stroke risk stratification and its validation using ultrasonic Echolucent Carotid Wall plaque morphology: a machine learning paradigm *Comput. Biol. Med.* **80** 77–96, with permission from Elsevier.

We acknowledge Toho Hospital, Tokyo, Japan, for support in providing patient datasets to AtheroPoint™ (Roseville, CA, USA). We thank our clinical team for the manual tracings of the lumen and cIMT borders. We also acknowledge Sumit K Banchhor, Research Scholar at NIT Raipur for support in formatting and proof-reading the manuscript.

Appendix A Grayscale features

Table A1. Features of the gray-level co-occurrence matrix (GLCM).

Feature name	Equation
Contrast (Con)	$\text{Con} = \sum_{n=0}^{L_g-1} n^2 \left\{ \sum_{i=1}^{L_g} \sum_{j=1}^{L_g} P_d(i, j) \mid \lvert i - j \rvert = n \right\}$
Energy (Eng)	$\text{Eng} = \sum_i \sum_j P_d(i, j)^2$
Entropy (Ent)	$\text{Ent} = -\sum_i \sum_j P_d(i, j) \log(P_d(i, j))$
Homogeneity (HOM)	$\text{HOM} = \sum_i \sum_j \frac{1}{1 + (i + j)^2} P_d(i, j)$

Table A2. Features of the gray-level run length matrix.

Feature name	Equation
Short run emphasis	$\text{SRE} = \frac{1}{l_t} \sum_{y=1}^{M} \sum_{y=1}^{L} \frac{p(x, y)}{y^2} = \frac{1}{l_t} \sum_{y=1}^{L} \frac{P_t(y)}{y^2}$
Long run emphasis	$\text{LER} = \frac{1}{l_t} \sum_{x=1}^{M} \sum_{y=1}^{L} (p(x, y) \cdot y^2) = \frac{1}{l_t} \sum_{y=1}^{L} P_t(y) \cdot y^2$
Gray-level non-uniformity	$\text{GLN} = \frac{1}{l_t} \sum_{x=1}^{M} \left(\sum_{y=1}^{L} (p(x, y)) \right)^2 = \frac{1}{l_t} \sum_{x=1}^{L} P_q(x)^2$
Run length non-uniformity	$\text{RLN} = \frac{1}{l_t} \sum_{x=1}^{M} \left(\sum_{y=1}^{L} (p(x, y)) \right)^2 = \frac{1}{l_t} \sum_{x=1}^{L} P_t(y)^2$
Run percentage	$\text{RP} = \frac{l_t}{l_q}$
Low gray-level run emphasis	$\text{LGRE} = \frac{1}{l_t} \sum_{x=1}^{M} \sum_{y=1}^{L} \frac{p(x, y)}{x^2} = \frac{1}{l_t} \sum_{y=1}^{L} \frac{P_q(x)}{x^2}$
High gray-level run emphasis	$\text{HGRE} = \frac{1}{l_t} \sum_{x=1}^{M} \sum_{y=1}^{L} (p(x, y) \cdot x^2) = \frac{1}{l_t} \sum_{y=1}^{L} P_t(y) \cdot x^2$
Short run low gray-level emphasis	$\text{SRLGE} = \frac{1}{l_t} \sum_{x=1}^{M} \sum_{y=1}^{L} \frac{p(x, y)}{x^2 \cdot y^2}$
Short run high gray-level emphasis	$\text{SRHGE} = \frac{1}{l_t} \sum_{x=1}^{M} \sum_{y=1}^{L} \frac{p(x, y) \cdot x^2}{x^2}$
Long run low gray-level emphasis	$\text{LRLGE} = \frac{1}{l_t} \sum_{x=1}^{M} \sum_{y=1}^{L} \frac{p(x, y) \cdot y^2}{y^2}$
Long run high gray-level emphasis	$\text{LRHGE} = \frac{1}{l_t} \sum_{x=1}^{M} \sum_{y=1}^{L} p(x, y) \cdot x^2 \cdot y^2$

Appendix B Statistical results

Table B1. Patient demographics of the 204 patients.

Population	157 males and 47 females
Mean age	69 ± 11 years ranging from 29 to 88 years
Lesion location in CCA	108 patients had proximal lesions, 67 patients had lesions in the middle and 29 had lesions in the distal locations of the CCA
HbA1c	6.30 ± 1.1 (mg dl^{-1})
LDL cholesterol	101.61 ± 31.55 (mg dl^{-1})
HDL cholesterol	50.66 ± 15.22 (mg dl^{-1})
Total cholesterol	175.82 ± 37.97 (mg dl^{-1})
Smokers	40% of the patients

Table B2. Distribution of high-risk (HR) and low-risk (LR) images in our population based on the LDT. Italics represent low risk while bold represents high risk.

Distribution of patients in HR and LR with change in manual LDT					
SN	LDT (mm) threshold	# of images in HR	# of images in LR	% of images in HR	% of images in LR
1	*8*	395	*12*	97.05	*2.95*
2	*7.8*	389	*18*	95.58	*4.42*
3	*7.6*	381	*26*	93.61	*6.39*
4	*7.4*	374	*33*	91.89	*8.11*
5	*7.2*	358	*49*	87.96	*12.04*
6	*7*	342	*65*	84.03	*15.97*
7	*6.8*	326	*81*	80.1	*19.9*
8	*6.6*	302	*105*	74.2	*25.8*
9	*6.4*	269	*138*	66.09	*33.91*
10	**6.2**	**234**	173	**57.49**	42.51
11	**6**	**198**	209	**48.65**	51.35
12	**5.8**	**165**	242	**40.54**	59.46
13	**5.6**	**121**	286	**29.73**	70.27
14	**5.4**	**95**	312	**23.34**	76.66
15	**5.2**	**71**	336	**17.44**	82.56
16	**5**	**46**	361	**11.3**	88.7

Table B3. Accuracy comparison for five different kernels for the three different partition protocols $K = 5$, $K = 10$ and $K = \text{JK}$, using $N = 407$ images.

Fold/Kernel	Linear	RBF	Poly-1	Poly-2	Poly-3
$K = 5$	93.44	91.27	98.54	98.74	95.03
$K = 10$	93.46	91.58	98.49	98.80	96.01
$K = \text{JK}$	98.77	94.35	98.77	99.02	96.56

Table B4. Percentage accuracy for different feature combinations for the different partition protocols, $K = 5$, $K = 10$ and $K = \text{JK}$, for 20 trials (T).

	Far wall			Near wall			Combined wall		
Features-combination	$K = 5$	$K = 10$	$K = \text{JK}$	$K = 5$	$K = 10$	$K = \text{JK}$	$K = 5$	$K = 10$	$K = \text{JK}$
FC1	88.13	88.15	88.27	78.69	78.74	78.64	74.90	74.93	75.03
FC2	89.57	89.58	89.56	83.05	83.04	83.06	76.39	76.41	76.40
FC3	90.58	90.57	90.63	84.06	84.07	84.03	77.27	77.24	77.29
FC4	91.09	91.15	91.20	87.26	87.28	87.33	79.66	79.71	79.76
FC5	91.71	91.75	91.86	90.97	91.00	91.05	82.51	82.60	82.59
FC6	93.32	93.37	93.38	93.40	93.48	93.55	89.40	89.48	89.47
FC7	95.34	95.46	95.59	94.30	94.40	94.41	93.51	93.61	93.69
FC8	96.04	96.15	96.22	96.51	96.61	96.61	96.90	96.97	97.04
FC9	96.93	97.02	97.01	97.41	97.50	97.54	97.00	97.16	97.24
FC10	97.36	97.44	97.47	97.86	97.94	97.99	97.56	97.70	97.85
FC11	97.62	97.78	97.83	97.97	98.11	98.33	97.91	98.08	98.10
FC12	98.15	98.32	98.50	98.09	98.22	98.31	98.20	98.29	98.36
FC13	98.45	98.50	98.59	98.63	98.70	98.80	98.62	98.72	98.71
FC14	98.59	98.61	98.68	98.61	98.68	98.79	98.79	98.90	99.00
FC15	98.60	98.66	98.74	98.78	98.85	98.89	98.91	99.04	99.14
FC16	98.74	98.80	98.82	98.96	99.03	99.05	99.16	99.25	99.31

Table B5. Automated versus manual mean accuracies for three partition protocols, $K = 5$, $K = 10$ and $K = \text{JK}$, using $N = 407$ images for 20 trials (T).

	sRAS: Automated IMT region and automated LD		
	$K = 5$	$K = 10$	$K = \text{JK}$
Far wall	95.01	95.08	95.15
Near wall	93.41	93.48	93.52
Combined wall	91.04	91.13	91.18
	mRAS: Manual IMT region and manual LD		
Far wall	93.96	94.07	94.16
Near wall	91.92	92.04	92.11
Combined wall	91.91	92.02	92.08

Table B6. Names of the features for various feature combinations for the far wall, LD = 6.4 mm.

Features set	Total no of features	Name of the features	ACC (%) $K = 5$	ACC (%) $K = 10$	ACC (%) $K = \text{JK}$
FC1	1	16	88.71	88.74	88.70
FC2	2	16,9	90.71	90.69	90.66
FC3	3	16,9,12	90.92	90.96	91.15
FC4	4	16,9,12,1	91.18	91.28	91.65
FC5	5	16,9,12,1,4	91.22	91.11	91.40
FC6	6	16,9,12,1,4,8	93.06	92.93	93.12
FC7	7	16,9,12,1,4,8,10	94.64	94.80	94.84
FC8	8	16,9,12,1,4,8,10,2	95.36	95.53	95.58
FC9	9	16,9,12,1,4,8,10,2,15	95.23	95.66	95.33
FC10	10	16,9,12,1,4,8,10,2,15,11	95.53	95.69	95.58
FC11	11	16,9,12,1,4,8,10,2,15,11,13	95.47	95.62	95.58
FC12	12	16,9,12,1,4,8,10,2,15,11,13,14	98.06	98.29	98.28
FC13	13	16,9,12,1,4,8,10,2,15,11,13,14,7	98.11	98.15	98.03
FC14	14	16,9,12,1,4,8,10,2,15,11,13,14,7,5	98.37	98.49	98.53
FC15	15	16,9,12,1,4,8,10,2,15,11,13,14,7,5,6	98.64	98.78	98.77
FC16	16	16,9,12,1,4,8,10,2,15,11,13,14,7,5,6,3	98.62	98.73	98.53

GLCM features: 1—entropy; 2—energy; 3—contrast; 4—homogeneity; GLRLM features: 5—short run emphasis (SRE); 6—long run emphasis (LRE); 7—gray-level non-uniformity (GLN); 8—run length non-uniformity (RLN); 9—run percentage (RP); 10—low gray-level run emphasis (LGRE); 11—high gray-level run emphasis (HGRE); 12—short run low gray-level emphasis (SRLGE); 13—short run high gray-level emphasis (SRHGE); 14—long run low gray-level emphasis (LRLGE); 15—long run high gray-level emphasis (LRHGE); 16: fractal dimension (FD) feature.

Table B7. Change in percentage mean accuracy for different data size for three partition protocols, $K = 5$, $K = 10$ and $K = \text{JK}$, and total trials ($T = 20$).

Data size (in %)	# of patient images	$K = 5$	$K = 10$	$K = \text{JK}$
10	40	79.21	80.46	97.17
20	80	85.70	87.00	96.66
30	120	88.14	89.44	96.24
40	160	92.51	93.42	96.79
50	200	94.54	95.16	97.15
60	240	96.54	96.77	97.54
70	280	97.31	97.48	97.86
80	320	98.61	98.74	98.75
90	360	98.54	98.61	98.62
100	407	98.72	98.81	98.82

Table B8. PoM for far, near and combined walls for three partition protocols: $K = 5$, $K = 10$ and $K = \text{JK}$ and total trials ($T = 20$) for three different dominant feature (D) conditions.

PoM	Far wall	Near wall	Combined
	PoM for $D < 10$		
$K = 5$	98.05	97.53	97.2
$K = 10$	98.05	97.57	97.11
$K = \text{JK}$	98.05	97.62	97.25
	PoM for $D > 10$		
$K = 5$	99.52	99.15	99.42
$K = 10$	99.62	99.21	99.44
$K = \text{JK}$	99.67	99.22	99.53
	PoM for all D		
$K = 5$	98.88	98.38	98.95
$K = 10$	98.92	98.43	98.99
$K = \text{JK}$	98.95	98.47	98.94

Table B9. Mean sensitivity (recall), mean specificity, precision (PPV) and mean AUC for automated RAS versus manual RAS for total feature combinations to 16.

	Automated LD											
	Far wall				Near wall				Combined wall			
	Sens.	Spec.	PPV	AUC	Sens.	Spec.	PPV	AUC	Sens.	Spec.	PPV	AUC
$K = 5$	97.05	94.65	98.27	0.96	98.39	94.77	99.06	0.97	97.41	97.40	99.07	0.97
$K = 10$	96.92	94.87	98.31	0.96	98.59	94.72	99.08	0.97	97.87	97.48	99.31	0.98
$K = \text{JK}$	96.78	95.26	98.43	0.96	98.63	94.50	99.11	0.97	98.28	97.58	99.38	0.98
	Manual LD											
	Far wall				Near wall				Combined wall			
	Sens.	Spec.	PPV	AUC	Sens.	Spec.	PPV	AUC	Sens.	Spec.	PPV	AUC
$K = 5$	97.45	90.79	97.74	0.94	97.05	94.65	98.27	0.96	97.62	90.55	98.64	0.94
$K = 10$	97.67	91.07	97.96	0.94	97.52	93.82	98.42	0.96	98.04	90.99	98.96	0.95
$K = \text{JK}$	97.88	91.41	98.15	0.95	97.93	94.74	98.79	0.96	98.10	91.16	98.98	0.95

Table B10. Comparison of various tissue characterization techniques from literature against our proposed work.

SN	Author (year)	Algorithm	Wall plaque/wall segmentation	Data size	Features	Classifier	Cross validation	Validation against GT	Performance evaluation
1	Acharya *et al* (2011)	Risk assessment in carotid plaque images (Atheromatic™)	Manual segmentation for plaque region	346	Total of 3 features: DWT-based average (Dh1), average (Dv1), energy (E)	SVM	ACC: 83.7% PPV: 81.8% Sn: 80%, Sp: 86.4%	N/A	N/A
2	Acharya *et al* (2012a)	Carotid plaque tissue characterization and classification (Atheromatic™)	Manual segmentation for plaque region	160	Total of 32 features: texture	SVM	ACC: 90.66% Sn: 83.33% Sp: 95.39%	N/A	N/A
3	Acharya *et al* (2012b)	Risk stratification using texture-based features (Atheromatic™)	(a) Manual segmentation for plaque region; (b) Automated segmentation for wall using AtheroEdge™	(a) 346 plaque (b) 342 wall	(a) Total of 8 features: $LBP_{18}Ent$ $LBP_{18}Ene$ $LBP_{216}Ent$ $LBP_{216}Ene$ $LBP_{324}Ene$ LTE_5Ene LTE_6Ene LTE_8Ene (b) Total of 4 features: $LBP_{324}Ene$ LTE_2Ene LTE_8Ene $IMTV_{poly}$	(a) SVM, GMM, DT, KNN, NBC, RBPNN, Fuzzy (b) SVM, KNN, RBPNN	(a) ACC: 83.0% Sn: 87.4% Sp: 79.7% (b) ACC: 89.5% Sn: 89.6% Sp: 88.9%	N/A	N/A

4	Acharya *et al* (2013a)	Classification of carotid plaque images by tissue characterization (Atheromatic™)	Manual segmentation for plaque region	146	Total of 7 features: texture features (3), DWT (2) and HOS features (2)	SVM	ACC: 91.7% Sn: 97% Sp: 80%	N/A	SACI*: 7.04 ± 0.223 and 6.67 ± 0.186
5	Acharya *et al* (2013b)	Segmentation and risk assessment in carotid plaque images (Atheromatic™)	Manual segmentation for plaque region	346 146	Total features: 16 (UK dataset) 12 (Portugal dataset) FGLCM: *E*, contrast, entropy, correlation, correlation, homogeneity FRLM: SRE, GLNU, ASM, mean, LRE, RLNU, RP	SVM DT Fuzzy	(a) ACC: 85.3% Sn: 84.4% Sp: 85.9% (b) ACC: 93.1% Sn: 99.0 % Sp: 80%	N/A	N/A
6	Pedro *et al* (2013)	Tissue characterization for stroke risk (AtheroRisk™)	Manual segmentation for plaque region	146	Total of 16 features: Rayleigh parameter (4th, 5th, 6th), GLCM, wavelet, percentile (10, 50), DoS, echogenic cap, appearance, mean, skewness, mixture components (5th, 6th, No.), and plaque disruption	Enhanced activity index based on Bayes factor	ACC: 77% Sn: 70% Sp: 80.13%	Done against GT	N/A

(*Continued*)

Table B10. (*Continued*)

SN	Author (year)	Algorithm	Wall plaque/wall segmentation	Data size	Features	Classifier	Cross validation	Validation against GT	Performance evaluation
7	Acharya *et al* (2015)	Tissue characterization for far wall (Atheromatic™)	Automated far wall segmentation	118	Total of 7 features: 6 HOS features and 2 wall features (IMT and IMTVpoly)	SVM, KNN, RBPNN, DT	ACC: 91.8% Sn: 83.3% Sp: 95%	N/A	N/A
8	Proposed method	Automated segmentation and risk assessment in carotid far wall and near wall	Automated segmentation for wall region	407	16 texture features: GLCM, GLRLM 1; Chaotic features: FDi with feature optimization	SVM	Far wall: 98% Near wall: 98% Combined wall: 99%	Done against GT	PoM: 95.86%

ACC = Accuracy; Sn: Sensitivity; Sp: Specificity.

References

[1] Stroke statistics: Internet Stroke Center http://strokecenter.org/patients/about-stroke/stroke-statistics/

[2] WHO CVD http://who.int/mediacentre/factsheets/fs317/en/

[3] Saba L, Gao H, Acharya U R, Sannia S, Ledda G and Suri J S 2012 Analysis of carotid artery plaque and wall boundaries on CT images by using a semi-automatic method based on level set model *Neuroradiology* **54** 1207–14

[4] Sanches J M, Laine A F and Suri J S 2012 *Ultrasound Imaging: Advances and Applications* (London: Springer)

[5] Saba L, Tallapally N, Gao H, Molinari F, Anzidei M, Piga M, Sanfilippo R and Suri J S 2013 Semiautomated and automated algorithms for analysis of the carotid artery wall on computed tomography and sonography a correlation study *J. Ultrasound Med.* **32** 665–74

[6] Ross R 1995 Cell biology of atherosclerosis *Annu. Rev. Physiol.* **57** 791–804

[7] Tracqui P, Broisat A, Toczek J, Mesnier N, Ohayon J and Riou L 2011 Mapping elasticity moduli of atherosclerotic plaque *in situ* via atomic force microscopy *J. Struct. Biol.* **174** 115–23

[8] Teng Z, Zhang Y, Huang Y, Feng J, Yuan J, Lu Q, Sutcliffe M P F, Brown A J, Jing Z and Gillard J H 2014 Material properties of components in human carotid atherosclerotic plaques: a uniaxial extension study *Acta Biomater.* **10** 5055–63

[9] Amato M, Montorsi P, Ravani A, Oldani E, Galli S, Ravagnani P M and Baldassarre D 2007 Carotid intima–media thickness by B-mode ultrasound as surrogate of coronary atherosclerosis: correlation with quantitative coronary angiography and coronary intravascular ultrasound findings *Eur. Heart J.* **28** 2094–101

[10] Kao A H *et al* 2013 Relation of carotid intima–media thickness and plaque with incident cardiovascular events in women with systemic lupus erythematosus *Am. J. Cardiol.* **112** 1025–32

[11] Eigenbrodt M L, Bursac Z, Rose K M, Couper D J, Tracy R E, Ewans G W, Brancati F L and Mehta J L 2006 Common carotid arterial interadventitial distance (diameter) as an indicator of the damaging effects of age and atherosclerosis, a cross-sectional study of the Atherosclerosis Risk in Community Cohort Limited Access Data (ARICLAD) *Cardiovasc. Ultrasound* **4** 1–10

[12] Eigenbrodt M L, Sukhija R, Rose K M, Tracy R E, Couper D J, Ewans G W, Bursac Z and Mehta J L 2007 Common carotid artery wall thickness and external diameter as predictors of prevalent and incident cardiac events in a large population study *Cardiovasc. Ultrasound* **5** 1–11

[13] Ikeda N, Kogame N, Iijima R, Nakamura M and Sugi K 2013 Impact of carotid artery ultrasound and ankle–brachial index on prediction of severity of SYNTAX score *Circulation* **77** 712–6

[14] Araki T, Ikeda N, Dey N, Acharjee S, Molinari F, Saba L, Godia E C, Nicolaides A and Suri J S 2015 Shape-based approach for coronary calcium lesion volume measurement on intravascular ultrasound imaging and its association with carotid intima–media thickness *J. Ultrasound Med.* **34** 469–82

[15] Araki T *et al* 2016 PCA-based polling strategy in machine learning framework for coronary artery disease risk assessment in intravascular ultrasound: a link between carotid and coronary grayscale plaque morphology *Comput. Methods Programs Biomed.* **128** 137–58

[16] Ogata T, Yasaka M, Yamagishi M, Seguchi O, Nagatsuka K and Minematsu K 2005 Atherosclerosis found on carotid ultrasonography is associated with atherosclerosis on coronary intravascular ultrasonography *J. Ultrasound Med.* **24** 469–74
[17] Ziembicka K A, Tracz W, Przewlocki T, Pieniazek P, Sokolowski A and Konieczynska M 2004 Association of increased carotid intima–media thickness with the extent of coronary artery disease *Heart* **90** 1280–90
[18] Elias-Smale S E *et al* 2012 Carotid intima–media thickness in cardiovascular risk stratification of older people: the Rotterdam Study *Eur. J. Prev. Cardiol.* **19** 698–705
[19] Polak J F, Pencina M J, Meisner A, Pencina K M, Brown L S, Wolf P A and D'Agostino R B 2010 Associations of Carotid Artery Intima–Media Thickness (IMT) With risk factors and prevalent cardiovascular disease comparison of mean common carotid artery IMT with maximum internal carotid artery IMT *J. Ultrasound Med.* **29** 1759–68
[20] Polak J F, Pencina M J, Herrington D and O'Leary D H 2011 Associations of edge-detected and manual-traced common carotid intima–media thickness measurements with framingham risk factors: the multi-ethnic study of atherosclerosis *Stroke* **42** 1912–6
[21] Cinthio M, Jansson T, Eriksson A, Ahlgren A R, Persson H W and Lindstrom K 2010 Evaluation of an algorithm for arterial lumen diameter measurements by means of ultrasound *Med. Biol. Eng. Comput.* **48** 1133–40
[22] Bots M L, Baldassarre D, Simon A, de Groot E, O'Leary D H, Riley W and Grobbee D E 2007 Carotid intima–media thickness and coronary atherosclerosis: weak or strong relations? *Eur. Heart J.* **28** 398–406
[23] Mirek A M and Wolińska-Welcz A 2012 Is the lumen diameter of peripheral arteries a good marker of the extent of coronary atherosclerosis? *Med. Biol. Eng. Comput.* **71** 810–7
[24] Delsanto S, Molinari F, Giustetto P, Liboni W, Badalamenti S and Suri J S 2007 Characterization of a completely user-independent algorithm for carotid artery segmentation in 2-D ultrasound images *IEEE Trans. Instrum. Meas.* **56** 1265–74
[25] Molinari F, Zeng G and Suri J S 2010 Intima–media thickness: setting a standard for completely automated method for ultrasound *IEEE Trans. Ultrason. Ferroelectr. Freq. Control* **57** 1112–24
[26] Molinari F, Zeng G and Suri J S 2010 An integrated approach to computer-based automated tracing and its validation for 200 common carotid arterial wall ultrasound images a new technique *J. Ultrasound Med.* **29** 399–418
[27] Molinari F, Zeng G and Suri J S 2010 A state of the art review on intima–media thickness (IMT) measurement and wall segmentation techniques for carotid ultrasound *Comput. Methods Programs Biomed.* **100** 201–21
[28] Suri J S, Yuan C and Wilson D L (ed) 2005 *Plaque Imaging: Pixel to Molecular Level* (Amsterdam: IOS)
[29] Gupta A *et al* 2015 Plaque echolucency and stroke risk in asymptomatic carotid stenosis: a systematic review and meta-analysis *Stroke* **46** 91–7
[30] Inzitari D, Eliasziw M, Gates P, Sharpe B L, Chan R K, Meldrum H E and Barnett H J 2000 The causes and risk of stroke in patients with asymptomatic internal-carotid-artery stenosis. North American Symptomatic Carotid Endarterectomy Trial Collaborators *N. Engl. J. Med.* **342** 1693–700
[31] Acharya U R, Faust O, Alvin A P, Sree S V, Molinari F, Saba L, Nicolaides A and Suri J S 2012 Symptomatic vs. asymptomatic plaque classification in carotid ultrasound *J. Med. Syst.* **36** 1861–71

[32] Araki T *et al* 2016 Reliable and accurate calcium volume measurement in coronary artery using intravascular ultrasound videos *J. Med. Syst.* **40** 1–20

[33] Pedro L M, Sanches J M, Seabra J, Suri J S, Fernandes E and Fernandes J 2014 Asymptomatic carotid disease a new tool for assessing neurological risk *Echocardiogrphy* **31** 353–61 .

[34] Acharya U R, Vinitha Sree S, Rama Krishnan M M, Molinari F, Saba L, Sin Yee S H, Ahuja A T, Ho S C, Nicolaides A and Suri J S 2012 Atherosclerotic risk stratification strategy for carotid arteries using texture-based features *Ultrasound Med. Biol.* **38** 899–915

[35] Acharya U R, Faust O, Alvin A P, Vinitha Sree S, Molinari F, Saba L, Nicolaides A and Suri J S 2012 Symptomatic vs. asymptomatic plaque classification in carotid ultrasound *J. Med. Syst.* **36** 1861–71

[36] Acharya U R, Vinitha Sree S, Rama Krishnan M M, Saba L, Gao H, Mallarini G and Suri J S 2013 Computed tomography carotid wall plaque characterization using a combination of discrete wavelet transform and texture features: a pilot study *J. Eng. Med.* **227** 643

[37] Acharya U R, Rama Krishnan M M, Vinitha Sree S, Afonso D, Sanches J, Shafique S, Nicolaides A, Pedro L M, Fernandes F J and Suri J S 2013 Atherosclerotic plaque tissue characterization in 2D ultrasound longitudinal carotid scans for automated classification: a paradigm for stroke risk assessment *Med. Biol. Eng. Comput.* **51** 513–23

[38] Acharya U R, Rama Krishnan M M, Vinitha Sree S, Sanches J, Shafique S, Nicolaides A, Pedro L M and Suri J S 2013 Plaque tissue characterization and classification in ultrasound carotid scans: a paradigm for vascular feature amalgamation *IEEE Trans. Instrum. Meas.* **62** 392–400

[39] Sharma A M, Gupta A, Kumar P K, Rajan J, Saba L, Nobutaka I, Laird J R, Nicolades A and Suri J S 2015 A review on carotid ultrasound atherosclerotic tissue characterization and stroke risk stratification in machine learning framework *Curr. Atheroscl. Rep.* **17** 955

[40] Saba L *et al* 2016 Carotid inter-adventitial diameter is more strongly related to plaque score compared to lumen diameter: an automated and first ultrasound study in Japanese diabetic cohort *J. Clin. Ultrasound* **44** 210–20

[41] Araki T *et al* 2016 Two automated techniques for carotid lumen diameter measurement: regional versus boundary approaches *J. Med. Syst.* **40** 182

[42] Jain A K, Duin R P W and Mao J 2000 Statistical pattern recognition: a review *IEEE Trans. Pattern Anal. Mach. Intell.* **22** 4–37

[43] Acharya U R, Sree S V, Molinari F, Saba L, Nicolaides A and Suri J S 2015 An automated technique for carotid far wall classification using grayscale features and wall thickness variability *J. Clin. Ultrasound* **43** 302–11

[44] Noor N M, Than J C, Rijal O M, Kassim R M, Yunus A, Zeki A A, Anzidei M, Saba L and Suri J S 2015 Automatic lung segmentation using control feedback system: morphology and texture paradigm *J. Med. Syst.* **39** 1–18

[45] Molinari F, Constantinos P, Zeng G, Nicolaides A and Suri J S 2012 Completely automated multi-resolution edge snapper ('CAMES')—a new technique for an accurate carotid ultrasound IMT measurement: clinical validation and benchmarking on a multi-institutional database *IEEE Trans. Image Process.* **21** 1211–22

[46] Molinari F *et al* 2012 Ultrasound IMT measurement on a multi-ethnic and multi-institutional database: our review and experience using four fully automated and one semi-automated methods *Comput. Methods Program. Biomed.* **108** 946–60

[47] Molinari F, Meiburger K M, Saba L, Zeng G, Acharya U R, Ledda M, Nicolaides A and Suri J S 2012 Fully automated dual snake formulation for carotid intima–media thickness measurement: a new approach *J. Ultrasound Med.* **31** 1123–36

[48] Molinari F, Meiburger K M, Saba L, Acharya U R, Ledda M, Nicolaides A and Suri J S 2012 Constrained snake vs. conventional snake for carotid ultrasound automated IMT measurements on multi-center data sets *Ultrasonics* **52** 949–61

[49] Araki T *et al* 2016 A new method for IVUS-based coronary artery disease risk stratification: a link between coronary and carotid ultrasound plaque burdens *Comput. Methods Programs Biomed.* **124** 161–79

[50] Saba L, Lippo R S, Tallapally N, Molinari F, Montisci R, Mallarini G and Suri J S 2011 Evaluation of carotid wall thickness by using computed tomography and semiautomated ultrasonographic software *J. Vasc. Ultrasound* **35** 136–42

[51] Shrivastava V K, Londhe N D, Sonawane R S and Suri J S 2015 Reliable and accurate psoriasis disease classification in dermatology images using comprehensive feature space in machine learning paradigm *Exp. Syst. Appl.* **42** 6148–95

[52] Shrivastava V K, Londhe N D, Sonawane R S and Suri J S 2015 Exploring the color feature power for psoriasis risk stratification and classification: a data mining paradigm *Comput. Biol. Med.* **65** 54–68

[53] Shrivastava V K, Londhe N D, Sonawane R S and Suri J S 2016 A novel approach to multiclass psoriasis disease risk stratification: machine learning paradigm *Biomed. Signal Process. Control* **28** 27–40

[54] Soh L K and Tsatsoulis C 1999 Texture analysis of SAR sea ice imagery using gray level co-occurrence matrices *IEEE Trans. Geosci. Remote Sens.* **37** 780–95

[55] Kalyan K, Jakhia B, Lele R D, Joshi M and Chowdhary A 2014 Artificial neural network application in the diagnosis of disease conditions with liver ultrasound images *Adv. Bioinform.* **2014** 708279

[56] Tang X 1998 Texture information in run-length matrices *IEEE Trans. Image Process.* **7** 1602–9

[57] Mandelbrot B B 1983 *The Fractal Geometry of Nature* (New York: Freeman)

[58] Vapnik V 1998 *Statistical Learning Theory* (New York: Wiley)

[59] Muller K R, Mika S, Ratsch G, Tsuda K and Scholkopf B 2001 An introduction to kernel based learning algorithms *IEEE Trans. Neural Netw.* **12** 181–201

[60] Kohavi R 1995 A study of cross-validation and Bootstrap for accuracy estimation and model selection *Int. Joint Conf. Artif. Intell.* **14** 1137–43

[61] Molinari F, Meiburger K M, Zeng G, Nicolaides A and Suri J S 2012 CAUDLES-EF: carotid automated ultrasound double line extraction system using edge flow *J. Ultrasound Imaging* **24** 129–62

[62] Saba L, Than J C, Noor N M, Rijal O M, Kassim R M, Yunus A, Ng C R and Suri J S 2016 Inter-observer variability analysis of automatic lung delineation in normal and disease patients *J. Med. Syst.* **40** 1–8

[63] Acharya U R, Faust O, Vinitha Sree S, Molinari F, Saba L, Nicolaides A and Suri J S 2012 An accurate and generalized approach to plaque characterization in 346 carotid ultrasound scans *IEEE Trans. Instrum. Meas.* **61** 0018–9456

[64] Acharya U R, Faust O, Alvin A P, Krishnamurthi G, Seabra J C, Sanches J and Suri J S 2013 Understanding symptomatology of atherosclerotic plaque by image-based tissue characterization *Comput. Methods Programs Biomed.* **110** 66–75

IOP Publishing

Vascular and Intravascular Imaging Trends, Analysis, and Challenges, Volume 1
Stent applications
Petia Radeva and Jasjit S Suri

Chapter 14

An improved framework for IVUS-based coronary artery disease risk stratification by fusing wall-based and texture-based features during a machine learning paradigm

Sumit K Banchhor, Narendra D Londhe, Tadashi Araki, Luca Saba, Petia Radeva, John R Laird and Jasjit S Suri

The planning of percutaneous interventional procedures involves pre-screening and risk stratification of the coronary artery disease (CAD). Current screening tools use stand-alone plaque texture-based features and therefore lack the ability to stratify the risk. This institutional research board (IRB) approved study presents a novel strategy for CAD risk stratification using an amalgamation of intravascular ultrasound (IVUS) plaque texture-based and wall-based measurement features. As it is a common genetic plaque make-up, the carotid plaque burden was chosen as a gold standard for risk labels during the training phase of the machine learning (ML) paradigm. A cross-validation protocol was adopted to compute the accuracy of the ML framework. A set of 59 plaque texture-based features was padded with six wall-based measurement features to show the improvement in stratification accuracy. The ML system was executed using a principle component analysis (PCA)-based framework for dimensionality reduction and uses a support vector machine (SVM) classifier for the training and testing phases. The ML system produced a stratification accuracy of 91.28%, demonstrating an improvement of 5.69% when wall-based measurement features were combined with plaque texture-based features. The fused system showed an improvement in mean sensitivity, specificity, positive predictive value and area under the curve (AUC) by 6.39%, 4.59%, 3.31% and 5.48%, respectively, when compared to the stand-alone system. In addition to meeting the stability criterion of 5%, the ML system also showed a high average feature retaining power and mean reliability of 89.32% and 98.24%, respectively. The ML system showed an improvement in risk stratification accuracy when the wall-based measurement features were fused with the plaque texture-based features.

14.1 Introduction

Atherosclerotic cardiovascular disease accounts for the largest number of deaths in the USA [1]. The disease of atherosclerosis over time causes calcium to build-up in the coronary arteries [2]. During the advanced stage of the disease, the combined risk of the patient includes higher plaque growth leading to plaque rupture. This also includes the risk of developing different plaque components such as fibro-fatty, macrophages, calcium and fatty tissue. When these components increase in size, there is a risk of an increase in stenosis and stress on the fibrous cap thickness, which can cause the risk of rupture leading to myocardial infarction (MI). All of the above can be categorized as the 'risk of arterial wall rupture' or 'risk of MI'. Thus, rupture of the arterial wall cap can cause calcium to dislodge, blocking the oxygen-rich blood flow in the arteries, leading to myocardial infarction or stroke [3]. Current screening methods such as computed tomography (CT) and magnetic resonance imaging (MRI) [4, 5] suffer from excess radiation and magnetic interference, respectively. Further, these devices take a long time to reconstruct the images, thus they lack a real-time interface [4]. IVUS screening, on the other hand, has low-radiation exposure, is economic compared to MR/CT, is ergonomic and offers real-time diagnosis [6, 7].

Prior to stenting and percutaneous interventional procedures, cardiologists are interested in performing pre-screening and risk stratification of CAD. Studies for risk stratification of cardiovascular events are mainly categorized into two groups. The first group attempts to predict the risk by quantifying the plaque characteristics (i.e. texture-based features) while the second group predicts the risk by quantifying wall-based measurement features [8–13]. Christodoulou *et al* [8], in 2003, proposed a neural network for carotid plaque classification. Ten dominant texture feature sets were selected from a total of 61 texture features showing a low accuracy of 73.10% on a data size of 230 images. Two years later, Kyriacou *et al* [9] showed a carotid classification system that used a neural network classifier with ten different textures and carotid wall-based features and achieved even a slightly lower accuracy 71.2% on a data size of 274 images. The same group in 2009 applied a SVM classifier on the same database using only the texture features and showed an improvement in accuracy of 2.5%. In a hybrid neural network approach on B-mode carotid ultrasound images, Mongiakakou *et al* [10] in 2007 used 21 statistical and law features on 108 images. The neural network was trained on the combined use of genetic algorithms and back-propagation with momentum and adaptive learning rate and showed an accuracy of 99.10%.

Our team, led by author JSS, has been working on the characterization of carotid plaque. Acharya *et al* [12], in 2012, proposed an Atheromatic™ system for plaque stratification into symptomatic and asymptomatic plaques showing an accuracy of 82.40% and 81.70%, using SVM and AdaBoost classifiers, respectively. The same group [13], in 2012, obtained an accuracy of 83% by fusing the plaque texture-based and wall-based measurement features using an SVM classifier. A year later, the same group [14] obtained a further high accuracy of 85.3% by fusing discrete wavelet transform, higher order spectra and textural features on a large data size consisting of 492 images. A year later, Pedro *et al* [15] fused the clinical and texture features for the classification of carotid plaque. An enhanced activity index was proposed and was correlated with the presence or absence of ipsilateral appropriate ischemic symptoms. Leave-one-patient-out was applied to 146 carotid plaques obtained from 99 patients and a cross-validation accuracy of 77% was obtained. Araki *et al* [16] showed a CADx system using the SVM that demonstrated a training and testing-based ML system using plaque texture features for coronary artery risk assessment. Later, the same group [17] modified and improved their CADx system by introducing the PCA-based polling technique for selection of the grayscale dominant features for improving the stratification accuracy. These prior studies had ignored how plaque growth affects the walls of the arteries and lacked the prominent features contributed by the wall-based parameters. This study is an extension of the above studies using an amalgamation of IVUS plaque texture-based and wall-based measurement features. This is motivated by the current strategy by JSS and his team in stroke imaging where carotid intima–media thickness (cIMT) variability was fused with carotid longitudinal grayscale features to improve the stroke risk stratification [18, 19]. But in our current study, circular wall parameters along with the plaque calcium are derived as measurement features from IVUS coronary walls. Thus, the objective is to demonstrate the importance of wall-based measurement features and their integration with plaque texture-based grayscale features for better ML system design.

Calcium accumulations always occur in the atheroma region which lies between the lumen (inner wall or internal elastic wall) region and vessel (outer wall or external elastic wall) region [20]. Therefore, an expansion of the walls is purely a reflection of the growth of calcium in the arteries. Moreover, due to the multi-focal nature of calcium [21], the wall thickness can vary along the circular walls of the coronary artery. Figures 14.1 and 14.2 show typical examples of images showing a grayscale ring, along with calcium, lumen, vessel and atheroma regional areas corresponding to five different low-risk and high-risk patients, respectively. Furthermore, our study is based on two hypotheses: (i) fusion of plaque texture-based and wall-based measurement features can offer an improvement in the coronary artery risk stratification; (ii) due to the genetic make-up of the plaque, carotid plaque burden, which is considered as a biomarker for stroke risk [22–28], can be used as a risk label for patients with coronary artery disease [16, 17].

The novelty of this study is to demonstrate an improvement in the accuracy of the CADx system built for the coronary artery risk assessment by fusing plaque texture-based features with wall-based measurement features compared to a stand-alone system consisting of only plaque texture-based features. Our objective in this paper is to predict the class label of the plaque type as high-risk or low-risk.

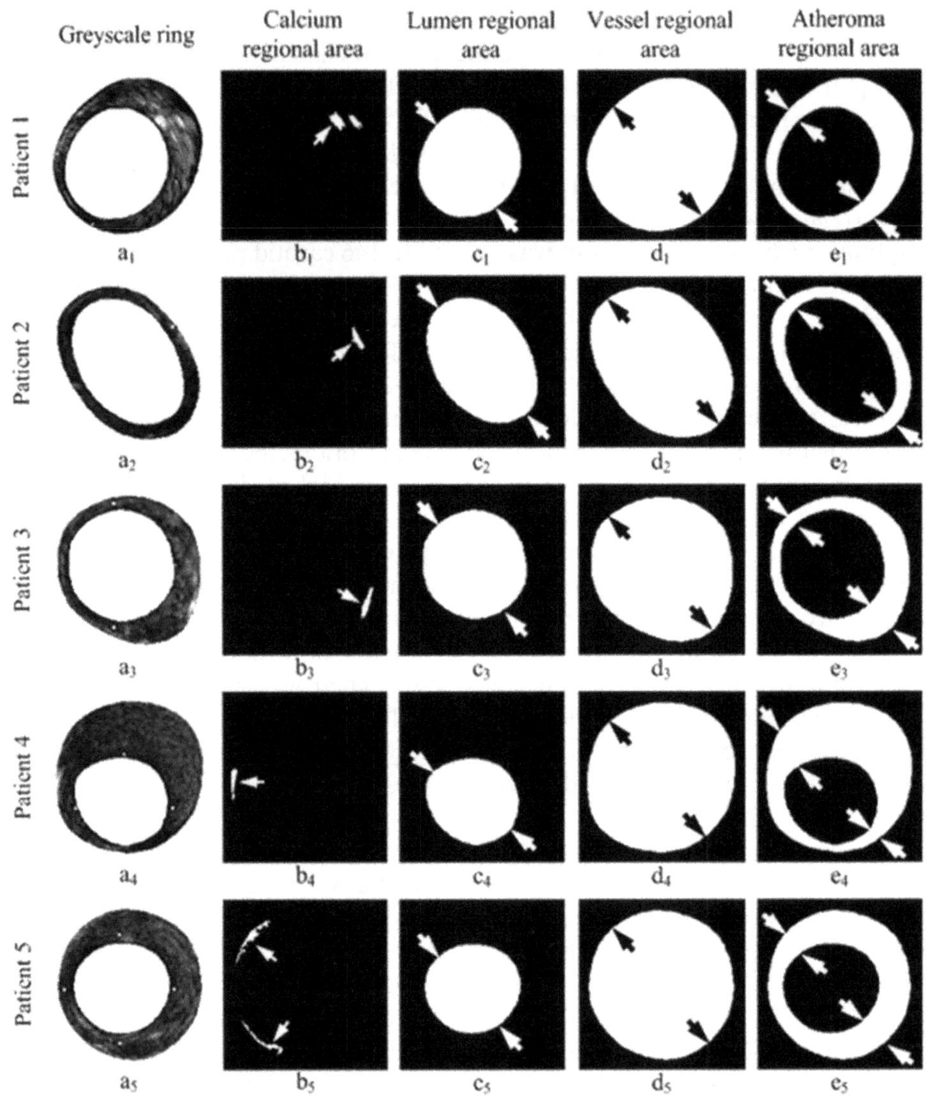

Figure 14.1. Typical examples of images showing the grayscale ring, calcium regional area, vessel regional area, lumen regional area and atheroma regional area from five different low-risk patients.

14.2 Patient demographics and data acquisition

14.2.1 Patient demographics

From a single case study, twenty-two patients with stable angina pectoris who underwent percutaneous coronary interventions between July 2009 and December 2010 were considered for this study. The study consisted of 22 patients (20 M 2 F) in the age group of 36–81 years (average 66 ± 12 years). In this database, ten patients had a calcified location on the left anterior descending, eight on the right, two on the

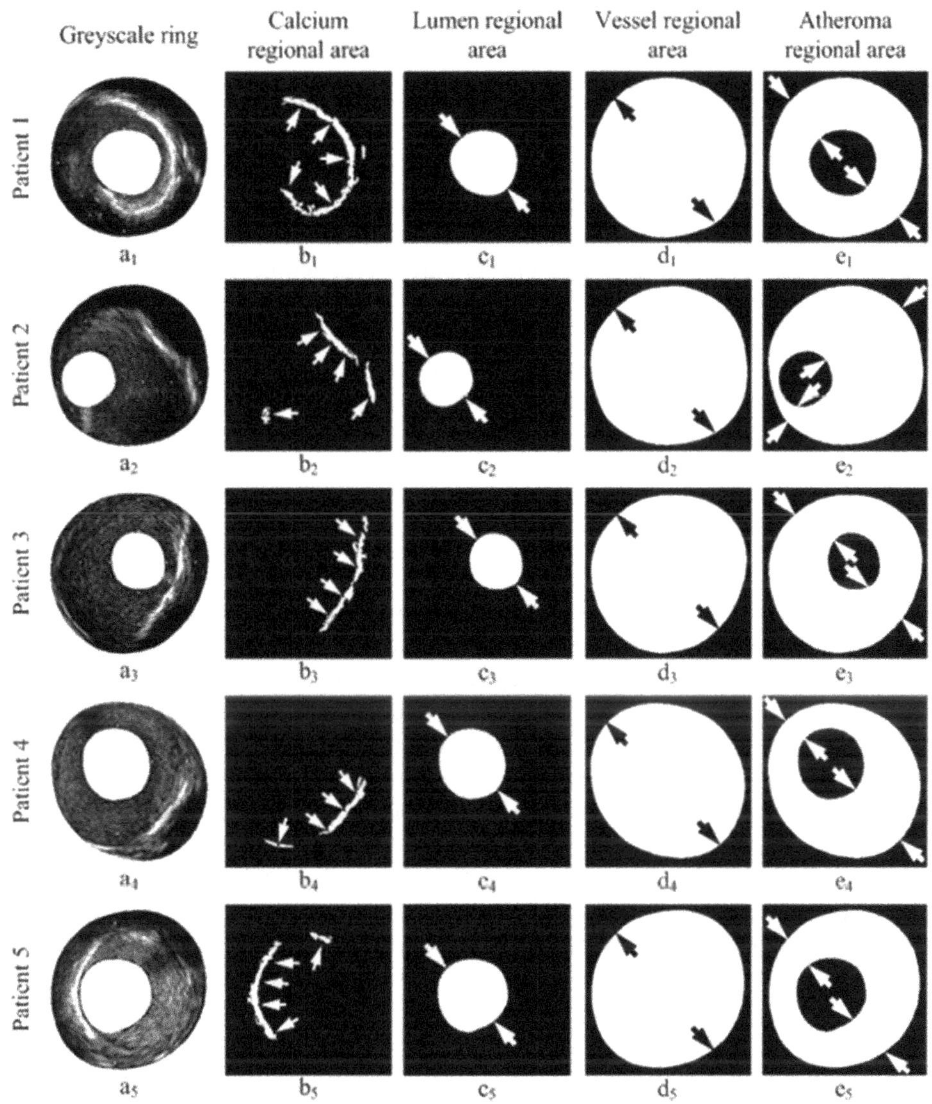

Figure 14.2. Typical examples of images showing the grayscale ring, calcium regional area, vessel regional area, lumen regional area and atheroma regional area from five different high-risk patients.

left circumflex and two on the left main coronary artery. Out of 22 patients, ten had proximal lesions, six in the middle, and six at a distal location. Five patients had a family history of CAD. Furthermore, one patient had a prior myocardial infarction while another had undergone a prior coronary artery bypass grafting. The mean hemoglobin, low-density lipoprotein (LDL), high-density lipoprotein (HDL) and total cholesterol were 5.6 g dL^{-1}, 94.4 mg dL^{-1}, 48.7 mg dL^{-1} and 168 mg dL^{-1}, respectively. Ten patients from the pool of 22 patients were smokers.

14.2.2 Data acquisition

The dataset was approved by the IRB and written informed consent was provided by all the patients. In this study, all the patients have undergone both carotid and coronary ultrasound examinations. Carotid examinations were performed with a scanner (Aplio XV, AplioXG, Xario, Toshiba, Inc., Tokyo, Japan) equipped with a 7.5 MHz linear array transducer. For coronary data acquisition, a 40 MHz IVUS catheter (Atlantis SR Pro; Boston Scientific, Marlborough, MA, USA) was used. For the carotid database, high-resolution images were acquired as recommended by the American Society of Echocardiography and, for the coronary database, the DICOM image format was used. Durng conversion into AVI movies, these DICOM images (16 bits per pixel) were further compressed to JPEG (8 bits per pixel) images. The mean pixel resolution for the carotid and coronary databases were 0.05 ± 0.01 mm/pixel and 0.0167 mm/pixel, respectively.

14.3 Methodology

14.3.1 IVUS data preparation

The coronary dataset consists of 22 patients with 2109 frames per patient. Our coronary data size preparation involves two assumptions: (a) the head and tail end frames did not contain any morphological information about calcium and (b) the artery is not a straight line and longitudinal and transversal displacements do exist between frames [29, 30]. In this database, the change in calcium was observed in every 10th frame. Using these two assumptions, we accumulated 4930 frames derived from 22 patients. Considering the carotid risk threshold [16, 17, 23], all the patients with a carotid plaque burden higher than or equal to 0.9 mm are categorized into the high-risk pool and the patients with a plaque burden lower than 0.9 mm are categorized in the low-risk pool. Accordingly, 14 patients were categorized as high-risk (~63.63%) and the other eight patients were in the low-risk pool (~36.36%). Note that our data size in the ML framework was not 22 subjects, but 4930 frames collected from 22 subjects, with pools consisting of 3043 high-risk frames and 1887 low-risk frames corresponding to 14 high-risk patients and eight low-risk patients, respectively.

14.3.2 Wall region of interest estimation

In this study for the region of interest (ROI) estimation, we have employed an ImgTracer™ system (courtesy of AtheroPoint™, Roseville, CA, USA) recently used by JSS and his team [20, 29–31]. Here, two experts (doctoral students with knowledge of coronary artery disease and IVUS imaging) generated the vessel wall region by manually tracing the internal elastic lamina (IEL) and external elastic lamina (EEL) borders. A typical example of manually traced IEL/EEL borders is shown in figure 14.3. In figure 14.3(a), the inner/outer yellow rings indicate IEL/EEL borders. The atherosclerotic wall region treated as the ROI is shown in figure 14.3(b).

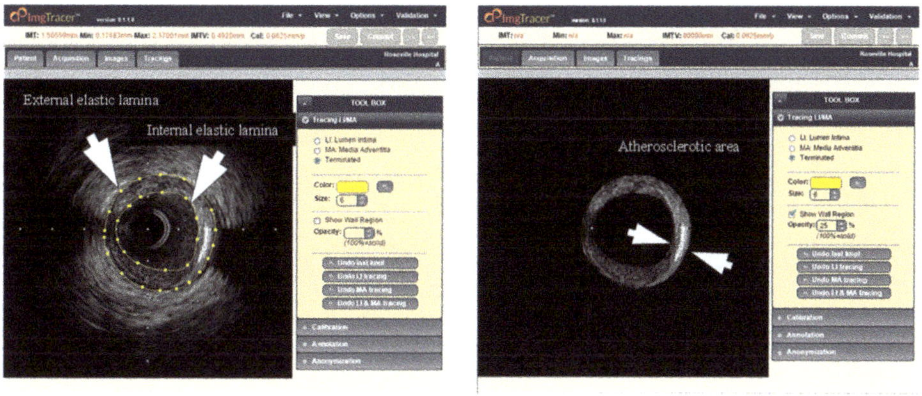

(a) (b)

Figure 14.3. (a) Manually traced internal elastic lamina and external elastic lamina indicated by the inner and outer yellow rings in the vessel wall region obtained by manually tracings using ImgTracer™. (b) Atherosclerotic grayscale ring image used as the ROI. (Courtesy of AtheroPoint™, Roseville, CA, USA. Source: Banchhor *et al* [29].)

14.3.3 Wall- and texture-based feature computation

In this study, we have computed six different wall-based measurement features, namely coronary calcium area, coronary vessel area, coronary lumen area, coronary atheroma area, coronary wall thickness and coronary wall thickness variability [20]. Coronary calcium area is computed using a well-established threshold-based segmentation technique [29, 31]. However, coronary vessel area, coronary lumen area and coronary atheroma area was computed by generating their corresponding binary mask images using the IEL/EEL borders manually traced by experts using the ImgTracer™ system [20]. Further, using the bidirectional concept of the polyline distance method [32, 33], we have computed the coronary wall thickness. Finally, coronary wall thickness variability is estimated by computing the standard deviation of the coronary wall thickness over all the frames. For this study, we have also extracted 59 different plaque texture-based features [16, 17], thus having a total set of 65 features. Detailed derivations of all the plaque texture-based features are as shown below.

14.3.3.1 Gray-level co-occurrence matrix (GLCM)

The GLCM matrix indicates the joint probability of the occurrence of the gray-level between neighboring pixels [34]. Let us assume a 2D image containing pixels with gray levels $(0, 1, \ldots, N-1)$. A GLCM indicates the probability of gray-level i occurring in the neighborhood of gray-level j. Here the (i, j)th entry of GLCM is denoted as $P_{\mathrm{df}}(i, j)$, which is normalized by dividing each element in the matrix by the sum of all the elements in the matrix. μ_i and μ_j represents the mean for the rows and columns at location $P_{\mathrm{df}}(i, j)$. Similarly σ_i and σ_j represent the standard deviation for the rows and columns at location $P_{\mathrm{df}}(i, j)$. The 18 features derived from GLCM are given in table 14.1 [35] which reflects the spatial distribution of intensity values of an image.

Table 14.1. Features of the GLCM.

Feature name	Equation
Mean (μ_i, μ_j)	$\mu_i = \sum_{i=0}^{N-1}\sum_{j=0}^{N-1}(i) \cdot P_{\text{df}}(i, j)$ $\mu_j = \sum_{i=0}^{N-1}\sum_{j=0}^{N-1}(j). P_{\text{df}}(i, j)$
Standard deviation (σ_i, σ_j)	$\sigma_i = \sum_{i=0}^{N-1}\sum_{j=0}^{N-1}(i - \mu_i) \cdot P_{\text{df}}(i, j)$ $\sigma_j = \sum_{i=0}^{N-1}\sum_{j=0}^{N-1}(i - \mu_j) \cdot P_{\text{df}}(i, j)$
Autocorrelation (ACorr)	$\text{ACorr} = \sum_{i=0}^{N-1}\sum_{j=0}^{N-1}(ij) \cdot P_{\text{df}}(i, j)$
Correlation (Corr)	$\text{Corr} = \dfrac{\sum_{i=0}^{N-1}\sum_{j=0}^{N-1}(ij) \cdot P_{\text{df}}(i, j) - \mu_i\mu_j}{\sigma_i\sigma_j}$
Contrast (Cont)	$\text{Cont} = \sum_{i=0}^{N-1}\sum_{j=0}^{N-1}(i - j)^2 \cdot P_{\text{df}}(i, j)$
Cluster prominence (CPro)	$\text{CPro} = \sum_{i=0}^{N-1}\sum_{j=0}^{N-1}(i + j - \mu_i - \mu_j)^4 \cdot P_{\text{df}}(i, j)$
Cluster Shade (CSha)	$\text{CSha} = \sum_{i=o}^{N-1}\sum_{j=0}^{N-1}(i + j - \mu_i - \mu_j)^3 \cdot P_{\text{df}}(i, j)$
Dissimilarity (D_{ij})	$D_{ij} = \sum_{i=0}^{N-1}\sum_{j=0}^{N-1}\lvert i - j\rvert \cdot P_{\text{df}}(i, j)$
Energy (Eng)	$\text{Eng} = \sum_{i=0}^{N-1}\sum_{j=0}^{N-1}P_{\text{df}}(i, j)^2$
Entropy (Ent)	$\text{Ent} = -\sum_{i=0}^{N-1}\sum_{j=0}^{N-1}P_{\text{df}}(i, j) \cdot \log\{P_{\text{df}}(i, j)\}$
Homogeneity (Homo)	$\text{Homo} = \sum_{i=0}^{N-1}\sum_{j=0}^{N-1}\dfrac{P_{\text{df}}(i, j)}{1 + (i - j)^2}$
Maximum probability (MPro)	$\text{MPro} = \max_{i,j} P_{\text{df}}(i, j)$
Sum of squares (SoS)	$\text{SoS} = \sum_{i=0}^{N-1}\sum_{j=0}^{N-1}(i - \mu)^2 \cdot P_{\text{df}}(i, j)$

Sum average (SAvg)	$\mathrm{SAvg} = \sum_{i=0}^{2(N-1)} i \cdot P_{x+y}(i)$
Sum entropy (SEnt)	$\mathrm{SEnt} = -\sum_{i=0}^{2(N-1)} P_{x+y}(i) \cdot \log\{P_{x+y}(i)\}$
Sum variances (SVar)	$\mathrm{SVar} = \sum_{i=0}^{2(N-1)} (i - \mathrm{SEnt})^2 \cdot P_{x+y}(i)$
Difference variance (DVar)	$\mathrm{DVar} = \sum_{i=0}^{N-1} (i - \mathrm{DVar}')^2 \cdot P_{x-y}(i)$
Difference entropy (DEnt)	$\mathrm{DEnt} = -\sum_{i=0}^{N-1} P_{x-y}(i) \cdot \log\{P_{x-y}(i)\}$
	where $P_{x+y}(k) = \sum_{i=0}^{N-1}\sum_{j=0}^{N-1} P(i, j),\ k = i + j = \{0, 1, \ldots 2(N-1)\}$ $P_{x-y}(k) = \sum_{i=0}^{N-1}\sum_{j=0}^{N-1} P(i, j),\ k = \lvert i - j\rvert = \{0, 1, \ldots 2(N-1)\}$

14.3.3.2 The gray-level run length matrix (GLRLM)

In the GLRLM, the gray intensity of the pixel is measured from the reference pixel and run length is defined as the set of pixels having the same gray levels in a specific direction. In this grayscale texture feature, $F(x, y)$ defines the set of pixels of successive runs of length y at reference gray level x. Here, GL defines the number of gray levels, RL defines the maximum run length, l_t is the total number of runs and l_q is the number of pixels in the image. From the GLRLM, 11 features are extracted, as shown in table 14.2 [35], which measure the joint distribution of gray-level and run length distribution.

14.3.3.3 Intensity histogram

In the intensity histogram, the following measurements are computed: mean energy, variance, entropy, skewness and kurtosis. Mean, variance and skew measure the brightness, contrast and the allocation of the gray level in an image. Entropy is the converse of skew. Here $I(j)$ defines the number of pixel intensities of value j. Table 14.3 shows the formulas for extracting seven features using the intensity histogram of a given image [35].

14.3.3.4 Gray-level difference statistics (GLDS)

The GLDS algorithm measures the absolute difference between the pairs of the gray levels for a given displacement γ. For any given displacement $\gamma = (\Delta x, \Delta y)$, let $I_\gamma(x, y) = \lvert I(x, y) - I(x + \Delta x, y + \Delta y)\rvert$ and PD_γ be the probability density function of I_γ. In this analysis, four features are extracted as shown in table 14.4 for displacement $\gamma = (0, 3), (3, 0), (3, 3),(3, -3)$ and their average values are considered [36].

Table 14.2. Features of the GLRLM.

Feature name	Equation
Short run emphasis (SRE)	$\mathrm{SRE} = \frac{1}{l_t}\sum_{y=1}^{\mathrm{GL}}\sum_{y=1}^{\mathrm{RL}}\frac{F(x, y)}{y^2} = \frac{1}{l_t}\sum_{y=1}^{\mathrm{RL}}\frac{F_t(y)}{y^2}$
Long run emphasis (LER)	$\mathrm{LER} = \frac{1}{l_t}\sum_{x=1}^{\mathrm{GL}}\sum_{y=1}^{\mathrm{RL}}(F(x, y)\cdot y^2) = \frac{1}{l_t}\sum_{y=1}^{\mathrm{RL}}F_t(y)\cdot y^2$
Gray-level non-uniformity (GLNU)	$\mathrm{GLNU} = \frac{1}{l_t}\sum_{x=1}^{\mathrm{GL}}\left(\sum_{y=1}^{\mathrm{RL}}(F(x, y))\right)^2 = \frac{1}{l_t}\sum_{x=1}^{\mathrm{RL}}F_q(x)^2$
Run length non-uniformity (RLNU)	$\mathrm{RLNU} = \frac{1}{l_t}\sum_{x=1}^{\mathrm{GL}}\left(\sum_{y=1}^{\mathrm{RL}}(F(x, y))\right)^2 = \frac{1}{l_t}\sum_{x=1}^{\mathrm{RL}}F_t(y)^2$
Run percentage (RPer)	$\mathrm{RPer} = \frac{l_t}{l_q}$
Low gray-level run emphasis (LGRE)	$\mathrm{LGRE} = \frac{1}{l_t}\sum_{x=1}^{\mathrm{GL}}\sum_{y=1}^{\mathrm{RL}}\frac{F(x, y)}{x^2} = \frac{1}{l_t}\sum_{y=1}^{\mathrm{RL}}\frac{F_q(x)}{x^2}$
High gray-level run emphasis (HGRE)	$\mathrm{HGRE} = \frac{1}{l_t}\sum_{x=1}^{\mathrm{GL}}\sum_{y=1}^{\mathrm{RL}}(F(x, y)\cdot x^2) = \frac{1}{l_t}\sum_{y=1}^{\mathrm{RL}}F_t(y)\cdot x^2$
Short run low gray-level emphasis (SRLGE)	$\mathrm{SRLGE} = \frac{1}{l_t}\sum_{x=1}^{\mathrm{GL}}\sum_{y=1}^{\mathrm{RL}}\frac{F(x, y)}{x^2\cdot y^2}$
Short run high gray-level emphasis (SRHE)	$\mathrm{SRHGE} = \frac{1}{l_t}\sum_{x=1}^{\mathrm{GL}}\sum_{y=1}^{\mathrm{RL}}\frac{F(x, y)\cdot x^2}{x^2}$
Long run low gray-level emphasis (LRLGE)	$\mathrm{LRLGE} = \frac{1}{l_t}\sum_{x=1}^{\mathrm{GL}}\sum_{y=1}^{\mathrm{RL}}\frac{F(x, y)\cdot y^2}{y^2}$
Long run high gray-level emphasis (LRHGE)	$\mathrm{LRHGE} = \frac{1}{l_t}\sum_{x=1}^{\mathrm{GL}}\sum_{y=1}^{\mathrm{RL}}F(x, y)\cdot x^2\cdot y^2$

14.3.3.5 The neighborhood gray tone difference matrix (NGTDM)

Essentially, NGTDM is a column matrix $K(i)$ wherein each ith value is the magnitude of the difference between the mean of the pixels in the neighborhood and the pixel under assessment. Here p_i is the probability of occurrence of gray-level value i. Busyness, contrast, complexity, coarseness and texture length are the five texture features that are derived from the NGTDM, as shown in table 14.5 [37, 38].

14.3.3.6 Invariant moment

In an invariant moment, the raw moments and the central moments were utilized for the feature extraction [39]. The seven features extracted using raw moments RM_{pq}, central moments CM_{pq} and central moments after scaling normalization M_{pq} for $p, q = 0, 1, 2, 3$ are shown in table 14.6. All the seven moments are invariant to scale, rotation and translation.

Table 14.3. Features of the intensity histogram.

Feature name	Equation
Mean (M)	$M = \sum_{j=0}^{N-1} j \cdot I(j)$
Energy (E)	$E = \sum_{j=0}^{N-1} I(j)^2$
Standard deviation (SD)	$\mathrm{SD} = \sqrt{\sum_{j=0}^{N-1} (i - M)^2 \cdot I(j)}$
Variance (Var)	$\mathrm{Var} = \sum_{j=0}^{N-1} (j - M)^2 I(j)$
Entropy (Ent)	$\mathrm{Ent} = \sum_{=0}^{N-1} I(j) \log_2 I(j)$
Skewness (Skew)	$\mathrm{Skew} = \pi^{-3} \sum_{j=0}^{N-1} (j - M)^3 I(j)$
Kurtosis (Kurt)	$\mathrm{Kurt} = \pi^{-4} \sum_{j=0}^{N-1} (j - M)^4 I(j) - 3$

Table 14.4. Features of GLDS.

Feature	Equation
Contrast (C_1)	$C_1 = \sum_{i=0}^{N-1} i^2 \cdot \mathrm{PD}_\gamma(i)$
Angular second moment (Φ_m)	$\Phi_m = \sum_{i=0}^{N-1} \mathrm{PD}_\gamma(i)^2$
Entropy (E_1)	$E_1 = -\sum_{i=0}^{N-1} \mathrm{PD}_\gamma(i) \cdot \log\{\mathrm{PD}_\gamma(i)\}$
Mean (M_1)	$M_1 = \sum_{i=0}^{N-1} i \cdot \mathrm{PD}_\gamma(i)$

14.3.3.7 The statistical feature matrix (SFM)

The values of the statistical properties of pixel pairs at various locations were stored in the SFM. CF is the normalization factor, usually considered to be 100 for coarseness computation. DM and CON represent the dissimilarity and contrast matrix, respectively. DV depicts the displacement vectors and Nms defines the

Table 14.5. Features of the NGTDM.

Feature name	Equation
Coarseness (Coar)	$\text{Coar} = \left[\sum_{i=0}^{N-1} p_i K(i)\right]^{-1}$
Contrast (Cont)	$\text{Cont} = \frac{1}{N(N-1)} \sum_{i=0}^{N-1}\sum_{j=0}^{N-1} p_i p_j (i-j)^2 \cdot \frac{1}{n^2}\sum_{i=0}^{N-1} K(i)$
Busyness (Bus)	$\text{Bus} = \frac{\sum_{i=0}^{N-1} p_i K(i)}{\sum_{i=0}^{N-1}\sum_{j=0}^{N-1}(ip_i - jp_j)}$
Complexity (Comp)	$\text{Comp} = \sum_{i=0}^{N-1}\sum_{j=0}^{N-1}\left\{\frac{\lvert i-j\rvert}{n^2(p_i + p_j)}\right\} \cdot \{p_i K(i) + p_j K(j)\}$
Texture strength (TS)	$\text{TS} = \frac{\sum_{i=0}^{N-1}\sum_{j=0}^{N-1}(p_i + p_j)(i-j)^2}{\sum_{i=0}^{N-1} K(i)}$

Table 14.6. Features of the invariant moment.

Feature name	Equation
I_1	$f_1 = M_{20} + M_{02}$
I_2	$f_2 = (M_{20} + M_{02})^2 + 4M_{11}$
I_3	$f_3 = (M_{30} - 3M_{12})^2 + (3M_{21} - M_{03})^2$
I_4	$f_4 = (M_{30} - M_{12})^2 + (M_{21} + M_{03})^2$
I_5	$f_5 = (M_{30} - 3M_{12})(M_{30} + M_{12})[(M_{30} + 3M_{12})^2 - 3(M_{21} + M_{03})^2] + (3M_{21} - M_{03})(M_{21} + M_{03})[3(M_{30} + M_{12})^2 - (M_{21} + M_{03})^2]$
I_6	$f_6 = (M_{20} - M_{02})[(M_{30} + M_{12})^2 - (M_{21} - M_{03})^2] + [4M_{11}(M_{30} + M_{12})(M_{21} + M_{03})]$
I_7	$f_7 = (M_{21} + M_{03})(M_{30} + M_{12})[(M_{30} + M_{12})^2 - 3(M_{21} + M_{03})^2] - (M_{30} - 3M_{21})(M_{21} + M_{03})[3(M_{30} + M_{12})^2 - (M_{21} + M_{03})^2]$
	where $\text{RM}_{pq} = \sum_{x=0}^{rw-1}\sum_{y=0}^{cl-1} x^p \cdot y^q \cdot f(x, y);\ \bar{x} = \frac{\text{RM}_{10}}{\text{RM}_{00}};\ \bar{y} = \frac{\text{RM}_{01}}{\text{RM}_{00}}$ $\mu_{pq} = \sum_{x=0}^{rw-1}\sum_{y=0}^{cl-1}(x - \bar{x})^p \cdot (y - \bar{y})^q \cdot f(x, y);$ $\eta_{pq} = \frac{\mu_{pq}}{\mu_{00}^{(1+(p+q)/2)}}$

number of elements in the set DV. M_{dm} represents SFM for the dissimilarity matrix, M_d represents the mean of M_{dm} and M_{dv} represents the deepest valley of M_{dm}. The fractal dimensions in the x and y directions are denoted by $\text{FD}_{\text{sf}}^{(x)}$ and $\text{FD}_{\text{sf}}^{(y)}$, as shown in table 14.7 [40].

Table 14.7. Features of statistical feature matrix.

Feature name	Equation
Coarseness (Coa)	$\text{Coa} = \frac{\text{CF}}{\sum_{(i,\,j)\in DV}\text{DM}(i,\,j)/\text{Nms}}$
Periodicity (Perio)	$\text{Perio} = \frac{M_d - M_{dv}}{M_d}$
Contrast (Cont)	$\text{Cont} = \sqrt{\sum_{(i,j)\in \text{DV}} \frac{\text{CON}(i,\,j)}{4}}$
Roughness (Roug)	$\text{Roug} = \frac{(\text{FD}_{\text{sf}}{}^{(x)} + \text{FD}_{\text{sf}}{}^{(y)})}{2}$

Table 14.8. Features of the MGFM.

Feature name	Equation
Mean grayscale value (μ_{GS})	$\mu\text{GS} = \frac{\sum_{i=0}^{N} X_i}{N}$
Mean grayscale standard deviation (σ_{GS})	$\sigma\text{GS} = \sqrt{\frac{\sum(X_i - \mu_{\text{GS}})^2}{N}}$

14.3.3.8 Mean grayscale feature matrix (MGFM)

Let X_i be a matrix of all the intensities of a grayscale (GS) image I, consisting of N number of elements. Then, the mean (μ_{GS}) and standard deviation (σ_{GS}) of the image I are as shown in table 14.8.

14.3.4 Principal component analysis with polling contribution

For this study, we have extracted 59 different plaque texture-based features [16, 17] along with six wall-based measurement features, thus having a total set of 65 features. However, since there are a large number of features (= 65), it is first necessary to extract the dominant features from the pool consisting of plaque texture-based features fused with wall-based measurement features. Since PCA is mainly used for dimensionality reduction, a PCA-based polling strategy is used in this study [41]. Here, we use eigenvectors to evaluate the significance of different feature components of the original samples. The algorithm of feature selection is as follows:

Step 1. First, we compute the covariance matrix of the dataset.

Step 2. Now, we compute the eigenvectors (V) and eigenvalues (λ) of the covariance matrix.

Step 3. Now, we select the largest eigenvalues and arrange the eigenvectors according to the selected eigenvalues.

Step 4. Now, we choose the number of principal components (n) using the condition:

$$\left(\sum_{j=1}^{n} \frac{\lambda_j}{\sum_{i=1}^{m} \lambda_i} \right) \geqslant X, \tag{14.1}$$

where X is the cut-off, varying from 0.90 to 0.99 with a step size of 0.01, and m represents the total number of eigenvalues.

Step 5. Now, we compute the contribution to the feature extraction result of each feature component as follows:

$$C_i = \sum_{k=1}^{n} |V_{ki}|, \tag{14.2}$$

where V_{ki} indicates the ith entry of V_k, $i = 1, 2, \ldots, m$ and $k = 1, 2, \ldots, n$. $|V_{ki}|$ shows the absolute value of V_{ki}.

Step 6. Finally, we sort the C_i in descending order and select the first n features components which will give the reduced number of dominant features without losing the feature values.

14.3.5 Support vector machine

For training the machine learning classifier to perform tissue classification, we have used a classifier based on SVM [16, 17]. SVM is a supervised learning model which performs classification by constructing a hyper-plane between the data points. This hyper-plane optimally separates the data into the desired number of classes [47]. The points near the hyper-plane are called support vectors and their distance from the hyper-plane is called the margin. The marginal hyper-planes are the two hyper-planes which are constructed on each side of the hyper-plane and the objective is to maximize the distance of the data points from these marginal hyper-planes [42, 43]. For performing the non-linear classification, kernel functions are used [44, 45]. Commonly used kernel functions are linear, the radial basis function (RBF) and polynomial (of different orders) [46]. The mathematical description of SVM is given below.

Let us consider a two-class classification task with the training sample of patterns $\{(m_i, n_i), i = 1, 2, \ldots, l\}$, where $m_i \in R^q$ represents input data for ith sample and $n_i \in \{-1, +1\}$ represents the corresponding target values, l is the total number of training samples and q is the dimension of the input space. The SVM model can be represented in feature space by the following equation:

$$p(x) = \omega^T \Phi(m) + \alpha, \tag{14.3}$$

where $\Phi(m)$ represents the kernel function which maps the input vector into higher dimensional space, α represents bias, ω is a weight vector which is normal to the hyper-plane and T denotes transpose. The decision rule is mathematically represented by the following equation:

$$\begin{aligned} \omega^T\Phi(m_i) + \alpha \geqslant +1 \qquad & \text{if } n_i = +1 \\ \omega^T\Phi(m_i) + \alpha \leqslant -1 \qquad & \text{if } n_i = -1. \end{aligned} \tag{14.4}$$

The non-linear kernel function finds the separating hyper-plane with a maximum margin $\frac{2}{\|\omega\|}$ between the classes in a feature space. To find the optimal separating hyper-plane, equation (14.3) is minimized as shown by the following equation:

$$€\sum_{i=1}^{l}\xi_i + \frac{1}{2}\|\omega\|^2, \tag{14.5}$$

where € is the trade-off parameter between the error and margin, and ξ is a slack variable. By using Lagrangian multipliers (£) in dual form, the equation (14.3) can be transformed into the following optimization problem:

maximize

$$\sum_{i=1}^{l}£_i - \frac{1}{2}\sum_{i=1}^{l}\sum_{j=1}^{l}£_i£_jn_in_jK_f(m_i, m_j) \tag{14.6}$$

subject to

$$\sum_{i=1}^{l}£_in_i = 0, \;\; £_i \geqslant 0 \;\forall\; i \tag{14.7}$$

where

$$K_f(m_i, m_j) = \Phi(m_i)^T \cdot \Phi(m_j). \tag{14.8}$$

Finally, the final decision function is mathematically represented by the following equation:

$$p(x) = \sum_{i=1}^{l}£_in_iK_f(m_i, m_j) + \alpha. \tag{14.9}$$

14.3.6 Machine learning (ML) paradigm for class prediction

Figure 14.4 shows the block diagram of the ML system used in this study using the fusion of plaque texture-based and wall-based measurement features (as shown by the arrows on the left and right). The patient population is divided into two components: the training population and the testing population. The training population is used for computing the learning parameters during the ML process. These parameters are computed using the training grayscale coronary wall region and corresponding carotid gold standard risk labels. This gold standard is derived from the concept of the second hypothesis, which states that atherosclerotic plaque has a common genetic make-up, as discussed before in step 1 [16, 17]. In the ML paradigm, one computes the offline grayscale plaque features and trains these features according to the gold standard risk labels derived from the carotid artery plaque burden. These offline parameters are then transformed by the online grayscale wall features computed from the test images to

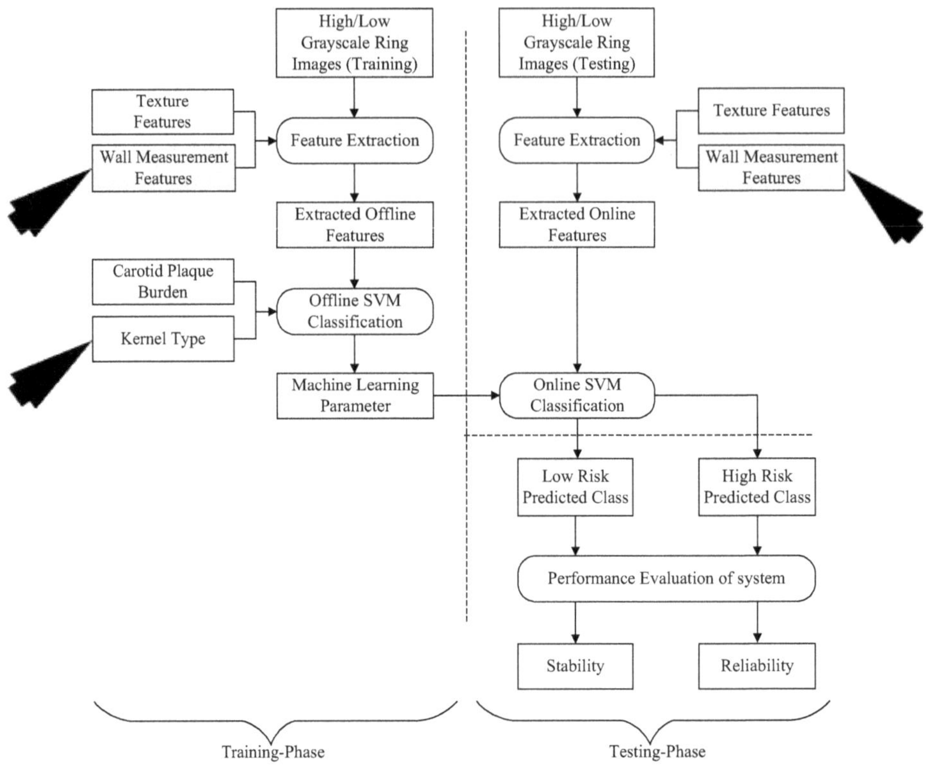

Figure 14.4. Improved coronary risk assessment system (cRAS) using the ML paradigm utilizing PCA with the fusion of plaque texture-based and wall-based measurement features. Gray boxes show novel wall-based measurement features.

predict its risk label. Finally, the process of ML is repeated for the cyclic combinations as per the *K*-fold combinations. Since there are ten parts (*K*10 protocol: 90% training and 10% testing), we therefore rotate this combination ten times to ensure that each set of 10% testing data gets a chance to become a training dataset. Each combination yields the stratification accuracy using the ML system. The mean value of the classification accuracy is then computed, which determines the final accuracy of the ML system. Furthermore, to separate the features in the SVM framework, we have adopted both a linear and four non-linear kernel functions [17], namely the RBF, and polynomial functions of order 1, 2 and 3. These kernel functions are used by the SVM during its training and testing phases.

14.4 Results

The main observations here are to see the effect of fusion of wall-based measurement features with plaque texture-based features on the stratification accuracy in the ML framework. These results will characterize (i) the PCA polling process, the best kernel design during the classification process and (iii) cut-off values between memorization versus generalization for a dataset size.

Table 14.9. Dominant features selected at each PCA-based cut-off using (a) stand-alone plaque texture-based features and (b) plaque texture-based features fused with wall-based measurement features.

Cut-offs	F1	F2	F3	F4	F5	F6	F7	F8	F9	F10	F11	F12	F13	F14	F15	F16
(a) Using stand-alone plaque texture-based features																
0.90	52	56	16	15	6											
0.91	52	56	16	15	6											
0.92	52	56	16	15	6											
0.93	52	56	55	26	24	4										
0.94	52	56	55	26	24	4										
0.95	52	56	55	26	24	4	31									
0.96	52	56	55	26	24	4	31									
0.97	52	44	56	55	26	42	43	4								
0.98	52	55	44	4	26	56	43	35	42	37						
0.99	55	52	26	56	44	4	43	28	37	42	35	31	24			
(b) Using plaque texture-based features fused with wall-based measurement features																
0.90	52	56	65	28	16											
0.91	52	59	61	56	26	55										
0.92	52	59	61	56	26	55										
0.93	52	65	59	26	61	55	44									
0.94	52	65	59	26	61	55	44									
0.95	52	65	55	61	44	56	59	26								
0.96	65	52	61	55	44	26	56	59	24							
0.97	65	61	52	55	44	26	59	4	56	21						
0.98	61	44	65	59	55	26	52	4	56	24	21	43				
0.99	44	61	65	55	26	59	52	43	4	37	24	21	54	35	28	42

The numerical numbers listed in the columns have unique feature names and these are as follows: 4—cluster prominence; 6—dissimilarity; 15—difference variance; 16—difference entropy; 21—gray-level non-uniformity; 24—low gray-level run emphasis; 26—short run low gray-level emphasis; 28—long run low gray-level emphasis; 31—variance; 35—skewness; 37—contrast (C_1); 42—contrast (C_0); 43—busyness; 44—complexity; 52—I7; 54—contrast (C_3); 55—complexity; 56—roughness; 59—coronary lumen area; 61—coronary calcium area; 65—coronary wall thickness variability, F—feature.

14.4.1 Dominant feature selection

The best dominant feature combination set can increase the accuracy of the SVM classifier. The objective of this experiment is to find the best matching set of features to yield the highest accuracy using a PCA-based polling strategy. This is achieved by taking different cut-offs ranging from 0.90 to 0.99 in increments of 0.01 for a fixed data size.

Table 14.9 shows the dominant features selected for different PCA-based cut-offs for (a) stand-alone plaque texture-based features and (b) plaque texture-based features fused with wall-based measurement features. In both cases, we can observe that the number of dominant features gradually increases with the increase in PCA-based cut-offs. In table 14.9, for the fusion of plaque texture-based and wall-based measurement features, the coronary calcium area (feature #61), coronary lumen area (feature #59) and coronary wall thickness variability (feature #65) are selected as the dominant features for different PCA-based cut-offs. The selection of dominant features taking different PCA-based cut-offs for both (a) stand-alone plaque texture-based features and (b) plaque texture-based features fused with wall-based measurement features is shown in figure 14.5.

14.4.2 Selection of the best kernel function

Since the hyper-plane for stratification is governed by the choice of kernel function used [47], we therefore choose five types of kernels [16, 17], such as linear, RBF, and polynomial of order 1, 2 and 3, respectively, for optimization in both paradigms: with and without wall-based measurement features.

For this protocol, we have fixed the data size. Using five different kernel functions, the accuracy of the SVM classifier for both (a) stand-alone plaque texture-based features and (b) plaque texture-based features fused with wall-based measurement features are shown in table 14.10. Figure 14.6(a) and (b) show the

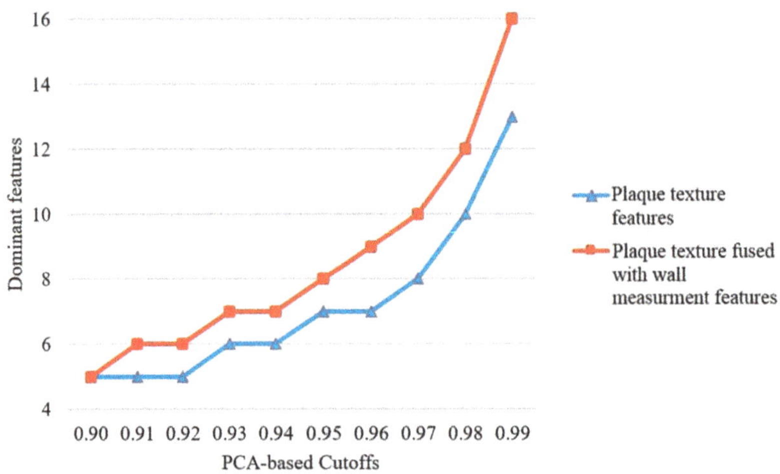

Figure 14.5. Numbers of dominant features versus PCA-based cut-offs using (a) stand-alone plaque texture-based features and (b) plaque texture-based features fused with wall-based measurement features.

Table 14.10. Classification accuracy using SVM with varying kernel function: (a) stand-alone plaque texture-based features and (b) plaque texture-based features fused with wall-based measurement features.

(a) Using stand-alone plaque texture-based features (in %)					
	Kernel functions				
Cut-offs	Linear	RBF	Poly-1	Poly-2	Poly-3
0.90	67.14	76.20	67.14	71.87	74.86
0.91	67.14	76.18	67.14	71.89	74.89
0.92	67.15	76.15	67.15	71.91	74.85
0.93	73.02	87.53	73.02	77.37	82.95
0.94	73.06	87.56	73.06	77.39	82.96
0.95	75.48	89.66	75.48	81.30	85.68
0.96	75.48	89.65	75.48	81.32	85.72
0.97	78.47	91.32	78.47	82.88	86.41
0.98	77.91	92.74	77.91	84.20	89.46
0.99	79.80	93.82	79.80	86.63	92.03
Average	73.47	86.08	73.47	78.68	82.98
SD	4.87	7.12	4.87	5.45	6.22
(b) Using plaque texture-based features fused with wall-based measurement features (in %)					
0.90	78.24	86.03	78.24	77.66	81.54
0.91	69.63	85.13	69.63	77.61	80.24
0.92	69.64	85.12	69.64	77.54	80.22
0.93	76.55	91.35	76.55	81.40	85.16
0.94	76.53	91.35	76.53	81.44	85.26
0.95	76.73	91.81	76.73	81.96	85.98
0.96	77.79	93.31	77.79	82.83	87.61
0.97	77.58	95.72	77.58	85.68	91.00
0.98	79.86	96.35	79.86	86.97	93.10
0.99	78.94	96.59	78.94	89.41	94.91
Average	76.15	91.28	76.15	82.25	86.50
SD	3.59	4.49	3.59	4.11	5.19

Poly—polynomial.

graphical representation of the accuracy of the SVM classifier for both (a) stand-alone plaque texture-based features and (b) plaque texture-based features fused with wall-based measurement features. We observe that for all the kernel functions, the mean accuracy of all the PCA-based cut-offs using the fusion of plaque texture-based and wall-based measurement features are higher compared to the stand-alone option where plaque texture-based features are only considered. Among all the kernel functions, RBF gave the highest accuracy for all the PCA-based cut-offs, hence is considered as the best among all four kernel functions. This is consistent with our other studies [16, 17].

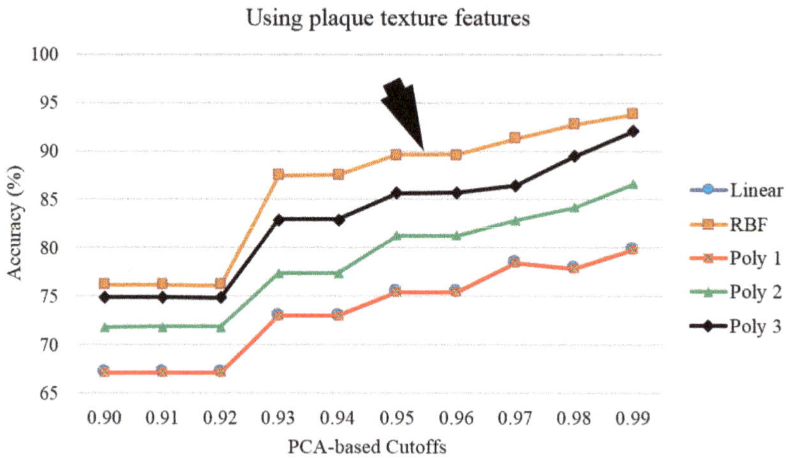

(a)

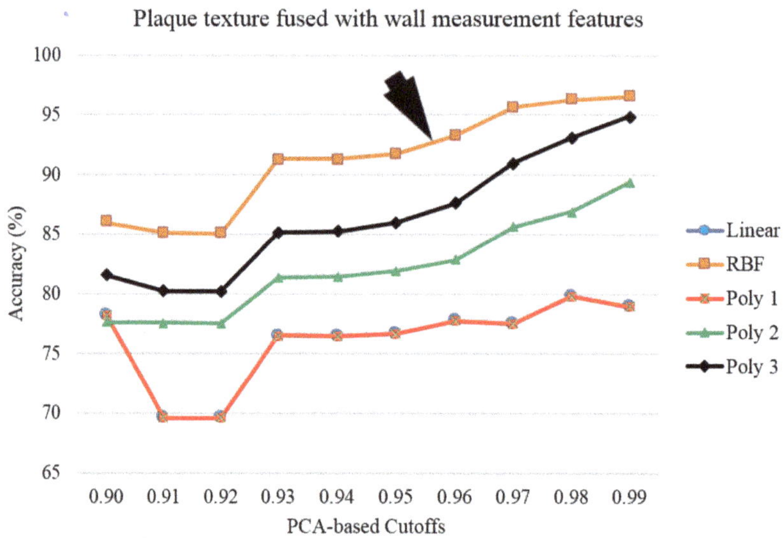

(b)

Figure 14.6. cRAS stratification accuracy versus PCA-based cut-offs for five different kernel functions (linear, RBF, polynomial-1, polynomial-2 and polynomial-3) using (a) stand-alone plaque texture-based features and (b) plaque texture-based features fused with wall-based measurement features.

14.4.3 Memorization versus generalization

Since the data size can affect the training coefficients, it is important to know when the generalization is achieved [16, 17]. In our study, we have varied the data size in ten intervals ranging from 493 to 4930 in the increment of 493 frames. These 493 frames are randomly selected and then added to the corresponding ongoing pool.

Since our cRAS is highly dependent upon the grayscale morphological characteristics that change from patient-to-patient, and further the calcium deposit varies along with the wall-based measurements, it is, therefore, imperative to establish the metrics by which we can evaluate the performance of our cRAS. We therefore choose the following evaluation parameters: (a) dominant feature retaining power; (b) receiver operating characteristic curve of the system; (c) reliability index; and (d) stability, respectively. The whole idea is to understand the absolute and relative performance along with the variations in changing parameters, which helps to understand the bounds of operation. For example, reliability reveals how accurate a system behaves for different databases. The stability of the system is evaluated if the deviation of the mean accuracy is within the tolerance limit (say 5%). We want to emphasize that performance evaluation is equally adopted for both (a) stand-alone plaque texture-based features and (b) plaque texture-based features fused with wall-based measurement features, demonstrating the comparative approach and showing the effectiveness of the wall-based measurement features in the cRAS.

Table 14.11 and figure 14.7 shows the variation of the SVM accuracy with varying data size for both (a) stand-alone plaque texture-based features and (b) plaque texture-based features fused with wall-based measurement features. We observe that for all the data sizes, the mean accuracy of all the PCA-based cut-offs, using the fusion of plaque texture-based and wall-based measurement features was higher compared to a stand-alone plaque texture-based feature paradigm, as now the dominant features are selected from a wider, diverse and strong pool of features.

14.5 Performance evaluation

14.5.1 Dominant feature retaining power of the cRAS

The dominant feature retaining power (DFRP) is the ability of the cRAS to retain the best dominant features responsible for producing a high accuracy for different PCA-based cut-offs. It is the ratio of similar dominant features between any two cut-offs, say m and n (SDF_{m-n}), and the number of dominant features selected taking the cut-off m (DF_m). Using the notation * for the product, we can mathematically compute DFRP in percentage as [17]

$$\text{DFRP}(\%) = \left(\frac{\text{SDF}_{m-n}}{\text{DF}_m}\right) * 100. \tag{14.10}$$

For this study, the DFRP taking different PCA-based cut-offs for both (a) stand-alone plaque texture-based features and (b) plaque texture-based features fused with wall-based measurement features is shown in table 14.12. The mean DFRP of all the PCA-based cut-offs, using the fusion of plaque texture-based and wall-based measurement features, is almost similar (= 89.32%) as compared to stand-alone plaque texture-based features (= 90.16%).

Table 14.11. Average accuracy of each data size using (a) stand-alone plaque texture-based features and (b) plaque texture-based features fused with wall-based measurement features.

(a) Using stand-alone plaque texture-based features (in %)										
	Data size									
Cut-offs	493	986	1479	1972	2465	2958	3451	3944	4437	4930
0.90	100.00	100.00	100.00	100.00	100.00	100.00	71.06	49.90	76.60	76.20
0.91	100.00	100.00	100.00	100.00	100.00	100.00	71.03	50.00	76.56	76.18
0.92	100.00	100.00	100.00	100.00	100.00	100.00	91.37	92.98	90.32	76.15
0.93	100.00	100.00	100.00	100.00	100.00	100.00	91.39	92.98	90.32	87.53
0.94	100.00	100.00	100.00	100.00	100.00	100.00	95.85	95.01	91.71	87.56
0.95	100.00	100.00	100.00	100.00	100.00	100.00	95.85	95.01	91.66	89.66
0.96	100.00	100.00	100.00	100.00	100.00	100.00	98.09	96.88	94.96	89.65
0.97	100.00	100.00	100.00	100.00	100.00	100.00	98.47	97.42	95.52	91.32
0.98	100.00	100.00	100.00	100.00	100.00	100.00	98.47	98.03	96.56	92.74
0.99	100.00	100.00	100.00	100.00	100.00	100.00	99.27	98.17	97.51	93.82
Average	100.00	100.00	100.00	100.00	100.00	100.00	91.08	86.64	90.17	86.08
SD	0.00	0.00	0.00	0.00	0.00	0.00	10.92	19.43	7.60	7.12
(b) Using plaque texture-based features fused with wall-based measurement features (in %)										
0.90	100.00	100.00	100.00	100.00	100.00	100.00	90.75	84.82	90.31	86.03
0.91	100.00	100.00	100.00	100.00	100.00	100.00	90.83	84.79	90.35	85.13
0.92	100.00	100.00	100.00	100.00	100.00	100.00	95.68	96.20	93.70	85.12
0.93	100.00	100.00	100.00	100.00	100.00	100.00	96.36	96.21	93.68	91.35
0.94	100.00	100.00	100.00	100.00	100.00	100.00	96.39	97.08	96.00	91.35
0.95	100.00	100.00	100.00	100.00	100.00	100.00	98.60	98.32	95.94	91.81
0.96	100.00	100.00	100.00	100.00	100.00	100.00	99.30	98.38	97.48	93.31
0.97	100.00	100.00	100.00	100.00	100.00	100.00	99.42	99.03	97.97	95.72
0.98	100.00	100.00	100.00	100.00	100.00	100.00	99.44	99.08	98.23	96.35
0.99	100.00	100.00	100.00	100.00	100.00	100.00	99.50	99.07	98.69	96.59
Average	100.00	100.00	100.00	100.00	100.00	100.00	96.63	95.30	95.24	91.28
SD	0.00	0.00	0.00	0.00	0.00	0.00	3.40	5.64	3.12	4.49

14.5.2 Receiver operating characteristics

The true positive rate (sensitivity) and false positive rate (100-specificity) are mostly used to measure the diagnostic capability of the analysis. It is a way to identify how well the classification methods can detect the true calcium. The true positive rate (TPR) and false positive rate (FPR) can be mathematically formulated as

$$\text{TPR} = \frac{\text{True positive}}{(\text{True positive} + \text{False negative})} \tag{14.11}$$

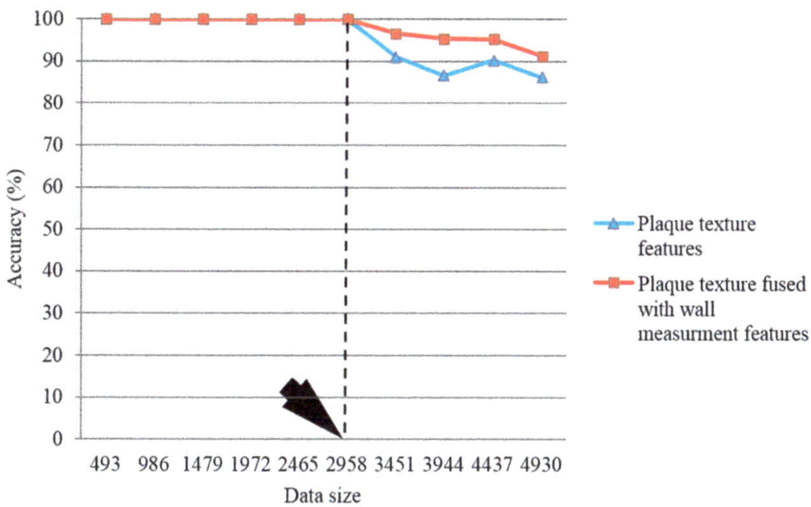

Figure 14.7. Average accuracy versus changing data size for $K = 10$ and $T = 20$ using (a) stand-alone plaque texture-based features and (b) plaque texture-based features fused with wall-based measurement features.

$$\text{FPR} = \frac{\text{True negative}}{(\text{True nagative} + \text{False positive})}. \tag{14.12}$$

True positive/False positive is defined as the number of times a high-risk patient is correctly/incorrectly identified with respect to the carotid plaque burden (gold standard) risk labels. Similarly, True negative/False positive is defined as the number of times a high-risk patient is incorrectly identified.

The receiver operating characteristic can be graphically represented using the true positive rate and false positive rate and is generally used to quantify the diagnostic accuracy of the analysis. Using the carotid plaque burden, we compute the receiver operating characteristic for the optimized PCA-based cut-off (i.e. 0.99) for both (a) stand-alone plaque texture-based features and (b) plaque texture-based features fused with wall-based measurement features, as shown in table 14.13, while the corresponding visual curves are shown in figure 14.8. Note that we computed sensitivity, specificity, positive predictive value and AUC for the optimized kernel only, which is the RBF. As can be seen, the ACU for plaque texture-based fused with wall-based measurement features was 0.91 compared to 0.86 for the stand-alone plaque texture-based cRAS system.

14.5.3 Reliability index of the cRAS

In this study, the behavior of the system is analyzed by computing the reliability index (RI) of the system for both (a) stand-alone plaque texture-based features and (b) plaque texture-based features fused with wall-based measurement features and is mathematically given as

Table 14.12. DFRP calculation for different PCA-based cut-offs using (a) stand-alone plaque texture-based features and (b) plaque texture-based features fused with wall-based measurement features.

Cut-offs (m and n)	Dominant features at m	Dominant features at n	Similar dominant features (SDF_{m-n})	Dominant feature retaining power (in %)
(a) Using stand-alone plaque texture-based features				
0.90 and **0.91**	5	5	5	100.00
0.91 and **0.92**	5	5	5	100.00
0.92 and **0.93**	5	6	2	40.00
0.93 and **0.94**	6	6	6	100.00
0.94 and **0.95**	6	7	6	100.00
0.95 and **0.96**	7	7	7	100.00
0.96 and **0.97**	7	8	5	71.43
0.97 and **0.98**	8	10	8	100.00
0.98 and **0.99**	10	13	10	100.00
(b) Using plaque texture-based features fused with wall-based measurement features				
0.90 and **0.91**	5	6	2	40.00
0.91 and **0.92**	6	6	6	100.00
0.92 and **0.93**	6	7	5	83.33
0.93 and **0.94**	7	7	7	100.00
0.94 and **0.95**	7	8	7	100.00
0.95 and **0.96**	8	9	8	100.00
0.96 and **0.97**	9	10	8	88.89
0.97 and **0.98**	10	12	10	100.00
0.98 and **0.99**	12	16	11	91.67

Table 14.13. Receiver operating characteristic for the highest PCA-based cut-off (= 0.99) and RBF kernel functions using (a) stand-alone plaque texture-based features and (b) plaque texture-based features fused with wall-based measurement features.

(a) Using stand-alone plaque texture-based features			
Mean sensitivity	Mean specificity	Mean PPV	Mean AUC
84.94 ± 8.44	87.92 ± 4.99	91.71 ± 3.96	0.86 ± 0.07
(b) Using plaque texture-based features fused with wall-based measurement features			
90.74 ± 5.22	92.14 ± 3.42	94.86 ± 2.39	0.91 ± 0.04

PPV—Positive predictive value, AUC—area under the curve.

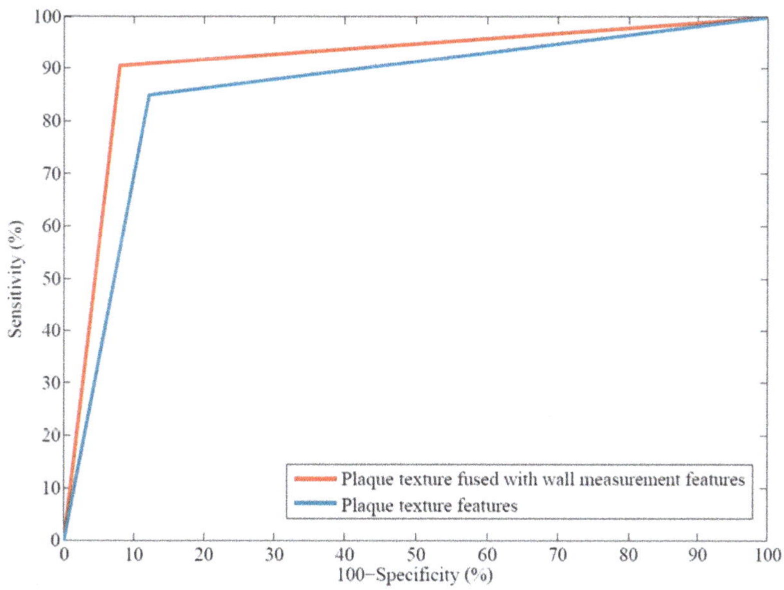

Figure 14.8. Receiver operating characteristic for the optimized PCA-based cut-off of 0.99 using (a) stand-alone plaque texture-based features and (b) plaque texture-based features fused with wall-based measurement features.

$$\mathrm{RI}_N(\%) = \left(1 - \frac{\sigma_N}{\mu_N}\right) * 100, \qquad (14.13)$$

where N is a set of ten datasets ranging from 493 to 4930 in increments of 493 frames, and σ and μ correspond to the standard deviation and mean of each dataset computed for different PCA-based cut-offs ranging from 0.90 to 0.99 for the optimized RBF kernel function. The overall reliability index using the fusion of plaque texture-based and wall-based measurement features was higher (= 98.24%) compared to stand-alone plaque texture-based features (= 94.86%), as shown in table 14.14.

Table 14.14. Reliability index (RI) at different data sizes (N) using (a) stand-alone plaque texture-based features and (b) plaque texture-based features fused with wall-based measurement features.

(a) Using stand-alone plaque texture-based features										
Data size	493	986	1479	1972	2465	2958	3451	3944	4437	4930	Average
RI$_N$ **(%)**	100.00	100.00	100.00	100.00	100.00	100.00	88.01	77.58	91.57	91.73	94.86
(b) Using plaque texture-based features fused with wall-based measurement features											
RI$_N$ **(%)**	100.00	100.00	100.00	100.00	100.00	100.00	96.48	94.08	96.73	95.08	98.24

14.5.4 Stability of the cRAS

In this study, we have also analyzed the stability of the system for both (a) stand-alone plaque texture-based features and (b) plaque texture-based features fused with wall-based measurement features. The deviation of the accuracy from the mean accuracy corresponding to all the PCA-based cut-offs for each data size was computed. The mean deviation for all the data sizes using the fusion of plaque texture-based with wall-based measurement features was under the tolerance limit of 5% compared to the stand-alone plaque texture-based cRAS, that turned out to be under the tolerance limit of 15%, as shown in table 14.15.

14.6 Discussion

14.6.1 Our system

This study demonstrated an ML risk assessment and stratification system, adopting a fusion of plaque texture-based features with wall-based measurement features. The ML system fusing plaque texture-based features with wall-based measurement features outperformed the equivalent using stand-alone plaque texture-based features. Thus, we validated our hypothesis. Because the atheroma region causes the IEL and EEL walls to expand bidirectionally [20], there was a clear motivation to use wall-based measurement features. Further, since the atherosclerotic calcium is multi-focal [2, 21, 48] and the detection process is well established [20], our cRAS leverages on this burden to improve the overall accuracy of the risk stratification. Note that our modeling assumes a negligible effect due to heart motion [49], thereby assuming it to be simple, pragmatic and ensuring high-speed processing due to the multiresolution approach for calcium detection. Our system demonstrated a high accuracy of stratification based on the training model that uses the concept of the genetic make-up of the carotid plaque burden. The carotid plaque burden (considered as a biomarker for stroke risk) can be used as a risk label for patients with coronary artery disease, which validated our second hypothesis. Finally, we want to emphasize that the cRAS did take advantage of a selection of the optimized features using a polling strategy in the PCA paradigm, ensuring best performance. From figure 14.5, it was observed that for different PCA-based cut-offs, the increase in the

Table 14.15. Deviation of accuracy from mean accuracy for different data sizes using (a) stand-alone plaque texture-based features and (b) plaque texture-based features fused with wall-based measurement features.

(a) Using stand-alone plaque texture-based features (in %)										
	Data size									
Cut-offs	493	986	1479	1972	2465	2958	3451	3944	4437	4930
0.90	0.00	0.00	0.00	0.00	0.00	0.00	20.02	36.74	13.57	9.88
0.91	0.00	0.00	0.00	0.00	0.00	0.00	20.05	36.64	13.61	9.9
0.92	0.00	0.00	0.00	0.00	0.00	0.00	0.29	6.34	0.15	9.93
0.93	0.00	0.00	0.00	0.00	0.00	0.00	0.31	6.34	0.15	1.45
0.94	0.00	0.00	0.00	0.00	0.00	0.00	4.77	8.37	1.54	1.48
0.95	0.00	0.00	0.00	0.00	0.00	0.00	4.77	8.37	1.49	3.58
0.96	0.00	0.00	0.00	0.00	0.00	0.00	7.01	10.24	4.79	3.57
0.97	0.00	0.00	0.00	0.00	0.00	0.00	7.39	10.78	5.35	5.24
0.98	0.00	0.00	0.00	0.00	0.00	0.00	7.39	11.39	6.39	6.66
0.99	0.00	0.00	0.00	0.00	0.00	0.00	8.19	11.53	7.34	7.74
Average	0.00	0.00	0.00	0.00	0.00	0.00	8.02	14.67	5.44	5.94
SD	0.00	0.00	0.00	0.00	0.00	0.00	6.92	11.75	5.00	3.38
(b) Using plaque texture-based features fused with wall-based measurement features (in %)										
0.90	0.00	0.00	0.00	0.00	0.00	0.00	5.88	10.48	4.93	5.25
0.91	0.00	0.00	0.00	0.00	0.00	0.00	5.80	10.51	4.89	6.15
0.92	0.00	0.00	0.00	0.00	0.00	0.00	0.95	0.90	1.54	6.16
0.93	0.00	0.00	0.00	0.00	0.00	0.00	0.27	0.91	1.56	0.07
0.94	0.00	0.00	0.00	0.00	0.00	0.00	0.24	1.78	0.76	0.07
0.95	0.00	0.00	0.00	0.00	0.00	0.00	1.97	3.02	0.70	0.53
0.96	0.00	0.00	0.00	0.00	0.00	0.00	2.67	3.08	2.24	2.03
0.97	0.00	0.00	0.00	0.00	0.00	0.00	2.79	3.73	2.73	4.44
0.98	0.00	0.00	0.00	0.00	0.00	0.00	2.81	3.78	2.99	5.07
0.99	0.00	0.00	0.00	0.00	0.00	0.00	2.87	3.77	3.45	5.31
Average	0.00	0.00	0.00	0.00	0.00	0.00	2.63	4.20	2.58	3.51
SD	0.00	0.00	0.00	0.00	0.00	0.00	1.98	3.50	1.52	2.55

number of dominant features is higher for the fusion of plaque texture-based and wall-based measurement features compared to the stand-alone plaque texture-based paradigm. Also, in table 14.9, the selection of coronary calcium area, coronary lumen area and coronary wall thickness as dominant features proves that wall-based measurement features are as important as plaque texture-based features in coronary artery risk assessment.

14.6.2 A note on population size

One of the requirements in the ML framework is large enough population size for achieving generalization while maintaining satisfactory accuracy for risk stratification. We had approached our design strategy based on the number of frames rather than the number of patients as the population pool during the cross-validation protocol design. In our ML system design, even though we have a low population size of 22 subjects, we had a total of 4930 frames. These 4930 frames were stratified into 3043 high-risk frames and 1887 low-risk frames derived from 14 high-risk patients and 8 low-risk patients, respectively. Our analysis demonstrated that our cRAS system has a sufficient pool of frames to design an accurate risk assessment system.

14.6.3 A note on kernel functions

In table 14.10, we can clearly observe that the lowest classification accuracy is obtained for linear and polynomial order 1 kernel functions as the optimum separating hyper-plane cannot separate all of the database into two distinct classes. The classification accuracy of both the linear and polynomial order 1 functions is the same as there is not much difference between their kernel functions. With the increase in the order of the polynomial kernel functions, we observe an increase in the classification accuracy, as now the size of the function class increases. Finally, because of its Gaussian contribution, it was observed that the highest classification accuracy is achieved with the RBF kernel function.

14.6.4 A note on performance evaluation of our cRAS

A prerequisite for an ML system is to understand the variability due to (i) PCA-based dominance feature selection and (ii) the type of cross-validation protocol used while fusing the wall-based features with grayscale morphological characteristics of the plaque region derived from the IVUS video frames. It is thus imperative to evaluate the cRAS by understanding the metrics which evaluate the dynamics of the performance evaluation. We therefore took special steps in computing four different performance parameters, namely (a) dominant feature retaining power, (b) receiver operating characteristic curves, (c) reliability index, and (d) stability under both (i) stand-alone plaque texture-based features and (ii) plaque texture-based features fused with wall-based measurement features. The results of these analyses are shown in tables 14.12–14.15, respectively. The above curves/tables demonstrate encouraging results for the design for risk assessment.

14.6.5 Comparison against current literature and benchmarking

IVUS is one of the speedily emerging medical imaging modalities showing promising signs towards high-resolution imaging [50]. This opens new doors for many medical image analysis methods and techniques to extract and quantify plaque [20, 23, 29] and finally, to risk characterize the plaque into low- and high-risk bins using ML-based strategies [16, 17]. Not much work has been done so far in the area of IVUS-based CAD risk stratification; however, several studies in the literature have reported on carotid plaque characterization and risk stratification. Table 14.16 shows the comparison between these techniques using eight different attributes such

Table 14.16. Survey of risk stratification techniques in the literature.

Year	Authors	Arterial type	Population size	Feature (s) type	Total features	Feature selection technique (s)	Classifier (s)	Cross-validation accuracy
2003	Christodoulou *et al* [8]	Carotid	230	Tex	61	Mean, SD, Distance	MNN	73.1%
2005	Kyriacou *et al* [9]	Carotid	274	Tex, Wall	10	N/A	NN	71.2%
2007	Mongiakakou *et al* [10]	Carotid	54	SF, Law's	21	ANOVA	HNN	99.1%
2009	Kyriacou *et al* [11]	Carotid	274	Tex	10	N/A	SVM	73.7%
2012	Acharya *et al* [12]	Carotid	346	Tex	4	*T* test	SVM, AdaBoost	SVM—82.4%, AdaBoost—81.7%
2012	Acharya *et al* [13]	Carotid	346	Tex, Wall	3	*T* test	SVM	83%
2013	Acharya *et al* [14]	Carotid	492	DWT, HOS, Tex	7	*T* test	SVM	91.7%
2014	Pedro *et al* [15]	Carotid	146	Rayleigh mixture	16	N/A	EAI	77%
2016	Araki *et al* [16]	Coronary	2865	Tex	56	N/A	SVM	94.95%
2016	Araki *et al* [17]	Coronary	2865	Tex	56	PCA	SVM	98.43%
2017	Araki *et al* [51]	Carotid	407	Tex	16	N/A	SVM	FW—98.00%, NW—98.00%
2017	Saba *et al* [52]	Carotid	407	Tex	16	PCA	SVM	FW—98.55%, NW—98.83%
2017	Proposed	Coronary	4930	Only Tex, Tex fused with wall	65	PCA	SVM	Only Tex—86.08%, Tex fused with wall—91.28%

Tex—plaque texture-based; Wall—wall-based; NN—neural network; SF—statistical feature; SD—standard deviation; MNN—modular neural network; HNN—hybrid neural network, SVM—support vector machine; EAI—enhanced activity index; PCA—principal component analysis; DWT—discrete wavelet transform; HOS—higher order spectra; NW—near wall; FW—far wall; N/A—not applicable.

as year, artery type, population size and feature type, the number of features, feature selection techniques, classifier and cross-validation accuracy.

It was very recently that Araki *et al* [51] in 2017 performed a risk stratification on a database of 407 carotid B-mode ultrasound images. Here, the SVM classifier trained by 16 texture features provides a cross-validation accuracy of 98% for both the near and far wall, respectively. The same group [52] upgraded their system by utilizing a PCA-based pooling strategy for the dominant feature selection and obtained high accuracies of 98.55% and 98.83% for the carotid near wall and carotid far wall, respectively.

While the above benchmarking used carotid plaque classification for risk estimation, our team has been attempting to model coronary plaque risk stratification by fusing the coronary and carotid atherosclerotic genetic make-up concepts [22–28]. This study brings a novel approach of introducing coronary wall-based measurement features along with grayscale coronary plaque texture-based features for risk stratification. We, therefore, showed the cRAS for both (a) stand-alone plaque texture-based features and (b) plaque texture-based features fused with wall-based measurement features. The fused system showed an improvement of 5.69%. To the best of our knowledge, this is the first ML-based CADx system which utilizes a fusion of plaque texture-based and wall-based measurement features for coronary artery risk stratification.

14.6.6 Carotid plaque burden as a gold standard for the training phase in ML design

One of the important components of the cRAS design is the choice of the gold standard during the training phase. The idea behind the choice of the gold standard is to ensure that we have an indicator which has a strong link to the coronary artery disease while maintaining the low-cost design of the cRAS. Surely, one can consider the histology-based [53] or the calcium score [54] using CT as a gold standard. However, the CT results are not real-time, and it is difficult to reconstruct them as a 3D image [55]. They are not easily affordable, being very expensive and tedious protocols. Furthermore, the focus of our paper is solely based on ultrasound. The second option is to adopt the concept of genetic make-up between carotid and coronary atherosclerosis disease, which is now well established [22–28]. Previous studies had proven that cIMT influences the disease and death rates, which proves the relationship between plaque burden and cIMT in the coronary and carotid arteries [56–61]. Ogata *et al* [62] also showed the correlation of cIMT with the plaque accumulation in the left main coronary artery. Establishing this concept, we thus leveraged our gold standard choice to be the carotid artery and its plaque burden. One way to establish this gold standard is to measure the media wall thickness as an indicator, which can be computed using cIMT measurements [51, 52]. JSS and his team have shown numerous studies for cIMT measurement and its link to various cardiovascular risk events, such as ankle–brachial index [25], syntax score [26], etc. Since this study collected dual information, such as cIMT and coronary IVUS images, we therefore used cIMT measurements as the risk label for our cRAS.

14.6.7 A note on time computation for online risk prediction

An ML system is characterized by its training (or offline) and testing (online) phases. The time complexity of the risk assessment system is based on the hardware components, such as processor speed and computer RAM. The PC configuration of our system had the following: HP Compaq Elite 8300 with an Intel Core i7–3770 Processor, 3.40 GHz and 2 GB RAM, MATLAB 2013a software and the Windows-7 Operating System. Typically, the offline system is not accounted for in the overall time complexity of the ML design, however, our single frame training and testing times of the proposed cRAS were 0.0435 s and 0.0083 s, respectively, which can be considered as reasonably fast by looking at the previous risk assessment systems designed for carotids and coronary applications [17].

14.6.8 Strength, weakness and extensions

We demonstrated a machine learning system for risk assessment based on grayscale plaque morphology combined with wall-based features. We can characterize the benefits into two categories: primary benefits and secondary benefits. The key benefit of our design is the generalized system for risk assessment which can be extended to a more complex design by adding meaningful features which are clinically more relevant. The successful main idea of coronary risk dependence based solely on genetic make-up can also be further extended into other designs, such as histology-based or CT-based biomarkers. This is another powerful strength of our cRAS. The ability to fuse the wall-based measurement features with grayscale morphologic plaque texture-based features provides another platform for fusion of the feature paradigm. The secondary benefits are the ability to obtain higher classification accuracy using an SVM-based classifier, integration of a PCA-based polling strategy for dominant feature extraction, the ability to optimize the best kernel function, the ability to optimize the data to obtain the best accuracy, and the high mean sensitivity, specificity, positive predictive value and AUC. The system also has a high average feature retaining power and is reliable and stable.

Despite the above strengths, the study suffers from some limitations. The study utilizes manual tracings of IVUS images for ROI generation. The dataset used in the current study is controlled as all the patients come from a diabetic cohort. Intra/inter-observer variability could have been tried but is outside the scope of the current study, as tracing all the frames is very expensive. DICOM images with gating and registration schemes can be incorporated with a large dataset for extensive evaluations. Optical coherence tomography (OCT) is a high-resolution optical imaging technology and provides more accurate arterial cross-sections compared to IVUS [63]. We understand that there is a need for further OCT/histology-based validation and automated segmentation of IVUS walls [7], however, the current results are encouraging.

14.7 Conclusion

The coronary artery disease risk stratification tool based on IVUS wall grayscale morphological characterization, when fused with wall-based measurement features, showed superior performance using ML-based techniques. The system computed six novel wall-based measurement features: coronary calcium area, coronary vessel area, coronary lumen area, coronary atheroma area, coronary wall thickness and coronary wall thickness variability, which were fused with grayscale features, gave an improvement of ~6% in the accuracy for predicting the class label of the plaque type as high-risk or low-risk. All performance parameters showed similar behavior. Our cRAS also showed improvement in stability and reliability. Since the ML system was automated, it can be adopted one step closer to clinical use for cardiovascular imaging laboratories

Acknowledgments

Reprinted from Banchhor S K, Londhe N D, Araki T, Saba L, Radeva P, Laird J R, Suri J S 2017 Wall-based measurement features provides an improved IVUS coronary artery risk assessment when fused with plaque texture-based features during machine learning paradigm **91** 198–212, with permission from Elsevier.

Funding

This research did not receive any specific grant from funding agencies in the public, commercial, or not-for-profit sectors.

Conflicts of interest

The authors declare no conflict of interest.

References

[1] Mozaffarian D *et al* 2016 Executive summary: heart disease and stroke statistics—2016 update: a report from the American Heart Association *Circulation* **133** 447–54

[2] Ross R 1995 Cell biology of atherosclerosis *Annu. Rev. Physiol.* **57** 791–804

[3] Libby P, Ridker P M and Hansson G K 2011 Progress and challenges in translating the biology of atherosclerosis *Nature* **473** 317–25

[4] Ramani K *et al* 1998 Contrast magnetic resonance imaging in the assessment of myocardial viability in patients with stable coronary artery disease and left ventricular dysfunction *Circulation* **98** 2687–94

[5] Schoenhagen P *et al* 2003 Coronary imaging: angiography shows the stenosis, but IVUS, CT, and MRI show the plaque *Cleve. Clin. J. Med.* **70** 713–20

[6] Schoenhagen P and Nissen S 2002 Understanding coronary artery disease: tomographic imaging with intravascular ultrasound *Heart* **88** 91–6

[7] Katouzian A *et al* 2012 A state-of-the-art review on segmentation algorithms in intravascular ultrasound (IVUS) images *IEEE Trans. Inf. Technol. Biomed.* **16** 823–34

[8] Christodoulou C I *et al* 2003 Texture based classification on atherosclerotic carotid plaques *IEEE Trans. Med. Imaging* **22** 902–12

[9] Kyriacou E *et al* 2005 Ultrasound imaging in the analysis of carotid plaque morphology for the assessment of stroke *Stud. Health Technol. Inform.* **113** 241–75

[10] Mougiakakou S G *et al* 2007 Computer-aided diagnosis of carotid atherosclerosis based on ultrasound image statistics, laws' texture and neural networks *Ultrasound Med. Biol.* **33** 26–36

[11] Kyriacou E *et al* 2009 Classification of atherosclerotic carotid plaques using morphological analysis on ultrasound images *J. Appl. Intell.* **30** 3–23
[12] Acharya R U *et al* 2012 Symptomatic versus asymptomatic plaque classification in carotid ultrasound *J. Med. Syst.* **36** 1861–71
[13] Acharya U R *et al* 2012 Atherosclerotic risk stratification strategy for carotid arteries using texture-based features *Ultrasound Med. Biol.* **38** 899–915
[14] Acharya U R *et al* 2013 Understanding symptomatology of atherosclerotic plaque by image-based tissue characterization *Comput. Methods Programs Biomed.* **110** 66–75
[15] Pedro L M *et al* 2014 Asymptomatic carotid disease—a new tool for assessing neurological risk *Echocardiography* **31** 353–61
[16] Araki T *et al* 2016 A new method for IVUS-based coronary artery disease risk stratification: a link between coronary and carotid ultrasound plaque burdens *Comput. Methods Programs Biomed.* **124** 161–79
[17] Araki T *et al* 2016 PCA-based polling strategy in machine learning framework for coronary artery disease risk assessment in intravascular ultrasound: a link between carotid and coronary grayscale plaque morphology *Comput. Methods Programs Biomed.* **128** 137–58
[18] Acharya U R *et al* 2015 An automated technique for carotid far wall classification using grayscale features and wall thickness variability *J. Clin. Ultrasound* **43** 302–11
[19] Saba L *et al* 2012 Carotid IMT variability (IMTV) and its validation in symptomatic versus asymptomatic Italian population: can this be a useful index for studying symptomaticity? *Echocardiography* **29** 1111–9
[20] Banchhor S K *et al* 2017 Relationship between automated coronary calcium volumes and a set of manual coronary lumen volume, vessel volume and atheroma volume in Japanese diabetic cohort: an intravascular ultrasound-based study *J. Clin. Diagn. Res.* **11** TC09–14
[21] Casscells W, Naghavi M and Willerson J T 2003 Vulnerable atherosclerotic plaque a multifocal disease *Circulation* **107** 2072–5
[22] Molinari F *et al* 2012 Automated carotid IMT measurement and its validation in low contrast ultrasound database of 885 patient Indian population epidemiological study: results of AtheroEdge™ Software *Int. Angiol.* **31** 42–53
[23] Saba L *et al* 2016 Accurate cloud-based smart IMT measurement, its validation and stroke risk stratification in carotid ultrasound: a web-based point-of-care tool for multicenter clinical trial *Comput. Biol. Med.* **75** 217–34
[24] Saba L *et al* 2017 Volumetric analysis of carotid plaque components and cerebral micro-bleeds: a correlative study *J. Stroke Cerebrovasc. Dis.* **26** 552–8
[25] Ikeda N *et al* 2013 Impact of carotid artery ultrasound and ankle–brachial index on prediction of severity of SYNTAX score *Circ. J.* **77** 712–6
[26] Ikeda N *et al* 2015 Improved correlation between carotid and coronary atherosclerosis SYNTAX score using automated ultrasound carotid bulb plaque IMT measurement *Ultrasound Med. Biol.* **41** 1247–62
[27] Araki T *et al* 2015 Calcium lesion volume measurement on intravascular ultrasound imaging and its association with carotid intima–media thickness *J. Ultrasound Med.* **34** 469–82
[28] Araki T *et al* 2015 A comparative approach of four different image registration techniques for quantitative assessment of coronary artery calcium lesions using intravascular ultrasound *Comput. Methods Programs Biomed.* **118** 158–72
[29] Araki T *et al* 2016 Reliable and accurate calcium volume measurement in coronary artery using intravascular ultrasound videos *J. Med. Syst.* **40** 51

[30] Banchhor S K *et al* 2016 Five multiresolution-based calcium volume measurement techniques from coronary IVUS videos: a comparative approach *Comput. Methods Programs Biomed.* **134** 237–58
[31] Banchhor S K *et al* 2017 Well-balanced system for coronary calcium detection and volume measurement in a low resolution intravascular ultrasound videos *Comput. Biol. Med.* **84** 168–81
[32] Suri J S, Haralick R M and Sheehan F H 2000 Greedy algorithm for error correction in automatically produced boundaries from low contrast ventriculograms *Pattern Anal. Appl.* **3** 39–60
[33] Saba L *et al* 2013 Inter- and intra-observer variability analysis of completely automated cIMT measurement software (AtheroEdge™) and its benchmarking against commercial ultrasound scanner and expert readers *Comput. Biol. Med.* **43** 1261–72
[34] Haralick R M 1979 Statistical and structural approaches to texture *Proc. IEEE* **67** 786–804
[35] Kalyan K *et al* 2014 Artificial neural network application in the diagnosis of disease conditions with liver ultrasound images *Adv. Bioinform.* **2014** 708279
[36] Weszka J S, Dyer C R and Rosenfeld A 1976 A comparative study of texture measures for terrain classification *IEEE Trans. Syst. Man. Cybern.* **6** 269–85
[37] Amadasun M and King R 1989 Textural features corresponding to textural properties *IEEE Trans. Syst. Man Cybern.* **19** 1264–74
[38] Niu L *et al* 2013 Surface roughness detection of arteries via texture analysis of ultrasound images for early diagnosis of atherosclerosis *PLoS One* **8** e76880
[39] Hu M-K 1962 Visual pattern recognition by moment invariants *IRE Trans. Inf. Theory* **8** 179–87
[40] Wu C M and Chen Y C 1992 Statistical feature matrix for texture analysis *CVGIP: Graph. Models Image Process.* **54** 407–19
[41] Song F, Guo Z and Mei D 2010 Feature selection using principal component analysis *Int. Conf. on IEEE System Science, Engineering Design and Manufacturing Informatization (ICSEM)* **vol 1** (Piscataway, NJ: IEEE) pp 27–30
[42] Burges C J 1998 A tutorial on support vector machines for pattern recognition *Data Min. Knowl. Discov.* **2** 121–67
[43] Sastry P 2003 An introduction to support vector machines *Computing and Information Sciences: Recent Trends* pp 53–85
[44] Muller K R *et al* 2001 An introduction to kernel based learning algorithms *IEEE Trans. Neural Netw.* **12** 181–201
[45] David V and Sanchez A 2003 Advanced support vector machines and kernel methods *Neuro Comput.* **55** 5–20
[46] Rodriguez J D, Perez A and Lozano J A 2010 Sensitivity analysis of *k*-fold cross validation in prediction error estimation *IEEE Trans. Pattern Anal. Mach. Intell.* **32** 569–75
[47] Vapnik V 1998 *Statistical Learning Theory* vol 1 (New York: Wiley)
[48] Tabas I, Williams K J and Borén J 2007 Subendothelial lipoprotein in retention as the initiating process in atherosclerosis: update and therapeutic implications *Circulation* **116** 1832–44
[49] Setarehdan S K and Singh S 2002 *Advanced Algorithmic Approaches to Medical Image Segmentation: State-of-the-art Applications in Cardiology, Neurology, Mammography, and Pathology* (London: Springer)
[50] Campos C M *et al* 2015 *Ex vivo* validation of 45 MHz intravascular ultrasound backscatter tissue characterization *Eur. Heart J. Cardiovasc. Imaging* **16** 1112–9

[51] Araki T *et al* 2017 Stroke risk stratification and its validation using ultrasonic echolucent carotid wall plaque morphology: a machine learning paradigm *Comput. Biol. Med.* **80** 77–96
[52] Saba L *et al* 2017 Plaque tissue morphology-based stroke risk stratification using carotid ultrasound: a polling-based PCA learning paradigm *J. Med. Syst.* **41** 98
[53] Scott D S *et al* 2000 Pathologic validation of a new method to quantify coronary calcific deposits *in vivo* using intravascular ultrasound *Am. J. Cardiol.* **85** 37–40
[54] Schamroth N, Gutstein A and Kornowski R 2017 Coronary artery calcium score: where do we stand? Current uses and implications in asymptomatic patients *Isr. Med. Assoc. J.* **19** 214–5
[55] Wahle A and Sonka M 2005 Coronary plaque analysis by multimodality fusion *Studies in Health Technology and Informatics, Plaque Imaging: Pixel to Molecular Level* ed J S Suri *et al* vol 113 (Amsterdam: IOS) pp 321–59
[56] Molinari F, Zeng G and Suri J S 2010 Intima–media thickness: setting a standard for a completely automated method of ultrasound measurement *IEEE Trans. Ultrason. Ferroelectr. Freq. Control* **57** 1112–24
[57] Sanches M J, Laine A and Suri J S 2011 *Ultrasound Imaging* (New York: Springer)
[58] Saba L *et al* 2014 *Multi-modality Atherosclerosis Imaging and Diagnosis* (New York: Springer)
[59] Saba L *et al* 2013 Association of automated carotid IMT measurement and HbA1c in Japanese patients with coronary artery disease *Diab. Res. Clin. Pract.* **100** 348–53
[60] Ikeda N *et al* 2014 Ankle–brachial index and its link to automated carotid ultrasound measurement of intima–media thickness variability in 500 Japanese coronary artery disease patients *Curr. Atheroscler. Rep.* **16** 1–8
[61] Nezu T *et al* 2015 Carotid intima-media thickness for atherosclerosis *J. Atheroscler. Thromb.* **23** 18–31
[62] Ogata T *et al* 2005 Atherosclerosis found on carotid ultrasonography is associated with atherosclerosis on coronary intravascular ultrasonography *J. Ultrasound Med.* **24** 469–74
[63] Akhtar M and Liu W 2016 Use of intravascular ultrasound vs optical coherence tomography for mechanism and patterns of in-stent restenosis among bare metal stents and drug eluting stents *J. Thorac. Dis.* **8** 104–8

Lightning Source UK Ltd.
Milton Keynes UK
UKHW050947190919
350069UK00004B/31/P

9 780750 319959